Tucholsky   Wagner   Zola   Scott   Sydow   Freud   Schlegel
Turgenev   Wallace   Fonatne
Twain   Walther von der Vogelweide   Fouqué   Friedrich II. von Preußen
Weber   Freiligrath   Frey
Fechner   Fichte   Weiße Rose   von Fallersleben   Kant   Ernst   Frommel
Richthofen
Engels   Fielding   Hölderlin
Fehrs   Faber   Flaubert   Eichendorff   Tacitus   Dumas
Eliasberg   Ebner Eschenbach
Feuerbach   Maximilian I. von Habsburg   Fock   Eliot   Zweig
Ewald   Vergil
Goethe   Elisabeth von Österreich   London
Mendelssohn   Balzac   Shakespeare   Dostojewski   Ganghofer
Lichtenberg   Rathenau   Doyle   Gjellerup
Trackl   Stevenson   Hambruch
Mommsen   Tolstoi   Lenz   Droste-Hülshoff
Thoma   Hanrieder
Dach   von Arnim   Hägele   Hauff   Humboldt
Verne
Karrillon   Reuter   Rousseau   Hagen   Hauptmann   Gautier
Garschin
Damaschke   Defoe   Hebbel   Baudelaire
Descartes
Hegel   Kussmaul   Herder
Wolfram von Eschenbach   Dickens   Schopenhauer   Rilke   George
Bronner   Darwin   Melville   Grimm   Jerome
Campe   Horváth   Aristoteles   Bebel   Proust
Bismarck   Vigny   Barlach   Voltaire   Federer   Herodot
Gengenbach   Heine
Storm   Casanova   Tersteegen   Grillparzer   Georgy
Chamberlain   Lessing   Langbein   Gilm   Gryphius
Brentano   Claudius   Schiller   Lafontaine
Strachwitz   Schilling   Kralik   Iffland   Sokrates
Katharina II. von Rußland   Bellamy   Raabe   Gibbon   Tschechow
Gerstäcker
Löns   Hesse   Hoffmann   Gogol   Wilde   Gleim   Vulpius
Luther   Heym   Hofmannsthal   Klee   Hölty   Morgenstern   Goedicke
Roth   Heyse   Klopstock   Kleist
Luxemburg   Puschkin   Homer   Mörike   Musil
La Roche   Horaz
Machiavelli   Kierkegaard   Kraft   Kraus
Navarra   Aurel   Musset   Moltke
Nestroy   Marie de France   Lamprecht   Kind   Kirchhoff   Hugo
Laotse   Ipsen   Liebknecht
Nietzsche   Nansen   Ringelnatz
Marx   Lassalle   Gorki   Klett
von Ossietzky   May   Leibniz   Irving
vom Stein   Lawrence
Petalozzi   Platon   Knigge
Sachs   Pückler   Michelangelo   Kock   Kafka
Poe   Liebermann   Korolenko
de Sade   Praetorius   Mistral   Zetkin

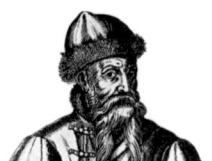
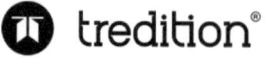

# Rural Hygiene

Henry N. (Henry Neely) Ogden

# Imprint

This book is part of the TREDITION CLASSICS series.

Author: Henry N. (Henry Neely) Ogden
Cover design: toepferschumann, Berlin (Germany)

Publisher: tredition GmbH, Hamburg (Germany)
ISBN: 978-3-8495-1367-2

www.tredition.com
www.tredition.de

# PREFACE

The following pages represent an attempt to put before the rural population a systematic treatment of those special subjects included in what is popularly known as Hygiene as well as those broader subjects that concern the general health of the community at large.

Usually the term "hygiene" has been limited in its application to a study of the health of the individual, and treatises on hygiene have concerned themselves almost entirely with discussing such topics as food, clothing, exercise, and other questions relating to the daily life of a person. Of late years, however, it has become more and more evident that it is not possible for man to live to himself alone, but that his actions must react on those living in his vicinity and that the methods of living of his neighbors must react on his own well-being. This interdependence of individuals being once appreciated, it follows that a book on hygiene must deal, not only with the question of individual living, but also with those broader questions having to do with the cause and spread of disease, with the transmission of bacteria from one community to another, and with those natural influences which, more or less under the control of man, may affect a large area if their natural destructive tendencies are allowed to develop.

Being written by an engineer, the following pages deal rather with the structural side of public hygiene than with [Pg vi] the medical side, and in the chapters dealing with contagious diseases emphasis is attached to quarantine, disinfection, and prevention, rather than to etiology and treatment. The book is not, therefore, a medical treatise in any sense, and is not intended to eliminate the physician or to give professional advice, although the suggestions, if followed out, undoubtedly will have the effect of lessening the need of a physician, since the contagious diseases referred to may then be confined to single individuals or to single houses.

It has not been possible, within the limits of this one book, to describe at length the various engineering methods, and while it is hoped that enough has been said to point the way towards a proper selection of methods and to a right choice between processes, the details of construction will have to be worked out in all cases, either by the ingenuity of the householder or by the aid of some mechanic or engineer.

Finally, it may be said that two distinct purposes have been in mind throughout, — to promote the comfort and convenience of those living in the rural part of the community who, unfortunately, while most happily situated from the standpoint of health in many ways, have failed to give themselves those comforts that might so easily be added to their life; and in the second place, to emphasize the interdependence of the rural community and the urban community in the matter of food products and contagious diseases, an interdependence growing daily as interurban communications by trolley and automobile become easy.

Cities are learning to protect themselves against the selfishness of the individual, and city Boards of Health have large powers for the purpose of guarding the health [Pg vii] of the individuals within their boundaries. The scattered populations of the open country are not yet educated to the point at which self-protection has made such authority seem to be necessary, and it is left largely to an exalted sense of duty towards their fellow-men so to move members of a rural community as to order their lives and ways to avoid sinning against public hygiene. In order to develop such a sense of honor, it is primarily necessary that the relation of cause and effect in matters of health shall be plainly understood and that the dangers to others of the neglect of preventive measures be appreciated. As a single example, the transmission of disease at school may be cited. Measles, scarlet fever, whooping cough, and diphtheria are all children's diseases, easily carried and transmitted, and held in check only by preventing a sick child from coming in contact with children not sick. No law is sufficient. The matter must be left to the mother, who will retain children at home at the least suspicion of sickness and keep them there until after all traces of the disease have passed away.

The health conditions in the open country, judged by the standard of statistics, are quite as good as those of the city. The comforts of country life are as yet inferior, and it is hoped that this book may do something to advance the standard of living in the families into which it may enter.

H. N. OGDEN.

Ithaca, New York,
November 1, 1910.

# CONTENTS

in air. Fresh-air inlet. Position of inlet. Foul-air outlet. Size of openings. Ventilation of stables. Cost of ventilation. Relation of heating to ventilation -

CHAPTER V

Quantity of Water Required for Domestic Use

Modern tendencies. Quantity of water needed per person. Quantity used in stables. Maximum rate of consumption. Variation in maximum rate. Fire stream requirements. Rain-water supply. Computation for rain-water storage. Computation for storage reservoir on brook. Deficiency from well supplies -

CHAPTER VI

Sources of Water-supply

Underground waters. Ordinary dug well. Construction of dug wells. Deep wells. Springs. Extensions of springs. Supply from brooks. Storage reservoirs. Ponds or lakes. Pressure or head -

CHAPTER VII

Quality of Water

Mineral matter. Loss of soap. Vegetable pollution. Animal pollution. Well water. Danger of polluted water -

CHAPTER VIII

Water-works Construction

Methods of collection. Spring reservoirs. Stream supplies. [Pg x] Dams. Waste weirs. Gate house. Pipe lines. Pumping. Windmills.

Hydraulic rams. Hot-air engines. Gas engines. Steam pumps. Air lifts. Tanks. Pressure tanks -

CHAPTER IX

Plumbing

Installation. Supply tank. Main supply pipe. Hot-water circulation. Kitchen sinks. Laundry tubs. Hot-water boiler. Water-back, wash-basin, bath-tub. Cost of plumbing installation. House drainage. Trap-vents. Water-closets -

CHAPTER X

Sewage Disposal

Definition of sewage. Stream pollution. Treatment of sewage on land. Surface application. Artificial sewage beds. Subsurface tile disposal. Automatic syphon. Sedimentation. Underdrains -

CHAPTER XI

Preparation and Care of Milk and Meat

Bacteria in milk. Effects of bacteria. Diseases caused by milk. Methods of obtaining clean milk. City milk. Dangers of diseased meat. The slaughter-house -

CHAPTER XII

Foods and Beverages

The human mechanism. Digestive processes. Teachings of the digestive operations. Balanced rations. Human appetite. Effect of individual habits. Cooking. Muscular and psychic reactions. Consump-

CHAPTER XVII

Typhoid Fever

Cause of the disease. The bacillus. Methods of transmission of typhoid. Construction of wells in reference to typhoid. Milk infection
by typhoid. Infection by flies. Other sources of typhoid fever.
Treatment of typhoid fever -


CHAPTER XVIII

Children's Diseases

After effects. Preliminary symptoms. Contagiousness. Quarantine
[Pg xii] for scarlet fever. Measles. Characteristic eruption of measles.
Whooping cough. Precautions against spread of whooping cough.
Chicken pox -


CHAPTER XIX

Parasitical Diseases

Malaria. Mosquitoes and malaria. Elimination of mosquitoes. Limitation of mosquito infection. Yellow fever. Characteristics of the
disease. Hookworm disease. Pellagra. Bubonic plague -


CHAPTER XX

Diseases controlled by Antitoxins

Smallpox. Value of vaccination. Characteristics of smallpox. Treatment of smallpox. Diphtheria. Cause of the disease. Production of
diphtheria antitoxin. Symptoms of diphtheria. Rabies. Tetanus -

# CHAPTER XXI

## Hygiene and Law

Principle of laws of hygiene. Self-interest, the real basis of law. Quality of water. Regulations governing foods. Basis of pure food laws. Protection of milk. Laws governing quarantine -

## LIST OF FIGURES

# RURAL HYGIENE

**CHAPTER I**

# *VITAL STATISTICS OF RURAL LIFE*

It is commonly supposed that good health is the invariable accompaniment of country life; that children who are brought up in the country are always rosy-cheeked, chubby, and, except for occasional colds, free from disease; that adults, both men and women, are strong to labor, like the oxen of the Psalmist, and that grandfathers and grandmothers are so common and so able-bodied that in practically every farmhouse the daily chores are assigned to these aged exponents of strong constitutions and healthy lives. If, however, we are honest in our observations, or have lived on a farm in our younger days, or have kept our eyes open when visiting in the country, we will remember, one by one, certain facts which will persistently suggest that, after all, life on the farm may not be such a spring of health as we have been led to believe. We will remember the frequency of funerals, especially in the winter, and the few families in which all the children have reached maturity. We will remember the worn-out bodies of men and women, bent and aged while yet in middle life. [Pg 2]

It is worth while, then, at the beginning, to find out, if we can, just what are the conditions of health in rural communities, in order to justify any book dealing with rural hygiene; for it is plain that if health conditions are already perfect, or nearly so, no book dealing with improved methods of living is needed, and the wisdom of the grandparents may be depended on to continue such methods into the next generation.

*Death-rate.*

The usual method of measuring the health conditions of any community, such as a city, town, county, state, or country, is to compute the general death-rate, as it is called; that is, the number of deaths occurring per 1000 population. For example, in 1908, with its estimated population of 8,546,356, there occurred in New York State 138,441 deaths, or 16.2 deaths for every 1000 population. Sixteen and two-tenths is, then, the general death-rate for the state for that year. This method of determining the health of a community is crude and should not be too strictly relied upon for proving the healthfulness implied. The rate is at best only an average, and takes no account of anything but death, one death being a greater calamity, apparently, than a dozen persons incapacitated from disease. Then, too, this death-rate is greatly affected by peculiarities of the community in age, sex, nationality, and occupation, and by local conditions of climate, altitude, and soil. The effect of these local conditions can best be explained after a consideration of the general death-rate and its definite values in different places.

In the United States, as a whole, or, more exactly, in that part of the United States which keeps such records of [Pg 3] deaths as to be reliable (about one half), the annual average death-rate for the five-year period 1901-1905 was 16.3, and this may be compared with the death-rate in other countries shown in the following table for the same period: —

**Table I. Death-rates in Various Countries**

| | |
|---|---|
| Australia | 11.7 |
| Austria | 24.2 |
| Belgium | 17.0 |
| Denmark | 14.8 |
| England | 16.0 |
| France | 19.6 |
| Germany | 19.9 |
| Italy | 21.9 |
| Japan | 20.9 |
| Netherlands | 16.0 |
| New York State | 17.1 |

| Norway | 14.5 |
| Spain | 26.1 |
| Sweden | 15.5 |
| United States | 16.3 |

*Ideal death-rates.*

There are special reasons why the Australian death-rate should be low, but, neglecting this one country entirely, it will be seen that Norway, Denmark, and Sweden have rates of 14.5, 14.8, and 15.5, respectively; rates which may be considered as good as any country can attain at the present time. But the United States, as a whole, has about one more death per 1000 than these countries, and New York State two more per 1000 population. This means that in New York State there are 16,000 more deaths each year than if the population were living in Sweden under Swedish conditions and laws. Or, expressed in another way, it means that in Sweden one out of every sixty-five persons dies each year, and in New York one out of every fifty-eight persons.

The rate in New York State is high because the state [Pg 4] contains a large number of cities, and concentration of population generally implies all kinds of bad and unsanitary conditions. As a rule, a higher death-rate may be expected in a densely populated community than in a sparsely settled one, and we should therefore expect a rural community to show a lower death-rate than a city or urban community. It is not a fair estimate of the health of any rural locality, such as a county where no large cities exist, to compare its death-rate with the average of the state, or with the average rate of some other county which contains a large city. This fact is plainly brought out by the statistics in Table II, from the several sanitary districts into which the state of New York is divided, as shown on the map, Fig. 1:—

**Table II. Showing Varying Death-rates in Different Parts of New York State**

| | Death Rate in |
| --- | --- |
| | |

| Sanitary Districts | 1901-5 | 1906 | 1907 |
|---|---|---|---|
| New York State | 17.1 | 17.1 | 17.5 |
| Maritime | 19.0 | 18.2 | 18.4 |
| Hudson Valley | 17.2 | 17.0 | 18.2 |
| Mohawk Valley | 15.5 | 16.3 | 16.6 |
| West Central | 15.0 | 15.6 | 16.6 |
| Lake Ontario and Western | 14.9 | 15.5 | 15.9 |
| East Central | 14.9 | 15.4 | 15.9 |
| Southern Tier | 14.4 | 14.7 | 15.6 |
| Adirondack and Northern | 13.9 | 15.1 | 15.3 |

[Pg 5]

*Death-rates in New York State.*

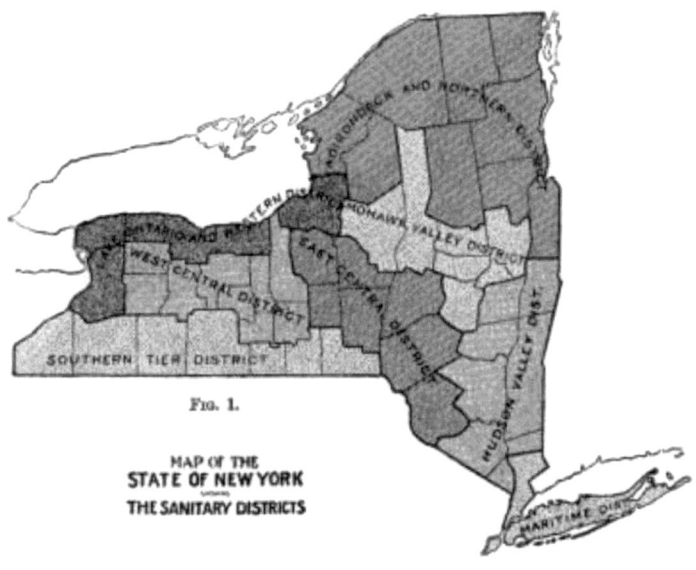

Fig. 1.

MAP OF THE STATE OF NEW YORK SHOWING THE SANITARY DISTRICTS

The Maritime District includes the four counties of New York City and comprises about half the population [Pg 6] of the state. Its population is almost entirely quartered under distinctly urban conditions, in some parts with a congestion not equaled in any other city of the country. It would naturally, therefore, have a high death-rate, and that it is no higher than it is makes it a matter for congratulation. And yet the rate in New York City is higher than in the other principal large cities of the world. For example, the rates for the five-year period 1900-1904 in Berlin averaged 18.3, in Paris 18.2, and in London 16.9, New York being 19.4 for the corresponding period. The excess in New York is due in part to local conditions and in part to a less active oversight in matters of public health. Similarly, the Hudson Valley District, which embraces the large cities along the Hudson, has a higher death-rate than the state average, whereas the other six districts have low rates, chiefly because of the large proportion of agricultural land and small towns. The last district should be noted particularly, since its rate is remarkably low and its number of cities very small, compared with the area included. The conclusion may be properly drawn, therefore, that statistics confirm the general impression that life in the country is healthier than life in the city.

*Accuracy of death-rate records.*

One factor must be considered, however, since it plays an important part in drawing conclusions from these kinds of statistics, and that is, the accuracy of the records. In a city in which every one must be buried in a public cemetery, and when the physician, the undertaker, and the sexton all have to keep records which must agree, it is not easy for any burial to occur without the fact being [Pg 7] recorded and later registered in the Census Office at Washington. But in the country, a person may be killed by accident, for example, and buried in a private lot without the undertaker recording it at all. The result is that the total number of deaths seems fewer and the death-rate seems smaller than the facts warrant, so that a false idea of the healthfulness of the community obtains. That errors of this sort have existed in the past can be seen by examining the death-rates for New York City and those for regions outside that city for the past ten years: —

**Table III. Death-rates in New York City and Elsewhere in New York State, 1898-1908**

|      | New York | Outside | Difference |
|------|----------|---------|------------|
| 1898 | 20.4     | 14.5    | 5.9        |
| 1899 | 19.6     | 14.9    | 4.7        |
| 1900 | 20.6     | 15.0    | 5.6        |
| 1901 | 19.9     | 15.1    | 4.8        |
| 1902 | 18.6     | 14.1    | 4.5        |
| 1903 | 17.9     | 15.2    | 2.7        |
| 1904 | 18.5     | 17.3    | 1.2        |

| 1905 | 18.3 | 15.8 | 2.5 |
|------|------|------|-----|
| 1906 | 18.4 | 15.7 | 2.7 |
| 1907 | 18.5 | 16.4 | 2.1 |
| 1908 | 16.8 | 15.5 | 1.3 |

The decrease in the city rate is to be expected, since with greater knowledge of sanitary matters, more precautions against disease would naturally be taken. But it is not likely that the country is becoming more careless, [Pg 8] although the tendency to concentrate population even in rural hamlets may have an effect. It is rather more likely that the reports are made more carefully and that the records are more complete now than formerly. The apparent increase in the number of deaths in rural communities is, therefore, due to greater attention in reporting deaths rather than to any real increase in the number.

If the difference between the rural community death-rate and the rate in all the cities of more than 8000 population in New York State be shown, the difference between the city rate and the country rate is even less than that shown in the table, being only 0.7 deaths in 1000 for 1908. This shows that the boasted superiority of the country over cities is not very great; that it is marked only in the case of a very large city like New York; that, as the size of the city decreases, the difference disappears, and that the country rate in the United States is high when compared with the general rate of other countries like Denmark or even England, where the general rate includes the large cities.

*Effect of children on death-rate.*

An interesting sidelight on the apparent tendency of the country to have an increasing death-rate, year by year, is shown by the meager figures which are available on the subject of the number of small children in the different towns. The Chief Clerk in the Census Office, Mr. William S. Rossiter, has investigated the proportion of children in two rural counties of New York State, Otsego and Putnam, and has discovered the startling fact that while the population in those counties has hardly [Pg 9] changed since 1860, the proportion of young children has decreased almost one third in the forty years ending with 1900, as shown by the following table: —

**Table IV. Table showing Percentage of Children in Otsego and Putnam Counties, 1860-1900**

| County | 1900 | | | 1860 | | |
|---|---|---|---|---|---|---|
| | Total White Population | Under 10 Years | Per Cent | Total White Population | Under 10 Years | Per Cent |
| Otsego | 48,793 | 7,121 | 14.5 | 49,950 | 10,988 | 22.0 |
| Putnam | 13,669 | 2,332 | 16.9 | 13,819 | 3,333 | 24.1 |
| Total | 62,462 | 9,453 | 15.0 | 63,769 | 14,321 | 22.5 |

This shows that while in 1860, when the total population was about 64,000, the number of children was about 14,000 or 22.5 per cent, in 1900, when the total population was 62,462 or nearly the same, the number of children was only 9453, or a reduction in numbers of nearly 5000 children. In many of the small cities of New York State, the fact that there is a constantly decreasing number of children in the community is well recognized, the greater proportion of the population being past middle life. The death-rate, therefore, is lower, from this very fact.

*Death-rates of children.*

That the general death-rate is directly affected by the number of children living in a community is shown by the following table: [Pg 10] —

**Table V. Showing Deaths from all Causes in the United States for the Years 1901-1905, at Various Age Periods**

| Age | No. at Each Age | Per Cent of Total Population |
|---|---|---|
| Aggregate | 529,630 | — — |
| Under 1 year | 100,268 | 18.93 |
| Under 5 years | 143,684 | 27.13 |

| | | |
|---|---|---|
| 5-9 years | 13,679 | 2.58 |
| 10-19 years | 23,234 | 4.38 |
| 20-29 years | 46,685 | 8.81 |
| 30-39 years | 49,501 | 9.34 |
| 40-49 years | 48,811 | 9.21 |
| 50-59 years | 51,787 | 9.77 |
| 60-69 years | 59,856 | 11.31 |
| 70-79 years | 56,544 | 10.68 |
| 80-89 years | 29,408 | 5.55 |
| 90 and over | 6,441 | 1.21 |

This table shows two things: first, that children have a hard time reaching five years, as nearly one third of all the children born in any year die under five years, and second, that from five to twenty years is the healthiest—that is, safest—time of a person's life, since after twenty the constitutional diseases make themselves felt so that death becomes almost uniformly distributed from twenty to eighty. It is plain, then, that in any community a change in the relative proportion of children born in any year would change the death-rate, since with a smaller number of infants there could not be so many to die.

No statistics are available to determine the number of small children in the country as compared with that in the city, but it is probable that they are in excess in the [Pg 11] latter, since the highest birth-rates are found in the congested districts of cities where foreigners congregate. If this is so, it will account for and justify a higher rate of death in the city because of the larger number of children, as has been explained above, and the lower rate in the country may be due, not to better sanitary surroundings, but solely to fewer children.

According to statistics, the death-rate of children is almost 50 per cent higher in cities than in rural districts, and it is a general impression that most deaths in the country are from old age. English statistics show, however, and those of the United States would probably show the same thing, that while a baby born in the city is more likely to die before its first birthday than a baby born in the country, they have equal chances to finish a month of life and that the city child has better chances to live out the first week. The advantages of the country, therefore, do not begin to operate until after the first month of the baby's life, and there is a decidedly greater chance of the child's living in the city the first week on account, probably, of better and quicker medical attendance.

*Typhoid fever and the death-rate.*

Turning now to special diseases and comparing the number of deaths caused by special diseases in the country and in the city, it is to be noted, first of all, that a greater difference exists in the case of certain special diseases in the country and in the city than was found in the general death-rate. In the case of typhoid fever, basing the comparison on the statistics of the Census Office of the United States, we find, first, that, at present, the difference in the death-rates from typhoid fever in cities and in rural districts [Pg 12] is very small. It is also to be seen (from the following table) that in both city and in rural districts, the rate is steadily decreasing, although in neither has the rate yet fallen to what would, in other countries, be considered a reasonable and proper death-rate. The first line of the table is the actual death-rate from typhoid fever per 100,000 population, based on the total population resident in all the United States where vital statistics are kept; the second line gives the same data for cities not included in registration states; [1] the third line is based on figures for cities in registration states;[**] and the fourth line is based on the statistics for rural districts and villages of less than 8000 population: —

**Table VI. Showing Death-rates per 100,000 Population from Typhoid Fever in Places Indicated**

| Year | 1900 | 1901 | 1902 | 1903 | 1904 | 1905 | 1906 | 1907 | 1908 |
|---|---|---|---|---|---|---|---|---|---|
| The registration area | 35.9 | 32.4 | 34.5 | 34.4 | 32.0 | 28.1 | 32.1 | 30.3 | 25.3 |
| Registration | 36.5 | 33.9 | 37.5 | 38.2 | 35.2 | 30.1 | 34.2 | 32.9 | 25.8 |

| cities | | | | | | | | | |
|---|---|---|---|---|---|---|---|---|---|
| Cities in registration states | 28.5 | 26.5 | 25.9 | 24.6 | 24.0 | 22.0 | 34.2 | 31.7 | 24.5 |
| Rural part of registration states | 34.6 | 28.8 | 27.0 | 24.7 | 23.8 | 23.0 | 28.6 | 26.0 | 24.3 |

This table shows that, taking the United States as a whole, the typhoid-rate in rural districts is generally less [Pg 13] than in cities and that in cities the rate is excessively high.

When it is remembered that by filtration of public water-supplies the typhoid-rate may be brought down to about 15 per 100,000, and that cities with pure water-supplies will not exceed that rate, it is plain how serious is the danger from typhoid in such cities as Cohoes or Oswego. The following table from statistics taken in New York State shows the same conditions as Table VI. —

**Table VII. Showing Death-rates from Typhoid Fever per 100,000 Population in New York State as Indicated**

| Year | 1900 | 1901 | 1902 | 1903 | 1904 | 1905 | 1906 | 1907 | 1908 |
|---|---|---|---|---|---|---|---|---|---|
| Cities average | 25.4 | 23.9 | 23.4 | 22.6 | 21.6 | 19.1 | 19.0 | 20.7 | 20.1 |
| Rural districts | 32.0 | 27.3 | 23.4 | 22.1 | 21.8 | 21.8 | 20.2 | 19.3 | 20.8 |
| Average of city population | — | 38.9 | 33.9 | 43.0 | 40.3 | 32.2 | 30.5 | 32.1 | 32.4 |
| Average of rural population | — | 20.3 | 24.1 | 23.2 | 21.3 | 22.3 | 21.3 | 19.9 | 20.8 |

The first line is the death-rate in cities, found by taking the ratio of all the deaths from typhoid in cities to the population in those cities, and the second line is a similar ratio for rural districts. If the actual rates of the several cities be averaged, a method which has the effect of giving the rate found for a city of 10,000 equal value in the average with one of 1,000,000, the third line of the table is obtained; and in the same way, by averaging the death-rates of the counties of the state, excluding cities, the fourth line is obtained. These last two lines show that the average [Pg 14] of the city rates is noticeably higher than the average of the rural rates, and that, while since 1900 the average of the rural districts has remained uniform, the death-rate in cities has been continually decreasing.

It is, then, not fair to say, despite frequent but careless statements by writers on typhoid fever, that this disease is a country disease, and that it is transmitted to the city by the vacationist who finds the disease lurking in the waters of the farm well. Some years ago it was pointed out that the period of maximum development of typhoid fever is in the fall, and the conclusion was drawn that the disease was particularly prevalent then because that season is the end of the vacation period. That this is not true, or at any rate not entirely true, may be seen from the consideration of two facts, viz. first, that the death-rate in the country districts is low compared with the rates in cities, and second, that those stricken with the disease on their return to the city are quite as apt to have traveled through other cities and to have taken water from other places than farm wells.

*Typhoid in small cities.*

As a matter of fact, the greatest danger from typhoid fever is neither in the country nor the large city, but in the village or small city. Here the growth and congestion of population has made necessary the introduction of a water-supply, and in many cases this has not been supplemented by the construction of a sewerage system. The ground becomes saturated with filth, percolating, in many cases, into wells not yet abandoned, and the introduction of the typhoid germ brought in from outside is all that is needed to start a widespread epidemic. [Pg 15]

**Table VIII. Mortality from Typhoid Fever in the Cities of New York State, showing Total Deaths from Typhoid Fever and Deaths per 100,000 Population**

| | | Rate per 100,000 | | | | | | | | | |
|---|---|---|---|---|---|---|---|---|---|---|---|
| | Average rate per 100,000 for ten years | 1899 | 1900 | 1901 | 1902 | 1903 | 1904 | 1905 | 1906 | 1907 | 1 |
| *Cities using unfiltered lake water:* | | | | | | | | | | | |
| ...urn | 23.0 | 23.4 | 39.5 | 22.9 | 9.7 | 25.8 | 28.8 | 15.9 | 12.1 | 6.0 | 4 |
| ...kirk | 40.2 | 17.5 | 51.6 | 32.4 | 76.5 | 29.0 | 41.3 | 39.3 | 31.4 | 71.8 | 1 |
| ...va | 29.3 | 49.2 | — - | 46.3 | 9.0 | 52.1 | 42.0 | 32.7 | 24.0 | 15.4 | 2 |
| *Cities using unfiltered river water:* | | | | | | | | | | | |
| ...es | 84.4 | 88.3 | 113.0 | 58.4 | 133.2 | 91.3 | 103.6 | 57.9 | 57.8 | 78.2 | 6 |
| ...port | 48.4 | 18.1 | 18.0 | 71.5 | 35.4 | 75.7 | 34.6 | 51.8 | 67.6 | 50.1 | 6 |
| ...ara Falls | 132.9 | 113.0 | 123.3 | 143.7 | 148.1 | 114.0 | 135.3 | 184.4 | 154.5 | 126.0 | 8 |
| ...h Tona-da | 30.9 | 23.1 | 11.0 | 32.3 | 10.5 | 41.1 | 30.2 | 39.3 | 19.3 | 47.2 | 5 |
| ...ensburg | 54.6 | 87.8 | 39.5 | 31.4 | 62.3 | 61.7 | 68.9 | 53.1 | 67.3 | 47.1 | 2 |
| ...ego | 49.4 | 22.6 | 45.0 | 22.4 | 17.5 | 53.5 | 62.3 | 84.1 | 58.0 | 66.0 | 6 |
| ...e | 22.7 | 26.1 | 6.5 | 12.2 | 25.2 | 18.6 | 24.5 | 42.3 | 28.2 | 17.0 | 2 |
| ...wanda | 30.1 | 13.5 | 13.4 | 13.3 | — - | 26.0 | 38.4 | 25.3 | 50.6 | 25.0 | 9 |
| *Cities using filtered river water:* | | | | | | | | | | | |
| ...ny | 28.7 | 87.0 | 40.3 | 21.1 | 30.2 | 19.7 | 18.5 | 19.3 | 20.3 | 20.0 | 1 |
| ...hamton | 22.2 | 25.5 | 42.8 | 52.4 | 27.1 | 9.7 | 9.6 | 12.0 | 9.1 | 18.2 | 1 |

| | | | | | | | | | | |
|---|---|---|---|---|---|---|---|---|---|---|
| ira | 41.0 | 33.6 | 47.6 | 25.4 | 39.7 | 80.0 | 51.6 | 28.8 | 44.7 | 28.0 |
| ughkeepsie | 46.5 | 25.1 | 45.7 | 41.1 | 20.3 | 44.2 | 59.7 | 43.3 | 39.4 | 112.0 |
| nsselaer | 61.9 | 107.3 | 93.7 | 61.6 | 91.2 | 31.8 | 89.4 | 37.3 | 18.6 | 58.3 |
| tertown | 71.9 | 85.7 | 101.4 | 35.6 | 64.7 | 71.0 | 211.0 | 23.6 | 50.0 | 37.1 |
| tervliet | 57.5 | 105.7 | 77.0 | 55.6 | 62.3 | 55.2 | 61.8 | 47.9 | 47.7 | 20.4 |

*Cities using well or spring water:*

| | | | | | | | | | | |
|---|---|---|---|---|---|---|---|---|---|---|
| rning | 46.4 | 27.7 | 54.2 | 43.2 | 24.9 | 48.0 | 46.1 | 30.0 | 43.1 | 69.0 |
| rtland | 29.2 | 55.8 | 33.2 | 116.2 | 10.1 | – – | 9.2 | 26.6 | 8.7 | 24.6 |
| ton | 33.2 | 25.0 | – | 24.0 | 11.8 | 93.2 | 34.8 | 22.6 | 56.5 | 22.0 |
| ıca | 51.7 | 7.8 | 45.6 | 44.6 | 7.3 | 357.0 | 27.9 | 13.7 | 6.8 | – |
| an | 19.5 | 21.6 | 10.5 | 20.8 | 30.7 | 30.3 | 20.0 | – – | 20.0 | 19.1 |
| estown | 28.9 | 40.5 | 39.3 | 25.5 | 4.1 | 24.1 | 62.7 | 23.0 | 33.8 | 18.2 |
| enectady | 31.6 | 3.3 | 44.2 | 40.5 | 26.0 | 33.5 | 22.6 | 8.6 | 17.8 | 8.7 |

*Cities using water from streams and reservoirs:*

| | | | | | | | | | | |
|---|---|---|---|---|---|---|---|---|---|---|
| sterdam | 19.4 | 19.8 | 14.3 | 23.2 | 18.1 | 44.0 | 17.1 | 16.7 | 24.8 | 15.9 |
| ns Falls | 37.6 | 24.6 | 47.6 | 61.4 | 14.9 | 28.9 | 49.2 | 20.4 | 46.5 | 45.3 |
| versville | 20.0 | 16.7 | 49.0 | 5.4 | 43.3 | 10.8 | 5.4 | 21.4 | 5.3 | 5.3 |
| nstown | 19.1 | 20.2 | 69.1 | – | 20.0 | 30.1 | – – | 10.2 | 20.4 | – – |
| wburgh | 39.6 | 48.4 | 44.1 | 23.7 | 47.0 | 34.7 | 42.0 | 37.1 | 41.3 | 41.0 |
| w Rochelle | 21.1 | 7.1 | 6.8 | 38.0 | 29.3 | 22.0 | 15.5 | 19.5 | 23.2 | 22.0 |
| ttsburg | 21.0 | 24.1 | 23.7 | 34.1 | 11.0 | 21.1 | – – | 39.2 | 28.7 | 27.6 |
| y | 49.2 | 65.1 | 101.2 | 55.7 | 48.8 | 32.8 | 44.4 | 46.8 | 36.2 | 25.8 |
| ca | 17.3 | 16.3 | 14.1 | 15.6 | 20.3 | 16.6 | 17.8 | 9.5 | 27.6 | 15.2 |

| | | | | | | | | | | |
|---|---|---|---|---|---|---|---|---|---|---|
| Jervis | 42.7 | 10.6 | 31.9 | 31.8 | 52.5 | 73.1 | 72.6 | 72.2 | 31.0 | 51.0 | - |
| Falls | 36.4 | 29.3 | 125.2 | 28.5 | 37.5 | 27.7 | 36.4 | —- | 44.7 | 8.8 | 2 |
| da | 17.2 | 26.5 | 13.3 | 25.9 | 38.0 | —- | 36.3 | —- | 11.8 | —- | 1 |
| *Cities using filtered surface water:* | | | | | | | | | | | |
| ell | 28.8 | 76.1 | 25.1 | 32.8 | 32.1 | 55.0 | 7.7 | 30.2 | 7.5 | 7.5 | 1 |
| son | 59.2 | 62.8 | 94.4 | 41.3 | 81.3 | 30.0 | 167.7 | 48.5 | 38.0 | 9.4 | 1 |
| ston | 19.4 | 28.9 | 8.1 | 12.1 | 16.0 | 19.9 | 11.8 | 31.3 | 15.6 | 27.0 | 2 |
| lleton | 24.5 | 21.0 | 13.7 | 13.8 | 55.1 | 13.8 | 6.9 | 41.3 | 18.8 | 18.8 | 4 |
| nt Ver- | 14.6 | 5.0 | 4.9 | 13.6 | 8.8 | 8.5 | 20.6 | 20.0 | 19.4 | 37.7 | 7 |
| onta | 37.9 | 28.7 | 27.9 | 13.6 | 66.5 | 26.0 | 50.8 | 24.8 | 48.6 | 23.8 | 6 |
| ers | 9.9 | 10.8 | 4.1 | 15.9 | 9.3 | 14.2 | 15.2 | 1.6 | 6.2 | 11.9 | 9 |

[Pg 18]

Another reason for the prevalence of this disease in small cities is that the organization of their health boards is much less effective than that of larger cities. Individuals have not yet learned to sacrifice their own wishes for the sake of the community, and the local health officer, however much he may desire to do his duty, is not upheld by public opinion, and is therefore powerless.

In order to show the condition existing in the small cities of the state of New York, the preceding table has been prepared, showing the average death-rate for the cities of the state for the past ten years, excluding, however, the cities of New York, Buffalo, Rochester, and Syracuse, all of which have well-organized health boards, and where no epidemic of typhoid fever may be expected. Remembering that a rate of 15 per 100,000 is a normal rate, it will be easily seen how excessive is the amount of typhoid fever in most of the cities of New York State.

**Table IX. Showing Deaths from Tuberculosis per 100,000 Population in the United States**

|  | 1900 | 1901 | 1902 | 1903 | 1904 | 1905 | 1906 | 1907 | 1908 |
|---|---|---|---|---|---|---|---|---|---|
| The registration area | 180.5 | 175.1 | 163.6 | 165.7 | 177.3 | 168.2 | 159.4 | 158.9 | 149.6 |
| Registration cities | 198.8 | 192.1 | 180.7 | 183.6 | 195.5 | 184.4 | 181.5 | 179.4 | 170.1 |
| Cities in Registration states | 204.1 | 194.9 | 177.7 | 179.7 | 189.4 | 178.5 | 184.0 | 181.5 | 169.1 |
| Rural part of Registration states | 138.0 | 133.8 | 121.1 | 120.7 | 131.4 | 126.2 | 121.9 | 123.8 | 117.3 |

[Pg 19]

*Tuberculosis death-rate.*

Turning now to tuberculosis, the death-rate in cities is very markedly higher than in rural districts, and the superiority of the country as a place to live is hereby plainly demonstrated. The preceding table shows the death rate from tuberculosis in cities for the years 1903-1907, the data being taken from the United States Census Reports.

The death-rate in the cities is evidently about 60 per 100,000 greater than in the rural districts, due, of course, to the crowding in city tenements. This is true for nearly all cities, although the difference is more marked in some parts of the country than in others. In Massachusetts, for example, the death-rate in rural districts is slightly higher than the death-rate in cities, but tuberculosis is much more prevalent in that state than in any other part of the country. In New York State the rate in cities is about 70 per 100,000 greater than in rural districts, due, presumably, to the larger number of manufacturing centers in this state. In New York City the rate is constantly more than 200, and in 1908 in the borough of the Bronx it was nearly 500.

*Diphtheria as affecting the rate.*

Diphtheria is another disease that exacts heavier toll from the cities than from the country, about three times as many deaths occurring in the former as in the latter.

*Influenza, and its effect on death-rate.*

Influenza is, on the other hand, markedly severe on people in rural districts, the death-rate there being more than twice as high as in the cities. It is easy to see why [Pg 20] this is. Lack of sidewalks, lack of protection, lack of uniform temperature in the houses, and the lack of care in the first stages of illness, all tend to increase the death-rate from this disease.

*Pneumonia.*

The death-rate from pneumonia, on the other hand, is higher in the city, the vitality and power of resistance of victims probably being reduced under average city conditions.

*Other diseases.*

Diseases that are induced by water, all referred to under typhoid fever, but extending into such complaints as diarrhœa and enteritis, are much more severe in cities than in the country. Such an excess of general intestinal diseases shows again that a polluted water-supply is not peculiar to the country, but is responsible for an excessive death-rate in the city. Most of the constitutional diseases also have higher death-rates in the city than in the country. Bright's disease, for example, for the five years 1903-1907, had an average rate in cities of 107.3 per 100,000, while for the same five years in the rural districts the rate was only 68.6.

*Old age and the death-rate.*

Further showing the advantage of country life, it is to be noted that the number of deaths from old age in rural districts is nearly double that in cities. For example, in the same period already referred to the death-rate in cities of persons over sixty was 27.6, while in the rural districts, for the same period, it was 49.3, — nearly double.

*The need for attention to rural hygiene.*

One must conclude, therefore, that the chances of living [Pg 21] are increased through residence in the country or in rural districts, and one is therefore led to ask why, if conditions there are superior to those in the city, is it necessary to deal with the question of rural hygiene, and why attempt to improve conditions which are already evidently superior to those in cities. The answer to this must lie in the statement that the death-rate does not tell the whole story of public health. So far as the real welfare of a community is concerned, the standard should be that of the efficiency of the lives in the different age periods rather than the length of those periods. By efficiency in such a connection is meant not merely a life that is free enough from disease to permit the full number of working days in the year, and the full number of years in the man's life usually devoted to toil, or all together a life that contributes something of value to the world, whether produce from the farm or books evolved from the brain; but efficiency here means that composite development of the whole man—body, mind, and spirit—which we believe must have been intended when man was created with this threefold nature. It is in this composite development that those living in the country are sadly lacking in efficiency.

Not to the same extent as twenty-five years ago, but still too often is the farmer so exhausted by bodily toil that he has left no strength for the cultivation of either mind or spirit. For the brief period of spring and summer, the good farmer in the Eastern States works himself harder than any slave of old. Up with the sun, or earlier, he follows through the long day the hardest kind of manual labor. When the end of the day comes, after fifteen hours' physical strain, his weary body demands sleep, and no [Pg 22] vitality is left for mental improvement. In the winter, on the other hand, a lack of exercise is enforced, and the resulting interference with normal functions is so great that he lives the winter through in a sort of hibernation. He is nearly poisoned by lack of ventilation in the small living room, where the one stove makes living possible; he gets fat and indolent, and then with relaxed muscles plunges into furious labor again when spring comes round.

"No wonder," says Woods Hutchinson, "that by forty-five he has had a sunstroke and 'can't stand the heat' or has a 'weak back' or his 'heart gives out' or a chill 'makes him rheumatic.'" Such a life is not efficient any more than a steam engine is efficient when half the time it is run at such high speed that it tends to shake itself to pieces and the other half of the time it stands idle. Nor are the conditions under which farmers' wives live any better. Statistics show that the highest percentage of insanity in any class of persons in the United States (due chiefly to overwork, overworry, and lack of proper amusements and recreation) is to be found among farmers' wives.

An ideal life is not one which merely rounds out the allotted span, but one which, during that span, is measurably free from ailments and disabilities and in a condition to claim a share in the joy of living which belongs to every human being by reason of his existence. Such lives, to be sure, are seldom found, and no system of statistics yet devised has been able to take account of those ailments. Insurance companies, which make good losses for inability to work and which return the cost of medicines and doctors' bills, give the only information on the subject. From these, it has been shown that for each [Pg 23] death in a community there are a little more than two years of illness. Or, expressed differently, for every death occurring in a village, there are two persons constantly ill during the year. Or, still differently, there are, on the average, thirteen days' sickness per year for every person in a community.

It is the aim of all hygienic efforts to prevent not merely premature death, but also the inefficiency of unhealthy living, and it is the latter condition rather than the former which generally prevails in rural communities. As we have seen, the death-rates in the country, except for pneumonia, are not noticeably higher than in the city. But by minor ailments, with the resulting loss of daily efficiency, the rural communities are sadly overburdened. As Irving Fisher says in his Report on National Vitality:—

"But prevention is merely the first step in increasing the breadth of life. Life is to be broadened not only negatively by diminishing those disabilities which narrow it, but also positively by increasing the cultivation of vitality. Here we leave the realm of medicine and enter the realm of physical training…. Beyond athletic sports in turn comes mental, moral, and spiritual culture, the highest product of health cultivation. It is an encouraging sign of the times that the ecclesiastical view of the Middle Ages, which associated saintliness

with sickness, has given way to modern 'muscular Christianity.'...
This is but one evidence of the tendency toward the 'religion of
healthymindedness' described by Professor James. Epictetus taught
that no one could be the highest type of philosopher unless in exu-
berant health. Expressions of Emerson's and Walt Whitman's show
how much [Pg 24] their spiritual exaltation was bound up with
health ideals. 'Give me health and a day,' said Emerson, 'and I will
make the pomp of emperors ridiculous.' It is only when these health
ideals take a deep hold that a nation can achieve its highest development. Any country which adopts such ideals as an integral part
of its practical life philosophy may be expected to reach or even
excel the development of the health-loving Greeks."

**FOOTNOTES:**

[1] States in which full credit is given by U. S. Census Office for Vital Statistics collected from all parts of the state.

[Pg 25]

## CHAPTER II

# *LOCATION OF A HOUSE — SOIL AND SUR-ROUNDINGS*

In attempting to develop a system of rural hygiene, by means of which the full value of the advantages of pure air and sunlight, of healthful exercise and sound sleep, may be realized, the first step should be a proper location of the house. For, while it is possible to have good health in houses not advantageously located, and while the influence of unsanitary surroundings is not as great as was formerly supposed, yet there can be no question but that some influences, whether they be great or small, must result directly from the situation of a dwelling. For example, it has been noticed that a house whose cellar was damp was an unhealthy house to live in, and early text-books on hygiene quote statistics at length to prove this fact.

The early theories connecting ill-health with conditions in and around the house have been handed down, and to-day some are accepted as true, although by the modern science of bacteriology most of the early notions have been upset. For example, it was considered dangerous to breathe night air in the vicinity of swamps, and in one of the Rollo Books, so much read by the children of [Pg 26] the last generation, Uncle George requires Rollo, on a night journey through the Italian marshes, to stay inside the coach with the windows closed in order not to breathe the night air and so contract malarial fever. We know to-day that malarial fever comes only from mosquitoes, that night air has nothing to do with disease, and we hear the general advice of doctors that, except where it means the admission of mosquitoes, we should always sleep with our windows open in order to breathe as much night air as possible, because the night air is purer than any other air. These early traditions have not only concerned themselves with damp cellars and night air, but they have insisted that even the vicinity of a swamp or pond might lead to disease, and the State Department of Health of New York is in constant receipt of complaints because of alleged danger to health on account of some pond or swamp in the vicinity of houses.

Again, one tradition says that a house should not be located in the midst of a dense growth of trees, because the shade of the trees, however welcome in summer, will generate and maintain a condition of dampness in the house and, therefore, be injurious to the health of the inmates.

Another tradition is that a house ought not to be located in a valley, but that a hilltop, or at least a sidehill elevation, is preferable, the possible dampness of the valley being alleged again as the reason.

To-day, so far as is known, there is no direct evidence of dampness being primarily responsible for any disease, although, heretofore, such diseases as typhoid fever, yellow fever, bilious fever, malarial fever, cholera, and [Pg 27] dysentery have all been attributed to miasms springing from damp soil. To-day we are assured by experts that none of these diseases are induced by dampness alone. One could spend his days immersed in water up to his chin and never contract any sickness of the types mentioned merely through that act. Later on, we shall show how the presence of swamps in the vicinity of a house is objectionable because of their providing breeding places for insects, but the dampness itself never has and never will cause disease. As a concrete example, it may be noted that the country of Holland, in large part lying below the level of the sea, with drainage canals and ditches everywhere in evidence, is, in spite of such manifest possibilities of dampness, one of the most healthy countries in the world, as already pointed out in Chapter I. This fact not only emphasizes the small effect of surface waters and damp soils in promoting disease, but also magnifies the value of cleanliness for which the Dutch people are so famous.

*Damp soils.*

Why is it, then, that damp soils and damp cellars are objected to? Chiefly, because of the inconvenience and discomfort they occasion. A damp cellar means conditions favorable to the development of mildew and rot; prevents vegetables from keeping a normal length of time; accounts for moldy, decaying odors throughout the house, and is generally disagreeable. One is tempted to say that such a condition is also unhealthy, and it is quite possible that a person living over a damp cellar which contains accumulations of decaying vegetables, and breathing air loaded with organic compounds, may gradually lose his [Pg 28] normal vitality, and become thereby more readily susceptible to specific diseases, but the diseases themselves will not come from the dampness alone.

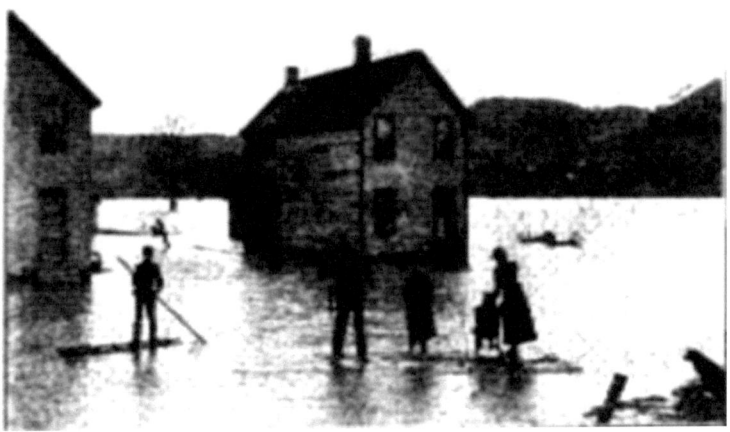

Fig. 2—Bad conditions about a dwelling.

The discomfort and inconvenience, however, are quite sufficient reasons to make it eminently desirable to have the house and the cellar dry. With this in mind, the selection of the house site should be carefully made. Instinctively, and with reason, the immediate neighborhood of low, swampy, marshy ground, of stagnant ponds, or of sluggish streams should be avoided. It should not be necessary to warn prospective builders that low land, subject to inundation, even though this may happen only occasionally, is not a wise choice of a building site. Figure 2 shows an inundation in a small village of

New York State in 1889. Floods are expected each spring and counted on as a part of the year's experience. [Pg 29] The resulting exposure and the inevitable effluvia following the receding waters are
both objectionable factors in hygienic living. Similarly, the vicinity
of a stream carrying organic matter, such as sewage from a town
above, should undoubtedly be avoided on account of possible odors
in summer. Not long ago, the writer was told by the owner of a
productive farm, situated below a small city in New York State, that
in the summer time the windows of his house had all to be kept
tightly shut at night, because of the effluvia from a stream a thousand feet distant, which carried the sewage from the city above.

*Location of house.*

A deep and narrow valley should be avoided, not so much because of the possible dampness in the valley, but because of the
noticeably lessened amount of sunlight which such a location involves. For such a house, the morning sun comes up much later,
and the afternoon sun disappears much earlier, and, since sunlight
is the best foe to disease, the more sunlight enters a house, the
healthier are those who live in it. On the other hand, the top of a hill
exposes a house to strong and cold winds, not desirable on any
account, and involving a large expense for heating in winter. Sloping ground, therefore, facing the south if possible, or better, some
knoll which rises above the general surface of a southern slope,
affords an ideal location. If the slope is toward the south, north
winds are kept off, and every ray of the life-giving winter's sun is
captured. If the house itself faces due south, the windows on the
north have no sunlight. If, on the other hand, the house faces southeast or southwest, then all sides of the house will receive direct sunlight at some time of the day. [Pg 30]

*Objections to trees.*

The vicinity of trees is not to be regarded as altogether evil, since
they provide both shade in summer and a screen against winds in
the winter. No disease comes from dampness because of their presence, and the worst thing which may be charged against a thick
growth is that it keeps out the sun. Practically two points may,
however, be urged against trees growing too close to a house. If
near enough for leaves to drop on the roof, rain troughs and leaders

become stopped up and cause trouble. A thick growth directly over a shingle roof allows organic matter to accumulate on the shingles, so that vegetation develops and the roof decays more rapidly than if exposed to sun and wind. Again, and it is no trivial matter, a house whose roof is easily accessible from trees is apt to become infested with squirrels, who get into the attic, run through the walls, and become a great nuisance. For these reasons, then, trees should be far enough away from the house to allow the sun to enter the windows freely and to keep away from the roof objectionable animals, large and small.

*Space between houses.*

It is a law or custom as ancient as the Romans that requires a proprietor to build his house so that the eaves should not overhang on the land of his neighbor. Our grandfathers, with the same idea, used to say that a man should be able to drive his team around his house on his own land. In our day it is highly desirable that a house should be built so as to leave as much land under control between the buildings and the lot line as possible. This, of course, does not apply to houses built on a farm of a [Pg 31] hundred acres or more, but rather to the house in a small village where a few hundred people live closely together, under rural conditions. In such a village the water-supply usually comes from wells, and the wastes of the household are discharged into privies and cesspools. There is no law, unfortunately, which restricts the location of either of these two essential structures, and it is quite possible for a well, built within a few feet of a property line, to be ruined in quality by a cesspool, built later, on the other side of the line. It seems very unjust that, after the trouble and expense of building a well, a neighbor may render it worthless by the location of his cesspool, and yet, unless one can prove a direct underground connection between well and cesspool, no law is applicable to prevent the construction of the latter.

Besides such a menace to health, there are other objections to the immediate vicinity of neighbors which can be avoided by a judicious interposition of space. For example, the writer listened through a long evening, recently, to a hearing before a City Commissioner of Health, where one householder and a crowd of witnesses complained of the noise made by a kicking horse in an adjacent stable. The one witness who was not disturbed by the noise, and who lived in the vicinity, was unexpectedly found to be deaf.

It is wisdom also to have a reasonable space between a house and the highway, chiefly because the dust of the road is thereby kept from the house. There are people who find much enjoyment in watching passers-by on the road, and with them front windows would be as close to the road as possible, but it is wiser to have a front yard of at least fifty feet depth when possible. [Pg 32]

Finally, the location on a sidehill, even when otherwise advantageous, is to be regarded with suspicion if the subsoil strata are horizontal and neighbors up the slope have cesspools in use. The writer knows of several cesspools, built in rock, which, so far as their owners were concerned, have worked successfully for many years, but the water leeching away through the rock was finally discovered to be the cause of continual dampness in neighboring cellars, on lower ground, to the manifest discomfort of those occupying the houses.

*Composition of soils.*

Having thus discussed the location of the house with reference to its surroundings, let us now more carefully examine the character of the soil or earth foundation on which the house shall be built. All soil is made up of varying proportions of mineral and vegetable matter in the interstices of which there are usually to be found more or less air, water, and watery vapor. The mineral substances of soil include almost all of the known minerals, although many of them are found in exceedingly small quantities. The most common and the most important mineral elements of the soil of New York State are carbon, silicon, aluminum, and calcium, which combine in various ways to make either sand, sandstone, clay, shale, limestone, or other rock. The particular form which these mineral elements assume is of interest in choosing a location for a house, for two reasons: —

In the first place, it has been asserted that the mineral constituents of a soil directly affect the health of persons living on that material. For instance, the earlier writers on hygiene gravely pointed out that very hard granite [Pg 33] rocks, when weathered and disintegrated, became permeated by a fungus and caused malaria. We are, however, now so sure of the cause of malaria that we only laugh at a theory upheld by scientists of only twenty years ago.

Some constitutional diseases, including goiter and cancer, have been supposed to flourish in localities where an excess of calcium exists in the soil, and it is true that these diseases do have an unusual prevalence in certain limited districts; but no modern scientist ventures to say whether the boundaries of those districts are determined by the character of the soil constituents or by some other predisposing factor. The truth is that, in matters not absolutely determined by science, many theories usually have to be evolved and proved worthless before the real cause is found.

In the matter of appendicitis, for instance, it was formerly asserted that the seed of grapes was responsible for the local inflammation, and that one could never have appendicitis if such seeds were not swallowed. This theory is to-day almost forgotten, and one eminent surgeon has asserted that the prevalence of this disease in a district depends on the calcium in the soil, since it is to that mineral that hard water is due, although this has not been substantiated. No information is to-day available by which the fitness of a soil for securing sanitary conditions of building can be determined.

*Cancer and soil conditions.*

In the case of cancer, however, while no final conclusions can be drawn, there is some definite indication that the soil conditions have connection with the occurrence and continued appearance of cancer. It is known that this [Pg 34] dread disease is abnormally prevalent in certain districts of the world where topography and climate are fairly alike. For example, the entire region between the Danube and the Alps from Vienna westward and between the Jura and Alps to Geneva furnishes the highest mortality from cancer in all Europe. The subsoil is clay with a thin covering of surface soil, the hillsides draining on to level valleys with meandering watercourses that frequently inundate and supersaturate the already moist soil.

This condition seems to prevail wherever cancer is abnormally prevalent. In England, in northwestern France, and in Spain the topography described in every case accompanies a high death-rate from cancer. It is of great interest to find that in New York State the two districts that are conspicuously affected by this disease have the same topography. The Unadilla Valley and some parts of the Allegheny Valley are noted for their cancer houses, and in both localities we find the same kinds of hillsides and water-soaked valleys as in Germany and France. It has also been noted that the older geological formations are free from the disease and that an occasional inundation does not seem to be a factor. Altogether there seems to be some ground for assuming a connection between cancer and soil conditions, at any rate until scientists have determined the real cause of the disease in those localities where it is now so markedly prevalent.

*Topography.*

The soil, however, with its mineral characteristics, does indirectly affect the health of the householder because different kinds of rock form themselves naturally into [Pg 35] different surface formations, some healthy and some unhealthy. For example, localities where granite rock abounds and comes near the surface are usually healthy because the surface slope is great enough to carry off all drainage water rapidly. The air therefore is dry and not influenced by the immediate vicinity of swamps. The drinking water is soft, and malarial breeding places are usually absent.

Limestone rock, on the other hand, is commonly laid down in horizontal strata, and while a succession of strata may frequently give rapid slopes, marshes are very common, existing even on the tops of the hills. The drinking water is always to be suspected as to quality because, in the first place, it is hard from absorption of lime, and in the next place, cavities and seams in the rock allow polluting material to travel for long distances.

Sandstone, being porous, may be considered a healthy foundation, and sands and gravels of all sorts are usually free from marshy land.

Gravel has always been assumed to be the healthiest soil on which a house could be built, provided the ground water reaches its highest stage three or four feet below the cellar bottom.

Sand is equally desirable except in the cases where vegetable matter has been mixed with the sand, rendering decay imminent. Water drawn from such sands in the form of springs will contain large quantities of nitrates which may lead to excessive development of vegetable life and may have on the human system the same laxative effect as comes from drinking swamp water.

Clays and heavy alluvial soils are not usually considered [Pg 36] desirable soils on which to build. Water does not run from such soils; they hold moisture, and hence are always damp, and marshes are very apt to exist in the vicinity.

*Effects of cultivation.*

It was formerly thought that extensive cultivation was objectionable from the standpoint of health, that manured fields in the vicinity of a house were undesirable, and that the turning up of a well-manured field with a plow in the spring was a very likely source of fever. It is a very common belief to-day that when water pipes are to be laid in city streets, thereby disturbing the soil and bringing fresh earth to the surface, typhoid or other fevers may be expected. There is, however, no ground for this belief, and the fact that laborers and their families live healthily in the midst of the thousands of acres of sewage-irrigated fields near Berlin, where the heavily manured fields are constantly being plowed, is a sure proof of this. The earlier text-books on hygiene all assert, however, the contrary; Parkes, for instance, says that irrigated lands, especially rice fields, which give a great surface for evaporation and also exhale organic matter into the air, are hurtful, and in northern Italy the rice grounds are required to be three quarters of a mile from the small towns to protect the village inhabitants against fevers. There is no ground, however, for such a requirement.

No evidence can be found that men who work in sewers and who breathe sewer air all the time are especially unhealthy. Statistics show that the laborers on the sewage fields of Paris and Berlin are actually healthier than the average person living within those cities.

No reason can be assigned, based on our present knowledge [Pg 37] of bacteriology, why upturned earth or manured fields should be unhealthy except as the breeding of insects may be encouraged thereby. The two essentials, however, which should be considered are: first, the topography or the formation of the soil in order that the surface water may run off freely, and second, the character of the soil so that ground water may not remain too near the surface. Whether the soil is rock or gravel makes very little difference.

*Made ground.*

One kind of soil, however, is distinctly objectionable, although, fortunately, in the country such a soil is unusual: That is, a soil made up of refuse, whether it be garbage, street sweepings from a near-by city, or factory refuse.

The writer has in mind one enterprising landowner and farmer who offered a near-by city the free privilege of dumping the city garbage on his land. This was done for several years, and the low-lying districts of his farm were all filled to a more advantageous level. This garbage was then covered with about a foot of dirt and the land sold in building lots to enterprising laborers determined to own their own homes. According to the old theories of hygiene, the occupants of such houses should have died like rats, but no particular excess of sickness in the one hundred houses so located could be observed. One must, however, believe, as we shall see later, that the repeated breathing of air drawn from such polluted soil must be unhealthy, even though the mortality records fail to show it.

It is interesting in this connection to note that the [Pg 38] organic matter in soil gradually disappears, just as a body buried in a grave will finally decompose. Experiments show that such organic matter as wheat straw or cloth in small pieces rots and decays in about three years. But this depends very largely on an excess of air. If the soil is open and the organic matter loose, oxidation takes place rapidly; but if a large pile of organic matter is buried in clay soil, it will take decades for it to disappear. The vegetable matter in soil is usually produced by the decay of plants which have either grown on the soil or have been washed down into its voids. A great deal was formerly written on the relation between this organic matter and the prevalence of malaria, and some earlier writers believed that the amount of malaria in a district was dependent upon the amount of vegetable débris in the soil. Since we have learned that malaria is carried by mosquitoes, we are less interested in the amount of organic matter in the soil. Its mere presence is not likely to be injurious.

*Water in the soil.*

Only the hardest rocks are entirely solid, the others containing a certain percentage of voids or interstices. These voids are filled with air or water, as the case may be, and we may stop for a moment to inquire the effect of the presence of this air and water. In loose sands the amount of voids is 40 to 50 per cent of the total volume, in sandstone about 20 per cent, and in other rock reduced amounts. The volume of air, therefore, in the soil under a cellar to a depth of four or five feet, amounts to a good many cubic feet and would not be worth inquiring into except for the fact that it is continually in a state of motion. When the ground water, perhaps normally five feet below [Pg 39] the cellar bottom, rises in the spring, this ground air is forced out, and in a cellar without a concrete foundation it rises into the cellar and penetrates into the house.

A house artificially warmed by stoves is continually discharging heated air from the tops of the rooms and colder air is being brought in from below to take its place. This air comes from the ground below, and in open soil may come from a great depth. A case has been noted where gas escaping from a main in a city street twenty feet from a cellar wall was, by the suction due to heat, drawn into the cellar and thence into the rooms of the house. It is possible that air from cesspools and broken drains in the vicinity of a house may, in this same way, contribute to the atmosphere breathed within the walls of the house. Gravelly and sandy soils, therefore, in order to maintain the superiority which they furnish for building construction, should not be polluted, since any pollution in the vicinity influences the quality of air which may get into the house. The method of preventing such ingress is plainly to water-proof the outside walls of the cellar and provide an air-tight floor over the cellar bottom. Methods of doing this will be discussed in the next chapter.

*Moisture in soils.*

The presence of water in the soil has usually been considered to be unhealthy because of the impression that it led to certain fevers. The writer has heard, for instance, of an attack of malaria being caused by a short visit to a damp vegetable cellar; and it is one of the triumphs of the century that the malarial parasite has been discovered, and the old theory of the dangers of moisture been done

49

away with. A damp cellar has always been considered to [Pg 40] be undesirable, but just why nobody knows. A damp cellar causes molds to form rapidly, thus destroying vegetables and other material which might naturally be stored there, but that the presence of moisture in a cellar in itself produces any organic emanation leading to disease is not true, although dampness is essential to the growth of certain organisms.

In the latter part of the nineteenth century, Dr. Bowditch, of Boston, showed that consumption developed most where the surrounding soil was moist, and generally it is the impression that dry air is the only proper air for a consumptive person to breathe. This theory, however, is being rapidly exploded, and patients now remain outdoors in any weather, and no kind of air is objected to by physicians, provided it is outdoor air. Some little time ago the writer was called by a Board of Health to investigate a certain swamp which had some odor, was considered a blot on the landscape in an unusually picturesque village, and was said to be responsible for a long list of contagious diseases. A house-to-house inquiry in the vicinity showed that among some dozen families, only one illness in the last few years could be remembered, and that was an old lady who had been on the verge of the grave for forty years.

It is curious to note the many examples which are cited by the earlier sanitarians to prove the dangerous effect of damp soil. For example, Pettenkofer, a very prominent German hygienist, says that in two royal stables near Munich, with the same arrangements as to stalls, feed, and attendance, and the same class of horses, fever affected the horses very unequally. In one stable, fever was [Pg 41] continually prevalent; in the other, no fever was found. Horses sent from the unhealthful to the healthful stables did not communicate the disease. The difference between the two places, says Pettenkofer, was that in the healthful stables the ground water was five to six feet below the surface, while in the unhealthful ones it was only two and a half feet from the surface. A system of drainage by which the ground water was brought to the same level under both stables made them equally healthful. The writer cannot help but feel that some other factor was involved, and while he has no doubt that excessive dampness in stables or cellars is undesirable, he does not believe that such dampness can be directly the cause of fevers of any sort.

It is not desirable, however, to live over a wet cellar nor to maintain a house in a constant condition of dampness, partly on account of its bad effect on the house and partly because such dampness may, by reducing the vitality of the household, become a predisposing factor in disease.

*Drainage.*

From whatever source dampness may come, it can be guarded against by giving to the surface of the ground in the vicinity of the house, on all sides, sufficient slope away from the walls so that there will be no tendency for water to accumulate against the cellar walls. On the top of a hill this is very easy to do, and the natural surface grade takes care of the surface water without difficulty. On a sidehill or in a valley artificial grading has to be resorted to, except on one side. [Pg 42]

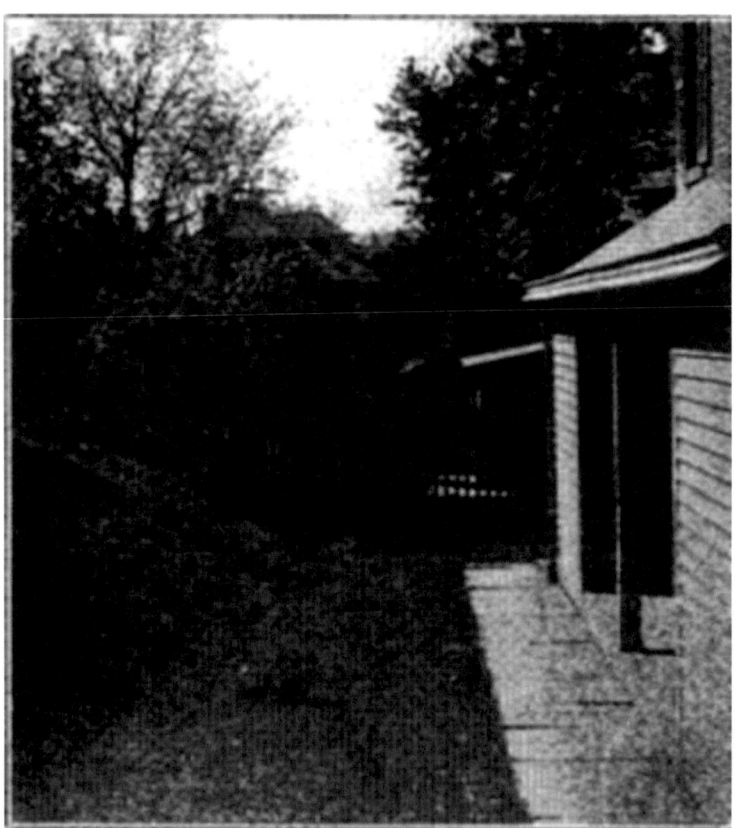

Fig. 3. — A grading that turns water away from the house.

Too much emphasis cannot be laid on the necessity for grading the ground surface away from the house. In some cases it may be sufficient to dig a broad shallow trench protected from wash by sods (Fig. 3). In other cases it may be desirable to pave the ditch with cobble stones or to build a cement gutter. In constructing such a surface drain, proper allowance must be made for the [Pg 43] accumulation of snow and the resulting amount of water in the spring, so that the distance in which the ground slopes away from the house ought to be, if possible, at least ten feet, so that there can be no standing water to penetrate the house walls. The slope necessary to carry surface water away need not be great. A fall of one foot in one hundred will be ample, even on grassy areas, and if the surface is that of a macadam road or the gutters of a drive, this grade may be cut in two. A slope of more than one foot in one hundred is permissible up to a maximum of seven or eight feet per hundred, more than this being æsthetically objectionable and tending to make the house appear too high. Whenever gutters are built in driveways or ditches to intercept water coming down the slopes, a suitable outlet must be provided to carry the water thus collected either into underground pipes, by which the water is led to some stream or gulley, or directly into some well-marked surface depression.

*Ground water.*

The soil always contains water at a greater or less depth, and the elevation of this "ground water," as it is called, varies throughout the year partly with the rainfall and partly with the elevation of the water level in the near-by streams.

It is not at all unusual for this ground water to rise and fall six feet or more within the year, high levels coming usually in the spring and fall, and low levels in the late summer and winter. It is easily possible, then, that a house cellar may seem dry at the time of construction in summer and may develop water to a foot or more in depth after occupancy. The presence of such an amount of [Pg 44] water in a cellar, whether injurious to health or not, is objectionable, and a subsoil trench should be provided in order to limit the height to which ground water may rise.

If a system of drainpipes is led around a house extending outward to include the surrounding yard, then the ground water will always be maintained at the level of those pipes, provided the system has a free outlet. Indeed, the question of an outlet for a drainage system is a most important factor, and no system of underdrains can be effective unless a stream or gulley or depression of some kind is available into which the drains may discharge. It is for this reason, quite as much as for any other, that the location of a house on a perfectly level bottom land is objectionable, since the ground there may be normally full of water with no existing depression into which it may be drained.

In the next chapter the proper method of laying drains close to the cellar wall, for the purpose of taking away the dampness from those walls, is described, but another system of drains is desirable, covering more area and more thoroughly drying the ground, provided the ground water needs attention at all. These drains should be laid like all agricultural drainage; and while substitution of broken stone, bundles of twigs, wooden boxes, or flat stone may be made, the only proper material to be used is burnt clay in the form of tile. These tiles are made in a variety of patterns, but the most common in use to-day is one which is octagonal outside and circular inside. They are about one foot in length and may be had from two to six inches inside diameter. The ordinary size for [Pg 45] laterals is four-inch diameter, while the mains into which these laterals discharge are generally of six-inch diameter. These tiles are laid in trenches about fifteen feet apart, although in porous soil, such as coarse sand or gravel, this distance may be increased to twenty feet. If the tiles are laid more than four feet below the surface, this distance may be increased, and if the tiles are five feet deep, the distance apart of the several lines may be fifty feet.

The grade of the line must be carefully taken care of, and while it is possible to lay a line of tile with a carpenter's level and a sixteen-foot straightedge, it is much safer to have an engineer's or architect's level and set grade stakes, as in regular sewer work. A fall of one fourth of an inch to the foot is a proper grade, although a greater slope is not objectionable. It is sometimes desirable in soft ground to lay down a board six inches wide in the bottom of a trench on which to rest the tile, but, unless the ground is very soft, this is not necessary. Care must be taken, however, if the board is not used, to have the bottom of the trench very carefully smoothed so that a perfectly even grade in the tile is maintained. There are three ways of laying out a line of trench as shown in the following sketches (Fig. 4). It is usually sufficient to run parallel lines of tile from fifteen to fifty feet apart over the area which it is desired to drain, and let the ends of these lines enter a cross line which shall carry off the water led into it. This cross line should be six inches in diameter as a general rule, unless there is more than a mile of small drains, in which case the size of the cross pipe ought to be increased to eight inches. This cross line then becomes the main outlet, and great care must be taken to see that it has a perfectly free delivery at all times of the year. In cities and sometimes in small villages it is possible to discharge this outlet pipe into a regular public sewer, provided the sewer is deep enough, and provided the municipal ordinances allow such a connection. Otherwise, the outfall must be carried to a natural depression. [Pg 46]

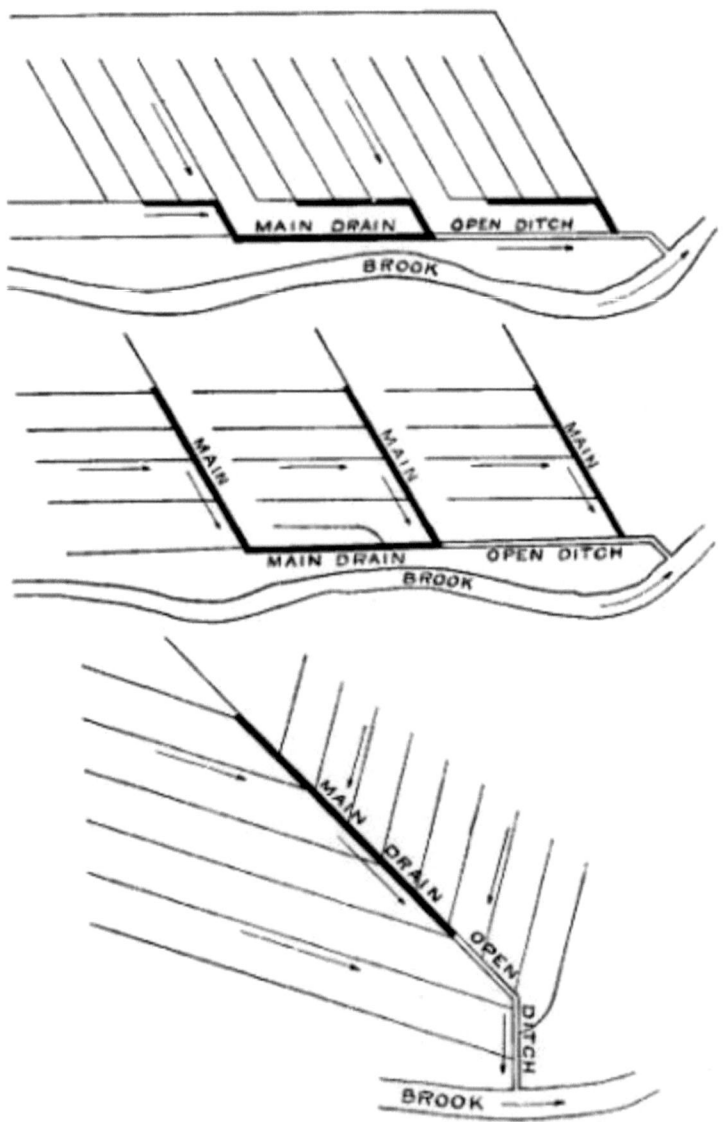

Fig. 4.—Modes of laying out drains.

[Pg 47]

56

In level ground, the problem of finding a suitable outlet is a serious one, and in many cases impossible of solution, so that the householder, being unable to find an outlet, must put up with the ground water and be as patient as possible during its prevalence. It does not do to trust one's eye to find a practicable outlet, since even a trained eye is easily deceived. An engineer with a level can tell in a few moments where a proper point of discharge may be found, and it is absurd to begrudge the small amount which it will cost, in view of the large expense involved in digging a long trench to no purpose.

Some years ago the writer was able to note the conditions in a house where the cellar excavation went three feet into limestone rock. The strata were perfectly level and the cellar floor of natural rock was apparently all that could be desired, smooth and flat, without involving any expense for concrete. One wall came where a vertical seam in the rock existed, and since this natural rock face was smooth and vertical and just where the cellar wall should go, it seemed unnecessary to dig it out and lay up masonry in its place. So it was left and the house built. When the spring rains came, however, the cellar was turned into a pond, water dripping everywhere from the vertical rock face, and coming up through the cellar bottom like [Pg 48] springs. It cost a great deal more then to make the changes and improvements necessary in order to secure a dry cellar than it would have done at the outset. This serves as an illustration of the need of taking every precaution at the beginning to insure a dry and well-drained soil around and below the cellar walls.

[Pg 49]

**CHAPTER III**

## *CONSTRUCTION OF HOUSES AND BARNS WITH REFERENCE TO HEALTHFULNESS*

Any liability to disease that may come from faulty construction of habitations is likely to spring from a polluted subsoil. Such pollution vitiates the air drawn from that soil and is a source of danger on account of the resulting impurity of the whole atmosphere within the house.

*Shutting out soil air.*

We have already seen (Chapter II) how it is possible for soil charged with organic matter to deliver, either through suction from a heated house or on account of a rising ground water, soil air into the cellar, and also that moist air may enter the house in the same way. In order to prevent this, it is plainly necessary to interpose some air-tight or water-tight layer between the house and the soil, and also, since perfection in this layer is impossible, to make provision for draining away any water which may accumulate against the walls. Ordinary builders do not lay much emphasis on the importance of either of these precautions, and while one may often see cellar walls roughly and carelessly coated on the outside, with tar or asphalt, a thoroughly water-tight coating is not a common [Pg 50] practice. Similarly, while draintile are often laid around a house, they are either laid so near the surface as to be useless or else they have no porous filling.

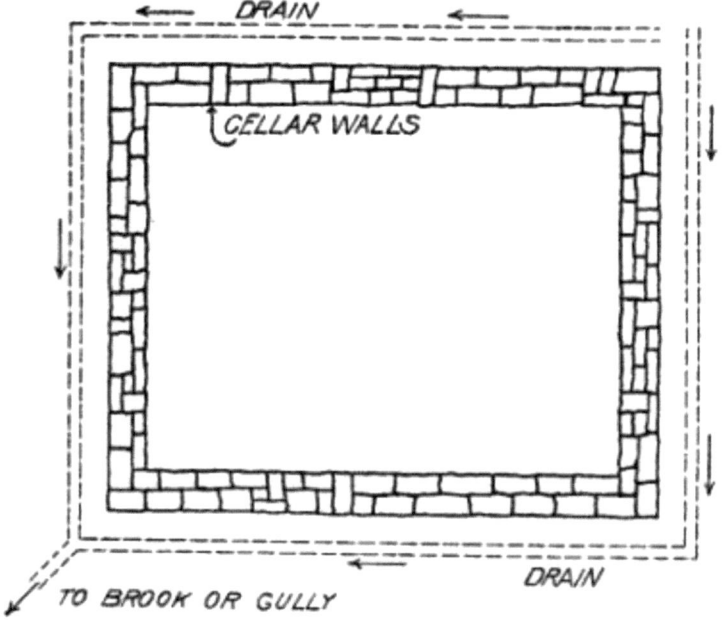

Fig. 5. — Exterior wall-drains.

To prevent moisture from entering the cellar, the first provision should be a tile drain (not less than four inches in diameter) laid completely around the house (see Fig. 5) on a grade of not less than six inches in one hundred feet. This drain at its highest point ought to be one foot below the bottom of the concrete floor of the cellar, and more than this, of course, at the lower end. This should be laid before or at the time the foundations for the house are being built, although it is possible to dig the necessary trenches and lay the tile after the house is built. If the available grade is small, this drain may be laid in two lines directly under the cellar floor as shown in Fig. 6. At the points A the bottom of the tile should be at least a foot below the dirt on which the cellar floor will be laid, and at the point B, about two feet. This drainpipe is best laid with regular sewer pipe and without cement in the joints. Then coarse gravel should be filled in around this tile so as to allow water to enter the pipe without carrying soil that later might settle in the pipe. [Pg 51]

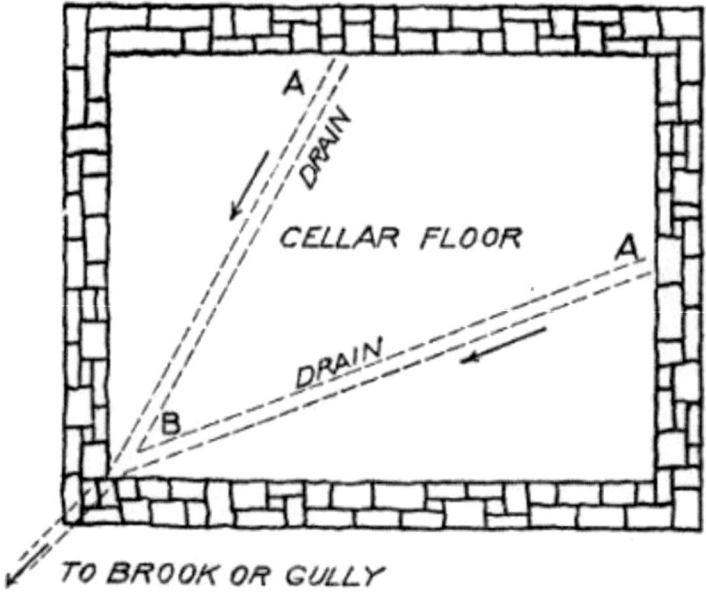

Fig. 6. — Interior cellar-drains.

[Pg 52]

*Position of outfall.*

There is always a question of where this drain shall end and into what it shall discharge, for in some soils this drainpipe may discharge continually. To allow the drain to empty on the ground means that its outer end will be broken; that if discharge takes place just before freezing weather, the drain will fill with ice and be broken, so that some other method must be devised. If the outer end can be laid into a brook where the velocity prevents the water from freezing, or where the outer end can be kept below water, a satisfactory disposal is found. Otherwise, it is better to discharge into a small covered cesspool, provided the soil is sufficiently porous to take care of the water, and provided the level of the ground water allows the construction of such a cesspool. In any case, it should be at some distance from the house, so that if it overflows, the water will not seep back to the cellar walls. By water-proofing the main wall and then backfilling against the wall with coarse gravel or broken stone, the same results as with open areaways are obtained and at a much smaller cost.

*Dampness of masonry walls.*

One fact peculiar to all kinds of masonry and known to all careful observers is that stone work, brick work, and concrete will allow dampness to permeate, whether it comes from water-bearing soil or a driving rain. One objection to concrete-block houses has been that a hard rain would cause moisture to form on the inside. Brick buildings have the same defect when the walls are built solid.

An air-space in the cellar walls is the only way of insuring a dry cellar, if the bottom of the cellar is below the [Pg 53] level of the ground water. A four-inch course of hollow brick may be used on the inside, or the wall may be actually divided into two walls with a space between.

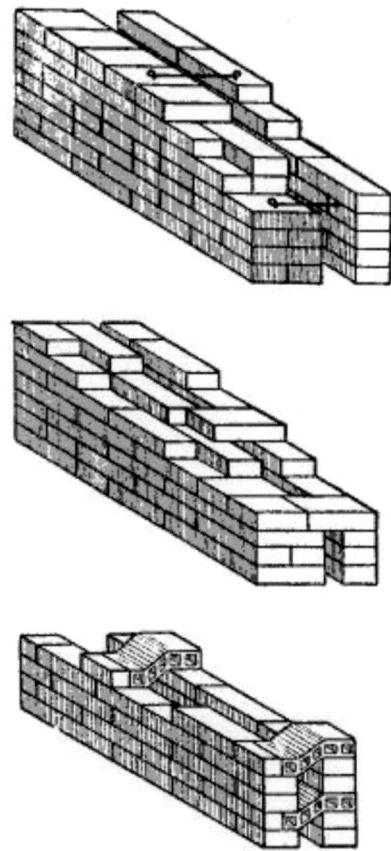

Fig. 7. — Wall modes of making air-space.

Figure 7 (after Warth) shows three different ways by which an air-space is secured and the two component parts of the wall held together. In the top view, the two walls, one eight-inch and one four-inch, are held together by wire ties, leaving an air-space of about four inches. In the middle drawing the walls are tied together by making the air-space three inches wide and then lapping the brick laid as headers over both walls. In the bottom view special terra-cotta blocks are used which pass through both walls. There can be no question of the value of such construction in eliminating dampness from the inside wall, but, it must be admitted, the cost of the walls is increased somewhat.

*Use of tar or asphalt on the wall.*

Instead of an open space, nowadays, it is more customary to thoroughly plaster the outside of the cellar wall, [Pg 54] and then paint it with a tar paint put on hot, which will adhere fairly well to the cement or masonry. Asphalt cannot be very readily used for this purpose unless it is an asphalt oil with but little bitumen paste. A paving asphalt, for example, even applied hot, does not adhere to the masonry, but slides down the walls as fast as it is applied. A successful method, however, of using such asphalt is to build the cellar wall in two parts, separated about half an inch, and filling in the intervening space with liquid asphalt. In this way, the asphalt is held in position, and is an absolute prevention of dampness.

Another method used successfully in the construction of one of the large railroad stations in Boston consists in painting the outside of the wall with tar and then pressing into the hot tar several layers of tar paper, the separate sheets overlapping in a special coating of tar. These sheets are thus made continuous around the building and under the basement so that no water can enter the building.

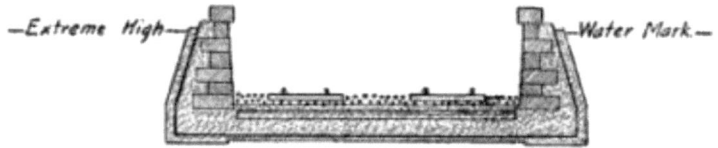

Fig. 8. — Water-tight wall.

A cross-section of one of the depressed tracks entering the Boston Station is shown in Fig. 8. The heavy black line represents ten thicknesses of tar paper, each one thoroughly painted with a thick paint of hot tar. It should be noticed that this water-tight coating is inclosed between masonry walls, so that the coating cannot be injured. [Pg 55]

It is possible theoretically by these methods to build an underground cellar so truly water-tight that it could be set down in a lake, where it might float like a boat and not leak a drop, and there may be some locations that require such construction, such as a low river valley or an old salt marsh or a city flat, where no adequate drainage is provided. But practically such construction will always be found expensive, and is, in most cases, unnecessary and ineffective, as already indicated, and where the percolating water cannot be tolerated, involves the installation of some kind of pump to throw out the water that will inevitably, in larger or small quantities, pass through the best water-proofing. It is, therefore, the part of wisdom to place reliance on draining the water away from the house rather than on water-proofing the cellar wall.

*Dry masonry for cellar walls.*

It may not be out of place to add a word of caution against the practice of building cellar walls of loose stone, without mortar. They make no pretense of being water-tight, they offer no resistance to the entrance of rats, and they soon yield to the pressure of the earth and present that wobbly, uncertain appearance of cellar walls seen in rural districts. Nor should the idea that the interior is to be visible and the exterior invisible blind the builder to the fact that it is far more important to have the outside smooth. If smooth, there are no projecting surfaces for water to collect in, no edges for the frozen earth to cling to and by expansion tear off from the wall. If smooth, the joints in the masonry can be pointed or filled with mortar, and thus a suitable surface for the tar or asphalt is provided. [Pg 56]

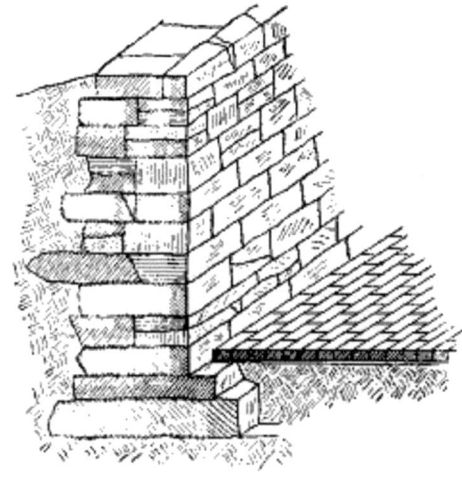

Fig. 9.—Rough-backed wall.

In Fig. 9 (after Brown) is shown a cellar wall with rough, irregular back, and it is easy to see how water would readily find its way down to one of the projecting stones and then along such a stone, through the wall into the cellar. With such a wall the action of the frost is more severe than with a wall with a smooth back, so that the wall in Fig. 9 is gradually pulled apart by alternate freezings and thawings. Figure 10 (after Brown), on the other hand, shows the cellar wall as it should be with smooth, even exterior, along which the water passes easily, with gravel backing, through which the water escapes to the drainpipe.

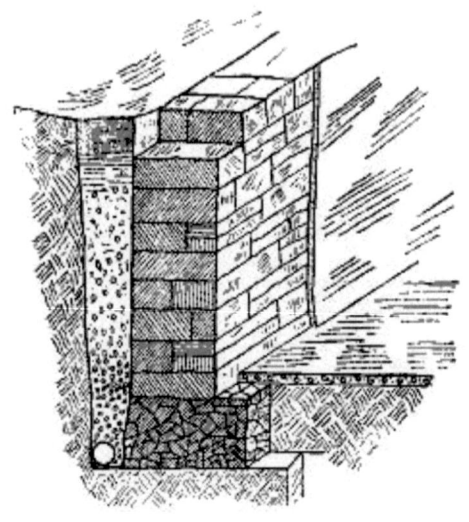

Fig. 10. — Even-backed wall.

*Damp courses in walls.* [Pg 57]

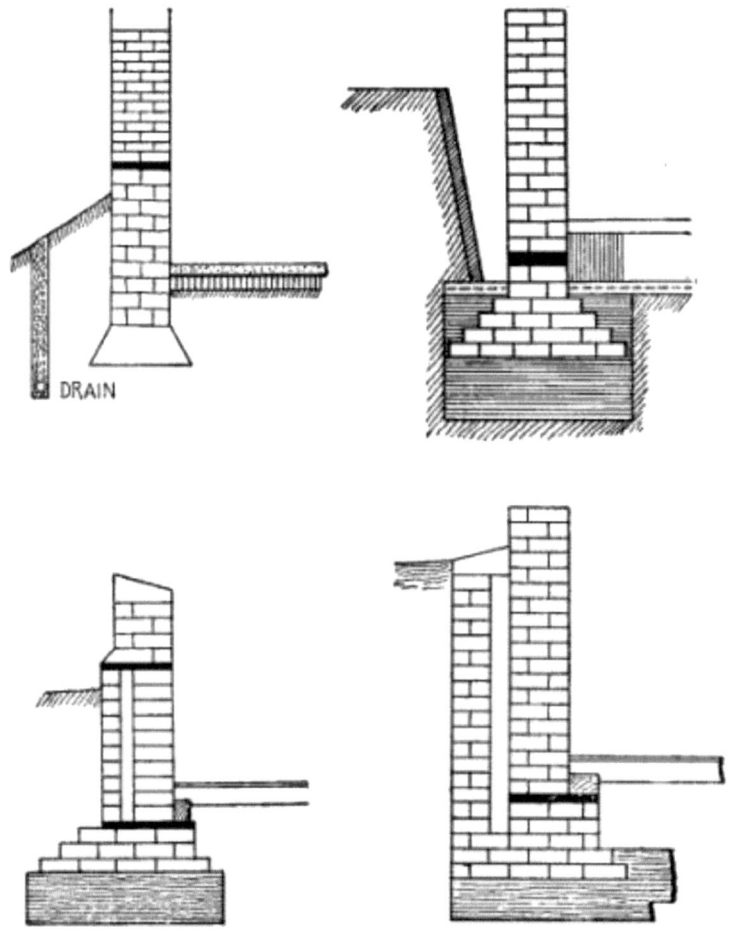

Fig. 11. — Four modes of making water-proof cellar walls.

Another important means of keeping moisture from the cellar walls is to provide what is called a damp course at about a level with the top of the cellar floor. Where the soil is naturally damp, and where the cellar wells are not adequately water-proof, a second damp course should be provided at the level of the ground so that moisture from the damp cellar walls may not pass up into the above ground portion, which is naturally dry. These damp courses, in their simplest form, consist in bringing the masonry level around the building, and painting the top surface with liquid coal tar. [Pg 58]

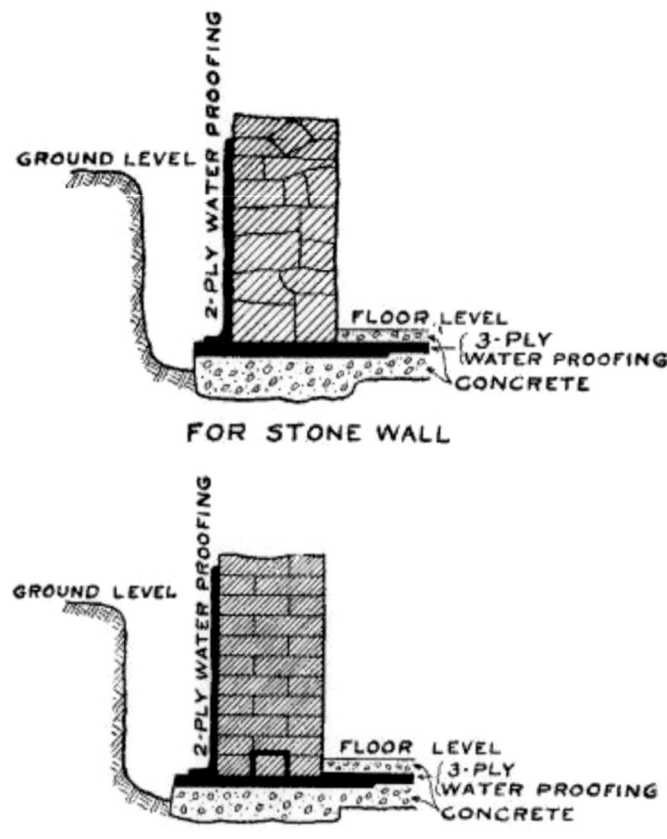

FOR STONE WALL

FOR BRICK WALL

Fig. 12.—Waterproofing of cellar walls.

[Pg 59]

Another method is to paint the masonry with liquid asphalt, and then imbed in this paint a thickness of asphalt-covered building paper which is again painted with asphalt. This may be done in the horizontal layer where it could not conveniently be done vertically.

Four different ways used in France for securing dry cellar walls are shown in Fig. 11. The heavy black line represents the damp course, which, when added to the effect of the interwall space, which is shown in all the drawings but the first, and there replaced by a deep drain, insures absolute freedom from all moisture within the cellar. Figure 12 shows sections recommended by Dr. George M. Price, and indicates clearly the location of the damp course.

*The cellar floor.*

The floor of the cellar, in the same way, must be kept from dampness, and this is best done by covering the cellar floor with a layer of concrete, one part cement, three parts sand, and six parts broken stone; or, one part cement and eight parts gravel may be used. Care should be taken, however, that the gravel does not contain an excess of sand, and it is always well in using gravel for concrete to check the proportion of these two materials. This may be done as follows: Sift the gravel through an ash sieve so that it is free from sand; fill a ten-quart pail even full with the gravel and then pour in water to the top of the pail, keeping account of the amount of water poured in. This volume of water gives the proper amount of sand to use with the gravel for concrete, and if more sand than this was present in the original gravel, it should be sifted out until the proper proportion is reached. [Pg 60]

Concrete is not water-tight, and the concrete floor of the cellar must be treated in some way to prevent water or moisture rising through this floor. One method is to cover the concrete thus laid with a denser mixture of cement and sand, put on three fourths of an inch thick, and made by mixing equal parts of sand and cement; or the asphalt layer already referred to in the cellar walls may be carried across the cellar, putting, as before, a paint layer on the concrete, then paper, then another paint layer, making it continuous and without a break from outside to outside. On top of this, to prevent wear and tear, a floor of brick, laid flat, or a two-inch layer of concrete may be laid.

*Cellar ventilation.*

The great importance of the cellar as that part of the house where, if anywhere, unhealthy conditions exist, justifies this prolonged discussion, and before leaving the subject, ventilation in the cellar should receive a word of encouragement. Too many cellars are damper than need be, are musty and close, full of odors of decaying vegetables and rotting wood, entirely from lack of ventilation. The cellar windows are small and always, closed. The cellar door is seldom opened, and never with the idea of admitting air. The impression on entering such a cellar is of a tomb.

The cellar, even in that part devoted to storing vegetables, needs ventilation as much as the house does, for the cellar air finds its way up into the house, and an unventilated cellar means a house with air deficient in oxygen and overloaded with carbonic acid, a condition which causes pale faces and anæmic bodies. Far better and [Pg 61] healthier is it to open all the cellar windows, covering them with coarse netting to keep out animals and with fine netting to keep out insects, and let the disease-killing oxygen and sunlight in. Malaria comes from the cellar, whenever the malarial mosquito can find there a breeding place. The writer has seen many cellars in which mosquitoes were living the year through in entire comfort, utilizing the moisture and warmth of the cellar to enjoy the winter months and up and ready for their mission at the first sign of spring. A cistern in the cellar is objectionable on this account, and if one exists, it should be covered with mosquito netting.

*The old-fashioned privy.*

Another source of ill-health as well as of temporary discomfort is the typical construction and continued use of an outside closet or privy. The physical shrinking from the use of the ordinary building is most reasonable. As generally constructed, great draughts of air (presumably for ventilation) are continually passing through the small building, and when the temperature of the outside air is at zero, or thereabouts, only the strongest physique can withstand the exposure involved without serious danger of consumption, influenza, and pneumonia, or at least inviting those diseases by reducing the vitality of the body. Two improvements suggest themselves and should be put into effect wherever this primitive construction must continue to be used.

In the first place, the building itself should not be fifty or a hundred feet away from the house, so that every one is exposed to rain, snow, slush, and ice in making the journey thither. But some corner of the woodshed or [Pg 62] barn should be utilized or the small building should be moved up by the back door and connected therewith by a roofed passage. The barn location is objectionable if it involves outdoor exposure in going from the house to the barn. A liberal use of earth in the privy vault will eliminate odors, and a water-tight box or bucket makes a frequent removal of the night soil practicable.

In the second place, a small stove ought to be provided to warm the closet in the coldest weather. Then the dislike to suffer from the cold, which leads so many to postpone nature's call, will be avoided, and the consequent digestive disorders which come from constipation and intestinal fermentations prevented.

*Cow stables.*

In matters of health, aside from ventilation, which is discussed in the next chapter, there is little to be said concerning the other buildings on the farm. Barns for hay are not involved. A few words may profitably be devoted to barns for stock, involving, as they do, by their construction, the health of the stock. One enthusiastic farmer writes that it is possible for farmers to keep their stock at all times under conditions which are an improvement upon the month of June. He believes that the cow stable should be as comfortable for the cows as the house is for the owner, subject to no fluctuations of temperature, and that, in this way, the health as well as the comfort and milk production of the cows would be maintained.

Light should be listed as the first essential of healthy stables, light to kill disease-producing bacteria, to make dirty corners and holes impossible, and to react on the [Pg 63] vitality of the animals. Compare this with some stables where fifteen, twenty, or thirty head are stabled in an underground dugout with two or three small windows not giving more than four square feet in all. Stable windows should be set, like house windows, in two sashes and capable of being raised or lowered at will. In winter a large sash may be screwed over the regular window to keep out frost and moisture, provided there is some independent method of ventilation.

For good healthy conditions, a cow needs about 500 cubic feet of space, with active ventilation. In old stables, with poor construction, as little as 200 cubic feet per cow was allowed, and when stables were made tight with matched boards and building paper, 200 cubic feet was found to be too small, and it was recommended that one cubic foot be allowed for each pound of cow. But when tried by wealthy amateurs, it was found that this was too large; the stables were damp and cold in winter and became a predisposing factor in the development of tuberculosis. Between the two extremes, 200 and 1000, is the practical average named above, namely, 500 cubic feet of air space for each cow.

For the health of the cow as well as for the good quality of the milk the stable should be built with special reference to being kept clean. The ceiling should be dust-tight, so that if hay is stored above, it will not sift through. The part of the barn where the cows are kept should be separated from the rest of the barn by tight partitions and a door into the cow stable. Nothing dusty or dirty should accumulate. The floor of all stables for cows, horses, hens, and pigs should be of concrete to insure the most [Pg 64] sanitary construction. Planks absorb liquids and wear out rapidly under the feet of the stock. Concrete can be kept clean, is nonabsorptive, and if covered with some non-conducting material, like sawdust, shavings, or straw, is a perfectly comfortable floor for the animals.

*Use of concrete.*

No development of recent times has tended more toward the improvement and greater comfort of house building than the use of concrete. In the earlier houses, the cellar walls were so badly built and the connection between the top of the cellar wall and the timber sill of the house was so poor that the winter's wind blew through above to the manifest discomfort of those in the house. The writer remembers sitting in the best room of a well-to-do farmer, and watching, with great interest, the carpet rise and fall with the gusts of wind outside. To avoid such unhappy consequences, farmers have been accustomed to bank up the house outdoors in the fall with dry leaves, spruce-boughs, or manure, usually to a point on the woodwork. This, of course, closes the cellar windows for the winter for the sake of keeping out the wind. A concrete wall, at the present price of cement, using gravel for the mixture instead of stone, need cost but little more than the price of the cement and the labor involved, and a tight cellar wall may thereby be obtained.

If the soil in which the cellar is dug is firm enough, the outside of the excavation can be made so that no form on that side will be required, but it is always better to make the excavation about two feet more than necessary, to put forms inside and outside, and, after their removal, plaster or wash the wall with a thick cream of cement [Pg 65] and water. In carrying the wall above the ground, forms must be used with great care to secure a smooth surface, and Fig. 13 shows two methods suggested by the Atlas Cement Company.

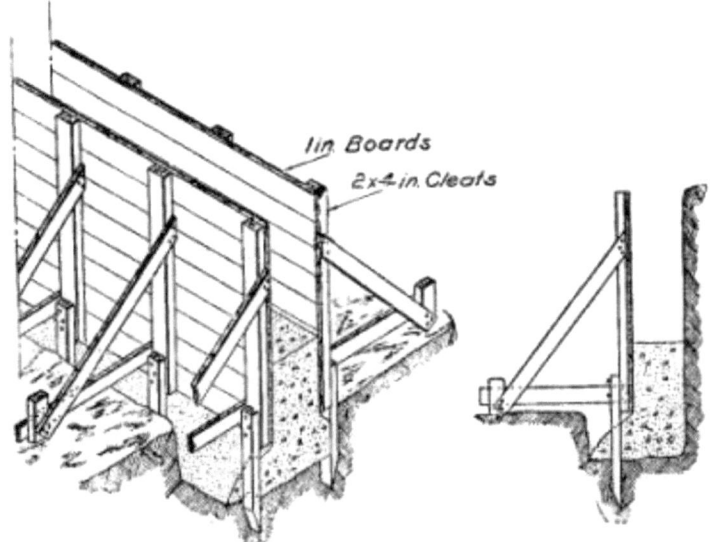

Fig. 13. — Cellar-wall forms.

There are so many forms of construction where concrete is not merely a convenience but a great advantage in the matter of health around the house, and particularly a house in the country, that there would be no end if one once began enumerating and describing the various methods and processes involved. Besides the cellar walls and cellar floor, there are outside the house, silos, manure bins, walks, curbing, steps, horse-blocks, hitching and other posts, watering troughs, and drainpipe, all successfully [Pg 66] made of this useful material. In the barn, the barn floor, the gutters, the manger and watering troughs, cooling tanks, and sinks are also made of cement. While it is possible to differentiate between the methods and the mixtures for these various purposes, it will not be greatly in error if the construction always follows the following principle.

Use enough cement to fill the voids in the gravel or in the sand and stone mixture employed, and have enough sand in the gravel or with the stone to fill the voids in the stone. This is readily determined, as already suggested, by the use of water. The water, which will occupy the voids in the stone, represents the necessary sand. When this amount of sand and stone is well mixed, the water then permeating the interstices represents the necessary cement, though it is a good plan to add about 10 per cent extra to allow for imperfect mixtures.

The mixing should always be done so thoroughly that when put together dry, no variation can be seen in the color of the mixture. It is surprising to see how readily a streak of unmixed dirt or of unmixed cement can be detected in a pile by the difference in the color which it presents. Such mixtures should always be made dry first and then the water added and again mixed until the result is of a perfectly firm consistency. Such a mixture can be applied to any of the purposes mentioned, and, in general, it is better to have too much water than not enough. The only difficulty with a very wet mixture is that the forms require to be made nearly water-tight, whereas with dry mixtures the same attention to the forms is not necessary.

If the concrete is to be used in thin layers, as in pipe or watering trough, where a smooth surface is wanted, better [Pg 67] results are usually obtained by using a dry mixture and fine gravel and tamping the mixture with unusual thoroughness. It is always unsafe to smooth up or re-surface a piece of concrete. The difference in texture of the surface coat causes it to expand and contract differently from the mass of concrete underneath, and inevitably a separation occurs. If it is desired to put on a sidewalk, for instance, a smooth top coat, the consistency of the two kinds of concrete should be alike, and the top coat should be applied almost immediately after the bottom layer is put in place. Where concrete is used to hold water, a coat of neat cement should always be put on with a broom or a whitewash brush, mixing the neat cement with water in a pail, and it does no harm to go over the surface three or four times, the object being to thoroughly close the pores in the concrete.

For floors of cellars or barns, the dirt should be evened off and tamped and then the cement concrete should be spread evenly over it, and tamped just enough to bring the water to the surface. When partially dry, a better finish is obtained by lightly troweling the concrete. In a cellar or barn, it is not necessary to divide up the area into squares or blocks as is done with sidewalk work, but the entire area may be laid in one piece. In order to keep the surface level, however, it may be found convenient to lay down pieces of 2" x 4" scantling, the tops of which shall be on the desired level of the finished floor. By filling in behind these scantlings, which can be moved ahead as the filling progresses, the exact level desired can be obtained. Usually four inches thick will be a proper depth of concrete for this purpose.

[Pg 68]

## CHAPTER IV

## *VENTILATION*

The average individual breathes in and out about eighteen times a minute, taking into his lungs the air surrounding him at the time and expelling air so modified as to contain large amounts of carbonic acid, organic vapor, and other waste products of the lungs. The volume of air taken in is about the same quantity as that expelled and amounts to eighteen cubic feet per hour. Fortunately, the air expired at a breath is at once rapidly diffused throughout the surrounding atmosphere, so that, even if no fresh air were introduced, the second breath inhaled would not be very different from the first. But after a certain length of time the air becomes so saturated with the waste products of the lungs that it is no longer fit to breathe, and it is evident that in order to keep the air in a room so that it can be taken into the lungs with any reasonable degree of comfort, there must be a continual supply of fresh air admitted with a proper provision for discharging polluted air. If this is not done, there is, so far as the lungs are concerned, a process established similar to that which is occasionally found when a village takes its water-supply from a pond and discharges its sewage into the same pond. [Pg 69]

Not long ago, the writer found in the Adirondacks a hotel built on the side of a small lake which pumped its water-supply from the lake, and discharged its sewage into the same lake only a few feet away from the water intake. That the hotel had a reputation of being unhealthy, and that it had difficulty in filling its guest rooms, is not to be wondered at, and yet individuals will treat their lungs exactly as the hotel treated its patrons.

*Effects of bad air.*

In order to establish a proper relation between the amount of impurities diffused through the air and the physiological effect on individuals breathing that air, certain observations have been noted and certain experiments have been made which prove without question the injurious effect of vitiated air.

Professor Jacob, late Professor of Pathology, Yorkshire College, Leeds, gives the following example on a large scale, to show the results of insufficient ventilation: "A great politician was expected to make an important speech. As there was no room of sufficient dimensions available in the town, a large courtyard, surrounded with buildings, was temporarily roofed over, some space being left under the eaves for ventilation. Long before the appointed time several thousand people assembled, and in due course the meeting began; but before the speaker got well into his subject, there arose from the vast multitude a cry for air, numbers of people were fainting, and every one felt oppressed and well-nigh stifled. It was only after some active persons had climbed on the roof and forcibly torn off the boards for a space about twenty feet square that the business of the meeting could be resumed." [Pg 70]

Remembering that the process of breathing is for the purpose of supplying oxygen to the blood and that the absorption of oxygen in the lungs is the same process which goes on when a candle burns, the following experiments were made by Professor King of the University of Wisconsin, to show the effect of expired air on a candle flame. He took a two-quart mason jar and lowered a lighted candle to the bottom, noting that the candle burned with scarcely diminished intensity. Through a rubber tube, he breathed gently into the bottom of the jar, with the result that the candle gradually had a reduced flame and was finally extinguished. He observed also that if the candle were raised as the flame showed signs of going out, the brilliancy of the flame was restored, while lowering the candle tended to extinguish the flame. Even when the candle was raised to the top of the jar, the flame was extinguished after sufficient air had been breathed into the jar. Clearly, then, he argued, air once breathed is not suitable for respiration, unless much diluted with pure air. He argued from this that if a candle using oxygen for combustion could not burn in expired air, therefore an individual using oxygen for the renewal of the blood could not be properly supplied in a room partially saturated with the expired products of the lungs.

Professor King also experimented with a candle burning in a jar on which the cover had been placed, and found that the candle was extinguished in thirty seconds, and he argued that if a candle was thus extinguished on account of the carbonic acid given off, so a person shut up in an air-tight chamber would similarly be extinguished in the course of time. [Pg 71]

To prove that expired air is poisonous to animal life, Professor King experimented on a hen, placing the same in a cylindrical metal air-tight chamber eighteen inches in diameter and twenty inches deep. The hen became severely distressed for want of ventilation and died at the end of four hours and seventeen minutes.

In the Wisconsin Agricultural Experimental Station, an experiment was conducted for fourteen days on the effect of ample and deficient ventilation on a herd of cows. The stable was chiefly underground and had two large ventilators which could be opened or closed at will. The food eaten, the water drunk, the milk produced, and weight of the cows were recorded each day. For a part of the time the cows were kept continuously in the stable with all openings closed, and then the ventilators were opened, the alternate conditions being repeated at intervals of four days. The amount of food consumed was practically the same under both conditions. The quantity of milk given was greater with good ventilation. The chief difference was in the amount of water consumed, since with the insufficient ventilation the cows drank on the average 11.4 pounds more water each, daily, and yet lost in weight 10.7 pounds at the end of each two-day period. Examination of the animals themselves also showed that a rash had developed on their bodies which could be felt by the hand and which was apparently very irritating, since it was so rubbed by the animals as to cause the surface to bleed. The evident teaching of the experiment is that under conditions of poor ventilation, it was impossible for the lungs to remove waste products to as great an extent as usual, and, therefore, the demand for [Pg 72] additional water was felt in order to stimulate greater action on the part of the kidneys to care for these waste products. That this was not a successful substitute was shown by the loss of weight in the animals, and by the irritation of the skin which evidently was trying to eliminate some of the remaining impurities through its surface.

*Modifying circumstances.*

Fortunately for mankind, it has not been customary, nor even possible, to build dwellings or stables approaching the air-tightness of a fruit jar. Air has great power of penetration, particularly when in motion, and a wind will blow air through wooden walls, and even through brick walls, in considerable quantity. It is practically impossible to build window casings and door frames so that cracks do not exist, through which air may find its way. When, however, in the wintertime, storm windows have been put on, or when, as occasionally happens, to keep out drafts, strips of paper are pasted carefully around all window casings, or when rubber weather strips are nailed tight against the windows and doors, conditions are obtained which resemble the mason fruit jar, and under those conditions, a person living continuously in such a room is experimenting on himself as Professor King did with the candle.

Another reason why it is difficult to make a room an air-tight chamber is that if a stove or fire-place be in the room, a strong suction is produced through the flame, and such suction requires the entrance of outside air. It is a common experience that a fire-place in a room otherwise tight will refuse to draw and will smoke persistently until a door or window is opened, when, a supply of air being provided, the fire is made bright and active. [Pg 73]

Fortunately, the vitiation of the air in a room is never so severe as that in an experimental chamber, and there are few examples which can be cited of men or women dying from lack of ventilation in an ordinary room. But the serious aspect of inadequate ventilation is not that it actually induces death, but that it decreases the powers and activities of the various organs of the body; that it interferes with their normal processes, that it loads up in the body an accumulation of organic matter which is normally oxidized by fresh air and which, if not oxidized, obstructs the activities of other organs of the body.

*Danger of polluted air.*

Unfortunately, it is not possible to detect by the physical senses that point at which the human organism suffers from insufficient ventilation. Some years ago, Dr. Angus Smith built an air-tight chamber or box in which he allowed himself to be shut up for various lengths of time in order to analyze his own sensations on breathing vitiated air. He found that, far from being disagreeable, the sensation was pleasurable, and he says, "There was unusual delight in the mere act of breathing," although he had remained in the chamber nearly two hours. On another occasion he stayed in more than two hours without apparent discomfort, although after opening the door, persons entering from the outside found the atmosphere intolerable. He placed candles in the box, which were extinguished in a hundred and fifty minutes, and a young lady, who was interested in the experiment, going into the box as the candles went out, breathed it for five minutes easily; she then became white, and could not come out without help. [Pg 74]

Nor is it possible to conclude from the experiments and observations cited that the body remains indifferent to polluted air until the latter has reached a certain definite saturated condition. There can be little doubt but that a degree of pollution far short of that necessary to produce death has a weakening effect on the human organism, and that by means of the increased functional activity of other organs doing work intended for the lungs the resistance to disease is much impaired. Life is a continual struggle of the bodily tissues against the attacks of the micro-organisms and their tendencies to destroy life; hence inadequate ventilation or any other condition which interferes with the normal action of the organs of the body causes weakness and affords opportunity for the attack of some disease-producing germ. It stands to reason that an individual whose lung tissues have become soft and incapacitated must be more liable to succumb to disease than another whose lung capacity is large and whose blood has been continually and sufficiently oxygenated.

Perhaps no more impressive proof of this is seen than in the ravages of consumption, which is so prone to attack those whose vitality is diminished by living in unhealthy and unventilated cellars or in crowded tenements. Statistics are very definite on the subject of tuberculosis among Indians, who rarely suffer from the disease when living in tents or on the open prairie, but when they become semi-civilized and crowd together in houses heated through the winter months by stoves, the germs of tuberculosis take firm hold, and the deaths from this disease are greater in proportion to population among this race than anywhere else. [Pg 75]

*Effect of change in air.*

This discussion illustrates another law of disease which makes the necessity for ventilation particularly great among rural communities where for nine months in the year outdoor life is freely enjoyed, namely, that when either an individual or people are brought under changed conditions, perhaps not unwholesome to those accustomed to them, those unaccustomed will suffer severely. So a lack of ventilation during the winter months in a farmhouse is very serious in its consequences to those who have had the full enjoyment of fresh air through the rest of the year.

Reference has already been made (in Chapter 1) to the prevalence of influenza in rural communities, and it is quite probable that this would be largely eliminated if the lungs were not deprived of their oxygen as they are in most houses on the farm.

*Composition of air.*

Ordinary air contains about 0.04 per cent of carbon dioxid; that is, four parts in ten thousand parts of air, the other nine thousand nine hundred ninety-six being made up of oxygen and nitrogen. Of course, it is not possible to express any definite value for the amount of carbon dioxid which is objectionable in air, because, in the first place, it is not certain that the carbon dioxid in itself is the cause of diminished vitality due to insufficient ventilation, and, in the next place, insufficient ventilation affects different people in different ways. But it is known that in the lungs the life-giving oxygen is changed to carbon dioxid, and that just as carbon dioxid gas will prevent the combustion of a candle flame, so carbon dioxid gas will destroy the life of man. [Pg 76]

When a deep well is to be cleaned out, the decomposition of organic matter in the bottom of the well will have, in all probability, caused the formation of this same carbon dioxid gas, and it is not uncommon for a man descending into such a well to be overcome by the gas, which, in some cases, even causes death. For this reason, it is common to lower into a well, before it is entered by a man, a candle or lantern, on the probability that if the lantern can stand it, certainly the man can, while if the lantern goes out, it is wise to avoid the risk of having a man's life put out in the same way.

*Organic matter in air.*

The stuffy and close feeling perceived in an ill-ventilated room is, however, due to the organic matter from the lungs, which is expired along with the carbon dioxid, and some chemists have argued that this amount of organic vapor ought to be measured instead of the carbon dioxid.

At the present time there is no simple and direct method of measuring organic vapor, and because this vapor increases in the atmosphere proportionately to the carbon dioxid gas, it is much simpler to measure the latter. Then it is impossible to fix a standard of carbon dioxid because a person whose lungs are well developed and whose blood is well oxygenated, or, as we say, one who has good red blood can stand, even if uncomfortable, a few hours of a bad atmosphere without suffering serious discomfort, while an anæmic or poor-blooded person would be affected to a greater degree. It is for this reason that in any house no living room, especially one heated by a coal stove, should be shut up tight against fresh air. This is the reason why the women of the family, who have to breathe [Pg 77] the same air over and over all day, are pale and weak and easily susceptible to disease, while the men, who are out of doors most of the time, and when indoors are made restless by the bad air, suffer much less from the ill effects.

Experiments seem to show that when the amount of carbon dioxid in the air has doubled, that is, when the expired air mixed with the air in the room has increased the proportion of carbon acid from four parts in ten thousand to eight parts in ten thousand, that the air is seriously affected, and that such ventilation ought to be provided that no greater amount than this could occur. This is such a condition that the room smells "close" or stuffy to a person coming in from outdoors, indicating organic emanations as well as an excess of carbonic acid gas. The question then is: how may this condition be avoided in an ordinary house, or in an ordinary stable, because the health of the cattle on a farm, judging at least by the character of the buildings provided, is quite as important as the health of the farmer's family.

We must take it for granted that no such elaborate schemes are possible as in public buildings or schools, where fans are provided, either to force air into the several rooms or else to suck it out. The ventilation of the house must be more simple and easily adjusted and must depend on the principle of physics that warm air rises and that if the warm air of a room is to be removed, air must in some way be supplied to take its place. The two essentials for ventilation are opportunity for the ingress and the egress of air — ingress for fresh air and egress for polluted air.

*Fresh-air inlet.*

In the construction, of a dwelling house, special and [Pg 78] adequate preparation for the admission of fresh air is seldom provided, so that the existing openings must be used for the purpose. This means that in the summertime an open window will furnish all the fresh air which a room receives and, when the temperature of the outside air is approximately that of the living room, such provision is ample and satisfactory. But in the wintertime, when the outside air is cold, the average person will prefer to suffer from the bad effects of impure air rather than admit cold air which may cause an unpleasant draft.

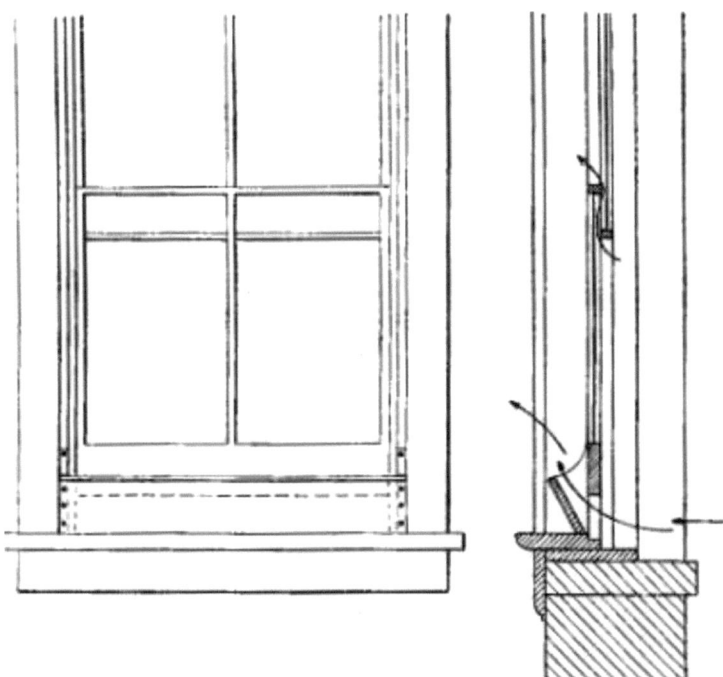

Fig. 14.—Letting in fresh air.

[Pg 79]

One of the simplest and best methods of providing an inlet for fresh air, without at the same time allowing blasts of wind to enter the room, is to fasten in front of the lower part of the window a board which shall just fill the window opening; then, raising the lower sash a few inches will allow fresh air to enter both at the bottom, where the board is placed, and at the middle of the window between the sashes (see Fig. 14). Persons sitting close by a window thus arranged may feel a draft even under these conditions, since the cold air thus admitted will sink at once to the floor and then gradually rise through the room to the ceiling, but unless one sits too near the window, this is an admirable method of admitting fresh air.

Another method, where steam or hot-water radiators are placed in the room, is to connect the outer air, either through the lower part of the window or through the wall of the room just below the window opening, with a space back of the radiator, so that the cold air entering will pass around and through the radiator and so be warmed as it enters.

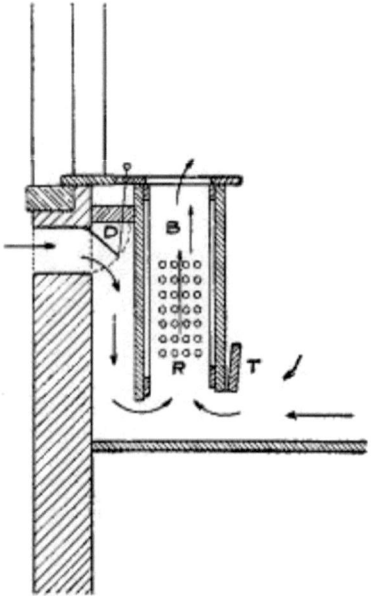

Fig. 15. — Ventilating device.

The picture (Fig. 15, after Jacobs) shows the arrangement of the radiators in one of the buildings of the University of Pennsylvania. A is the opening in the wall [Pg 80] below the window; D is a valve which regulates the amount of air entering through the opening; R is the radiator; B is a tin-lined box which surrounds the radiator; T is a door in front of the box, which when raised allows the air of the room to be heated and to circulate through the radiator. By adjusting the two valves D and T, air of any desired temperature can usually be obtained. Figure 16 (after Billings) shows an English device intended for the same purpose. The valve D in this case operates to admit air, either through the radiator or to the space between the radiator and the wall, in order to vary the temperature of the entering air. The valve T may be open or closed, and its position, together with that of the valve *F*, determines the proportion of the room air which is reheated.

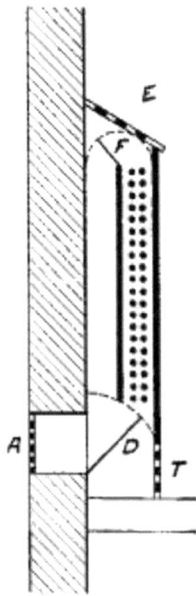

Fig. 16. — Ventilating device.

The writer remembers one schoolhouse where these methods were used successfully, the radiators being placed directly in front of the window and inclosed at the back, sides, and top, except for an opening to the outer air through the wall, properly controlled by a damper. In the writer's own office the radiators are by the side of the window and are boxed in, the connection being made with the outside air through a wooden box entering under the radiator. This is an admirable method, provided the radiator has sufficient surface to warm the fresh air admitted.

Another excellent arrangement is to provide a narrow [Pg 81] screen similar to that used for protection against flies, but with the screening material of muslin cloth instead of wire cloth. This muslin will break up the current of air so completely that no draft is felt by persons sitting even close to the open window.

*Position of inlet.*

The inlet for fresh air, if connecting directly with the outside air, should not be at the top of the room, since then the inlet would not serve to admit air, but rather to allow the warm air of the room to escape, and a burning match would inevitably show a draft outward instead of inward.

Neither is it desirable to have the fresh-air inlet near the floor of the room unless the entering air is warm, because cold air admitted will flow across the floor and remain there, not disturbing the warm upper layers. The effect then is not to improve the ventilation, but only to chill the feet of persons sitting in the room. The position of the window lends itself, therefore, to admission of fresh air, since it is neither at the top nor at the bottom of the room, but at the level most suitable for such admission.

*Foul-air outlet.*

Very few houses have any provision for the outlet of spent air, and if ventilation is thought of at all, the only idea usually is to provide, in part at least, for the admission of air and to make no adequate arrangement for its egress. Whenever a stove or fire-place is in use, the mere burning of fuel requires the consumption of air, and in cases where apparently no air is admitted to the room, insensible ventilation is at work bringing into the room, through the walls and through cracks around the doors and windows, the necessary air for combustion. [Pg 82]

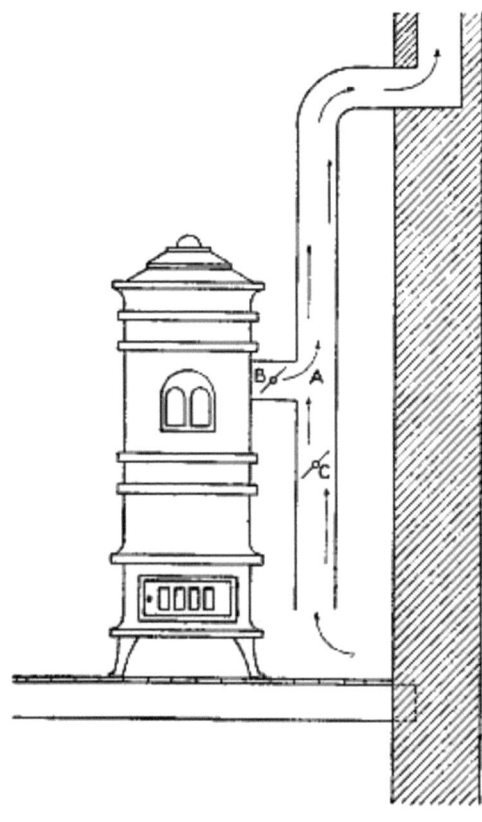

Fig. 17. — Ventilation by means of coal stove.

It may be proved by the laws of physics that a coal stove burning freely in a room causes adequate ventilation; and that only where the dampers of the stove are closed, so that not merely is the supply of fresh air diminished, but also the products of combustion are thrown out into the room, is there danger from lack of ventilation. The stovepipe in this case furnishes the necessary outlet for the impure air, and the following suggestion has been made in order to utilize this outlet, even when the fire is not burning freely or when the damper in the stovepipe is closed. If the stovepipe from a stove is carried horizontally, as it usually is, an elbow must be provided to raise the pipe to the stove hole in the chimney. Then providing a

T connection at the point marked *A* in Fig. 17 (after Billings), the lower part of the *T* may be carried to within a foot of the floor with a damper at the points *B* and *C*. [Pg 83] When the fire is burning freely, the damper at *C* is closed, and ventilation is secured through the stove, the damper at *B* being open. When the damper at *B* is closed and the fire checked, then the damper at *C* may be opened and the impure air drawn up the chimney from the level of the floor. This, it is said, is an effective arrangement for drawing off the polluted air of a room.

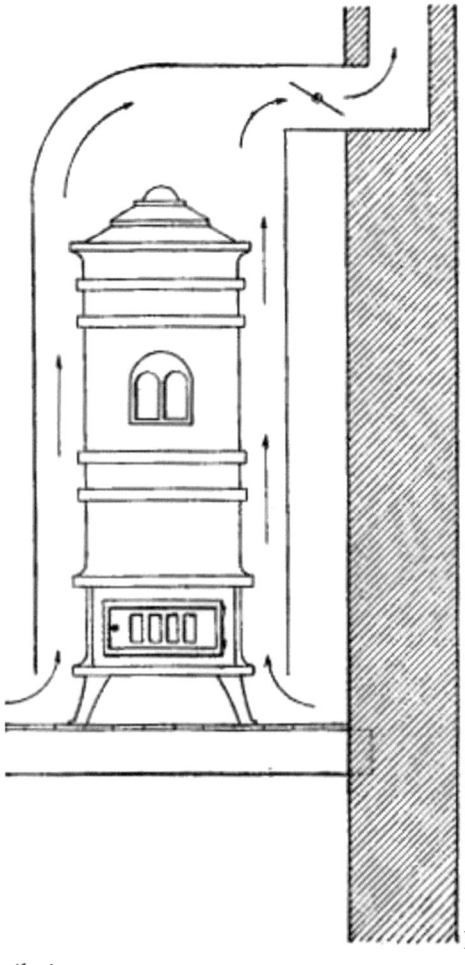

Fig. 18. — Coal-stove ventilation.

Another method is to surround the stove with a sheet-iron casing, as shown in Fig. 18 (after Billings), the top of the casing having a pipe leading into the chimney independently from the stovepipe. The casing becomes warm and heats the room by radiation, just as the stove does, but if the damper in the flue from the casing be opened partly, a strong draft along the floor and into this casing will be developed and the foul air thereby discharged into the chimney. It will be easily [Pg 84] possible, of course, to carry away all the heat from the stove in this method, and the damper in the flue of the casing must be carefully regulated to carry away only the desired amount of foul air.

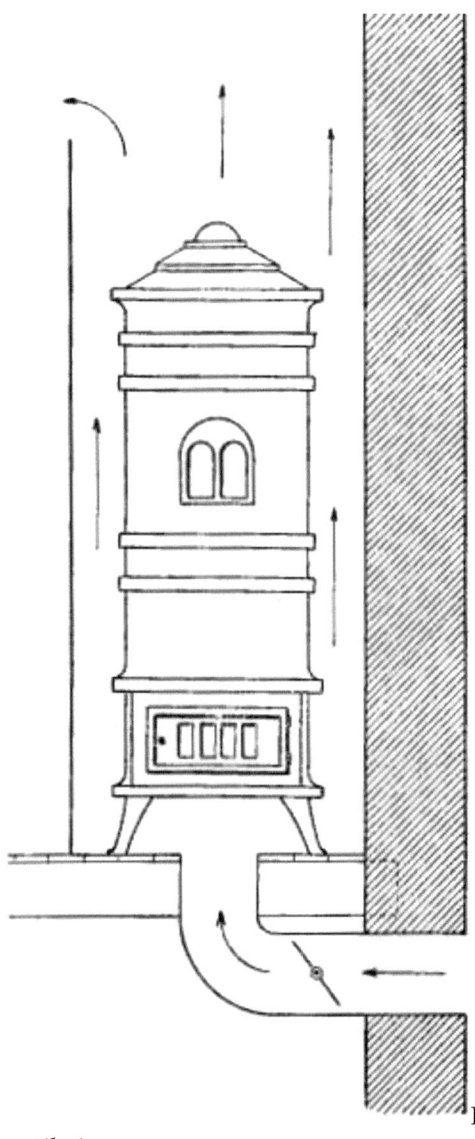

Fig. 19.—Coal-stove ventilation.

Still another method of using the heat of a stove to secure ventilation is shown in Fig. 19 (after Billings). Here the stove is surrounded with a sheet-iron jacket extending from the floor to about six feet above that level. A pipe is carried from the outside air up through the floor directly under the stove. By regulating the damper in this pipe the supply of fresh warmed air entering the room can be regulated. Doors in the casing must, of course, be provided for the purpose of taking care of the fire, [Pg 85] and of allowing air from the room near the floor to be heated instead of the outside air.

A most objectionable method of providing an outlet for polluted air from a room is to have a register in the ceiling with the ostensible purpose of warming the room above. It was the writer's misfortune once to stay a week in the country, in a room over the kitchen where this method of heating was employed, and the odors of cabbage, onions, and codfish which permeated the upper room, and clung there all night, still remain as a most unpleasant memory.

*Size of openings for fresh air.*

As an indication of the size of the openings needed, it has been said that in order to provide the necessary air movement, and yet to restrict the velocity of the moving air so that no objectionable drafts will be experienced, at least twenty-four square inches sectional area should be allowed as an inlet for each person, so that one square foot is required for six persons. This is, perhaps, a theoretical requirement. Certainly, it is more area than is likely to be obtained in actual ventilation. The space between two windows, for instance, is about one inch by thirty inches, — barely enough, according to this rule, for one person, and yet that opening is sufficient to appreciably improve the quality of the air in a room occupied by three or four persons.

Taking into account the necessary air required by lamps or gas burners, the inlet flue should have at least ten square inches area for each person, so that the ordinary single register should provide the necessary amount of air for a living room. When, as happens in houses where a studied [Pg 86] effort is made to preserve the health of the inhabitants, an outlet is cut into the wall and a flue carried up through the roof, the flue should be preferably near the floor and on the side of the room opposite the window or inlet. With such an arrangement (see Fig. 20) the air entering rises at first, but sinks at once because of the temperature, so that the direction of the air currents are diagonally across the room from the ceiling to the floor, thus renewing and changing all the air particles except those directly over the outlet. Where the air is introduced mechanically, that is, forced into the room, it is better to have the inlet and outlet on the same side, so that the entering air is shot in at the top, flowing across the room, then sinking and coming back, just below the point where it entered.

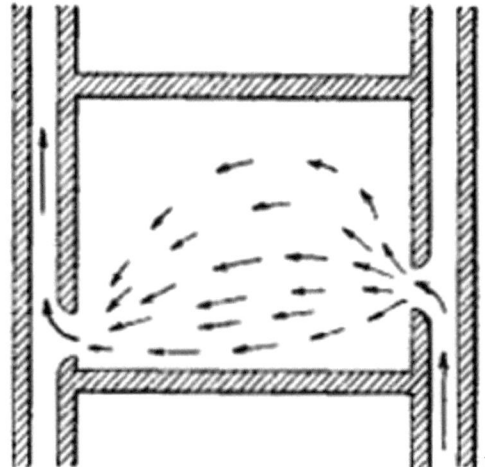

Fig. 20. — Outlets into the walls.

*Ventilation of stables.*

All that has been said on the subject of ventilation in houses applies equally well to the ventilation of stables, and a little book by Professor King of the University of Wisconsin, entitled "Ventilation," deals most thoroughly with the principles and practices of ventilation, not merely for dwellings but also for stables. Professor King proves by his experiments that the condition of cattle is much improved and that the milk-giving qualities are increased by a proper supply of fresh air, and in the book referred to, he gives a number of examples of the proper construction to provide adequate ventilation. It is most convincing [Pg 87] to see how unscientific is the old-fashioned underground stable, the sole idea of which was to conserve the animal heat by crowding together the cows and by absolutely excluding the outside air. For further details of his work, its principles and practices, the reader is referred to the book, which may be obtained from the author at Madison, Wisconsin.

*Cost of ventilation.*

To ventilate a house is expensive, and to ventilate a barn requires not only a certain expenditure of money but also a considerable amount of judgment. It is evidently cheaper to heat the same air in a room over and over than to be continually admitting cold fresh air, which will have to be warmed. This extra cost is, however, not excessive, when the movement of the air currents is properly controlled. The cost of warming the air necessary for ventilation for five persons should not be, at the rate of 1000 cubic feet of air to each person, more than ten cents a day in zero weather, with coal at five dollars a ton. Enough coal will have to be burned in addition to compensate for radiation, or, in other words, it requires a certain amount of coal to keep an empty room warm in winter without any question of ventilation, and in some badly built houses this amount is large.

*Relation of heating to ventilation.*

It does not follow because much heat is lost in this way that the ventilation is good, since the heated air may ascend to the ceiling and there escape without influencing the ventilation. In fact, one of the first principles of ventilation is that as soon as regular inlets and outlets are provided, all other openings ought to be rigidly closed. Then and then [Pg 88] only can the warmed pure air be admitted as desired, at the points intended, and the full value of the heat utilized. Especially is this control of openings important in ventilating barns. Here each animal is a natural heater, warming the air by direct contact and by rapidly breathing in and out large volumes of air which are thereby changed to a temperature of over ninety degrees Fahrenheit. The air around their bodies being warmed rises to the ceiling and spreads out to the two sides and is there gradually cooled and at the same time mixed with fresh air which enters at the top, so that the cow is constantly supplied with freshened air. A flue is needed to carry the foul air up through the roof, and fresh-air inlets in the outer walls on both sides are required, and with these openings carefully controlled and with no others interfering, the stable may be well ventilated, as shown in Fig. 21 (after King).

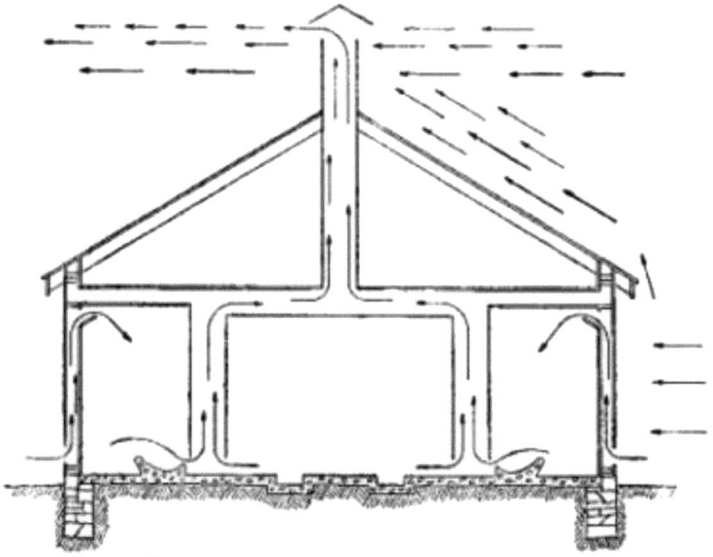

Fig. 21.—Cow-barn ventilation.

[Pg 89]

In all cases where ventilation is to be practiced, the walls and ceiling should not merely be tight in themselves, but they should be double, and the strictest attention paid to limiting the amount of heat lost by radiation. All the heat used ought to be concerned in ventilation, and in that only. To secure air-tight walls and ceiling, the studding and joists should be boarded in, both on the inside and out, and the space between should be filled with shavings, straw, dry moss, or any similar fibrous substance. The outside sheathing must be well laid and must be water-tight in order that rain shall not penetrate to the inside of the wall, and the roof must be tight so that the ceiling filling does not get wet and rot.

The choice, therefore, so far as ventilation of either house or barn goes, lies between a poorly built, loose-jointed structure without artificial ventilation and with poor economy in heat, and a well-built, air-tight structure, with ample ventilating pipes, carefully and intelligently planned and built. The first is healthy so far as pure air is concerned, but drafty and uncomfortable. The second is more expensive to build, but insures lasting health and comfort. Then the choice cannot but fall on the building which is easy to warm, healthful to live in, and readily ventilated. [Pg 90]

# CHAPTER V

*QUANTITY OF WATER REQUIRED FOR DOMESTIC USE*

Until the last few years it has been a sad commentary on the intelligence of the average farmer that but few attempts have been made to supply the farmhouse with running water, adequate to the needs of domestic use. The men of the farm long ago realized that carrying water for stock in pails was both laborious and time-consuming, and very few barnyards have not had running water leading into a trough to supply the needs of cattle. In many cases this supply has been extended into the barn, and in some cases into individual stalls, so that the farmer has long since eliminated the necessity of hauling water for his stock. Perhaps, because the farmer did not himself carry the water, but rather his wife, he has until recently not concerned himself with any extension of the water-supply into the house, and so long as the well in the yard did not run dry, he felt that his duty had been done. To be sure, bringing water from the well to the house in mid-winter involves much exposure and sometimes real suffering; occasionally the farmer has been moved on this account to have the well located in the woodshed or on [Pg 91] the back stoop, avoiding the long outdoor trip, but increasing the dangers of pollution to the water. It would be interesting to make a census of the farm water-supplies in any county for the purpose of estimating the intelligence of the farm-owners, since one cannot but feel that such a primitive water-supply argues, in most cases, an undeveloped or one-sided intelligence on the part of the property owner.

*Modern tendencies.*

Happily, such primitive methods of bringing water to the house are being superseded by satisfactory installations, and one by one, each farmhouse is being provided with running water in the kitchen sink and with a bath-room containing all the modern conveniences. One cannot deny that this costs money, both because of the pipe line necessary to bring the water to the house and because of the plumbing fixtures required in the house. Again, a water-supply in the house involves a well-heated house, since pipes not kept warm will, in the winter, inevitably freeze, ruining the pipe line and perhaps the ceilings and walls of the house itself. But if the owner of a house has any money to expend in improvements, surely no better way of adding to the comfort and health of his family can be found. An abundant supply of water increases the self-respect of the whole family and has been known even to change the temper of an entire household. For another reason, also, it is a good investment, inasmuch as the quality of the water supplied from a spring on a hillside is, generally speaking, better than that of a well surrounded by barnyards and privies.

It has been said that the civilization of a community is [Pg 92] measured by the amount of soap that it consumes, and it is almost the same thing to say that the refinement of a household is measured by the amount of water it uses. The poorer a family, the greater struggle it is to keep up the appearance of cleanliness, and no surer sign of rapid progress on a downhill road can be found than neglect of those practices which tend toward personal neatness. As the life of the farmer, then, becomes easier, as his condition becomes more prosperous, and as his family make more requirements, so, inevitably, is there in the farmhouse a greater demand for water in the kitchen, in the laundry, and in the bath-room.

*Quantity of water needed per person.*

Just how much water is needed in any house is not easy to predict, unless, at the same time, it is known, not merely the present habits of the family, but also their capacity to respond to the refining influence of unlimited water.

It has been shown by measuring the amount of water used in families of different social standing in cities of New England that the amount of water varies directly with the habits and social usages of the family. For example, in Newton, Massachusetts, where there are a large number of small houses with the water-supply limited to a single faucet, it was found that the water used amounted to seven gallons per day for each person in the house, while in houses supplied with all modern conveniences, the consumption of water was at the rate of twenty-seven gallons per day for each person. In Fall River, the conditions were much the same except that the poorer houses generally had one bath-tub and one water-closet, the amount of water used being eight and a half gallons [Pg 93] per head per day, while the most expensive house in the city used twenty-six gallons per head per day. In Boston, the poorest class apartment houses used water at the rate of seventeen gallons per head per day, the moderate class apartment houses at the rate of thirty-two gallons, first-class apartment houses at the rate of forty-six gallons, and the highest class apartment houses at the rate of fifty-nine gallons per head per day. The difference in these rates is easily understood by considering the habits of the individuals who make up the different classes referred to. In the poorer class of houses, the workers of the family are gone all day, and are too tired when home to spend much time in bathing. The children of such households are washed only occasionally, and the external use of water is generally regarded as an unnecessary trouble. In those families, on the other hand, where the necessity for daily toil is not so pressing, where bathing is more frequent, and where ablutions during the day are more often repeated, the amount of water used is much larger.

Another factor that affects the measured amount of water used in a family is the number of plumbing fixtures. At first sight, it would not seem possible that because there were two wash-basins in a house, an individual should use more water than if there were only one basin. Nor would it seem possible that an individual would take more baths with three bath-rooms available than if only one existed, and yet the number of fixtures does influence the individual who washes his hands frequently. With a wash-basin on the same floor, for instance, he washes often, whereas if it were always necessary to go upstairs for the purpose, his hands would go unwashed. Also, the more [Pg 94] fixtures there are, the greater is the amount of leakage, since every faucet will, in the course of time, begin to leak unless the packing is continually replaced. The amount of leakage is, therefore, in direct proportion to the number of fixtures.

The amount of water used then, per head per day, varies from seven to sixty gallons, but only by an intimate knowledge of the habits of the household can one predict the amount of water likely to be used. Perhaps as an average in a house having a kitchen sink and a bath-room containing a wash-basin, bath-tub, and water-closet, a fair estimate of the water used would be twenty-five gallons per head per day. This amount must be multiplied by a maximum number of persons to be in the house at any time, and then this number must be increased by the amount of water used in the barn and in the yard, if these are to be supplied from the same source as the house.

*Quantity used in stables.*

The amount of water used in the barn is even more than that used in the house, a variant depending on the habits of the manager. The minimum quantity needed per day is determined by the number of pailfuls of water which each head actually drinks multiplied by the number of head. But besides this there are many other uses to which water may reasonably be put in connection with stock.

On a dairy farm, there is the water needed to wash cans and bottles and in some cases to furnish a running stream of cold water for the aerator. In some stables a large amount of water is used for washing harnesses and carriages; in others, but a small amount goes for such purposes. [Pg 95] Some farmers have concrete floors in cow stables and pig pens and use a hose frequently to wash these floors clean. Other stables never see a stream of water and only see a shovel at infrequent intervals. The amount of water used outside the house is too uncertain a quantity to estimate on the average, but its influence and importance must not be overlooked.

*Maximum rate of water-use.*

It should now be noted that the quantity of water already referred to is the average quantity used through the twenty-four hours and does not mean the rate at which the water comes from the faucet. For example, three persons in a house use water, according to the above statement, at the rate of seventy-five gallons per day, but a whole day has 1440 minutes, and if seventy-five gallons be divided equally among the number of minutes, it means one gallon in every twenty minutes, or one quart in five minutes. It is obvious that no water-supply system for a house, designed to supply water at the average rate for the twenty-four hours would be satisfactory, since no person would care to wait all day for the amount. To wait five minutes to draw a quart of water would try the patience of any one, and while the total amount of water used in the house will be seventy-five gallons, provision must be made by which it can be drawn in small amounts at much higher rates. Practically all of the amount is used in the daylight hours or in twelve hours out of the twenty-four, so that the rate would be twice the average rate, and with this correction, two quarts of water could be drawn in five minutes.

But even this is too slow, and if one were to take a quart [Pg 96] cup to a kitchen faucet and note the time necessary to fill the measure with the water running at a satisfactory rate, he would find that unless the cup was filled in about ten seconds it would be considered too slow a flow. Since it is possible for more than one fixture to be in use at the same time, the pipes ought to be able to deliver the total amount running from different faucets open at the same time, and if it is considered possible for three faucets to run at once, as, for instance, the kitchen faucet, bath-room faucet, and barn faucet, then the supply pipe must be able to deliver, under our assumption, three quarts in ten seconds, or at the rate of about six thousand gallons a day. It is necessary, therefore, to distinguish carefully between the total quantity of water used per day and the rate at which such water is used.

The first of these requirements governs the size of the reservoir from which the water comes or the yield of the well or spring, or the capacity of a pump from a pond to a distributing tank; the other requirement governs the size of the pipe or faucet or the capacity of a pump which supplies direct pressure. It should be noted also that with ordinary fixtures, the rate of delivery and the corresponding sizes of the fixtures are not affected by the number of persons in the house, whereas the first requirement, that is, the total quantity of water used per day, is directly affected by the number of persons.

*Variation in maximum rates of water-use.*

The quantity of water used, however, is not uniform throughout the day or the week. It is commonly known, for instance, that on Monday, or wash-day, when the well is the only supply, a great deal more water has to be carried [Pg 97] on that day than on any other day in the week, and this same increased demand for water is made when the water comes in pipes into the house. Probably about half as much water again is used on Monday as on other days.

Again, in the hot weather of summer, more water is used for bathing and laundry purposes than in cold weather. But, on the other hand, there is a great tendency in cold weather to let the water run in a slow stream from faucets in order to prevent freezing. This has been found to just about double the amount of water used. It is only a reasonable safeguard, therefore, if it has been decided that the family needs are such as to require twenty-five gallons per head per day, to provide for double that amount in order to meet the demands of excessive daily consumption or of the hot and cold weather extremes.

*Fire streams.*

If a water-supply is to be installed for any house, the possibility of providing mains of sufficient size for adequate fire protection should always be considered, although it may not be found to be a necessary expenditure. In case of a fire a large amount of water is needed for a few hours, entirely negligible if it is computed as an average for the year, but a controlling factor in determining the size of mains or the amount of storage.

A good-sized fire stream delivers about 150 gallons per minute, and for a house in flames, four streams are none too many. The rate of delivery, therefore, for a fire should be at least 600 gallons per minute or a rate of nearly a million gallons per day, and if it is assumed that the fire might burn an hour before being [Pg 98] extinguished, 36,000 gallons of water would be used. If a spring or tank is the source of supply, the storage should be 36,000 gallons, and the pipe line from the tank to the hydrants must be large enough to freely deliver water at the rate of 600 gallons per minute. If the distance is not over 500 feet, a four-inch pipe is sufficiently large; but if the distance involved (from the reservoir or tank to the farthest hydrant) is more than about 500 feet, four-inch pipe is not large enough. This is because the friction in a large line of pipe is so great that the water cannot get through in the desired quantity. A four-inch pipe, discharging 600 gallons a minute, would need a fall of one foot in every four feet, while a six-inch pipe would need a fall of only one in thirty. Of course, if the reservoir from which the water comes is at such an elevation that the greater fall is obtainable, the smaller pipe may be used. It is more than likely, though, that the reservoir is about 3000 feet or more away, and the entire fall available only about thirty feet or one foot in one hundred. Then an eight-inch pipe would have to be used.

Whether fire-protection piping, therefore, is a wise investment or not, depends largely on the cost of installation. A four-inch cast-iron pipe laid will cost about forty cents per running foot, while an inch pipe, large enough for everything except fires, will cost about ten cents, so that the excess cost per foot for the sake of fire protection is thirty cents, for a distance up to 500 feet (when the grade is 1 to 4) or $150. If the grade is not 1 to 4, then the pipe must be six-inch, and the excess cost is fifty cents or the cost for 500 feet will be $250. If the distance is greater than 500 and the fall not great, so that [Pg 99] an eight-inch pipe has to be used, the excess cost is sixty-five cents a foot, or $650 for a 1000-foot line.

It is sometimes possible to economize by building a large tank containing about 36,000 gallons and using only a small pipe to fill, but always keeping the tank full. Such a tank would contain 4800 cubic feet or would be twenty-two feet square and ten feet deep, or it may be twenty-five feet in diameter and ten feet deep. This tank would have to be erected in the air, higher up than the top of the buildings, and would require heavy supports and a great expenditure. Unless, therefore, a convenient knoll or sidehill is available on which to build a concrete tank, the large pipe direct from the water-supply must be provided for fire protection. Whether it is worth while depends on the cost of insurance and whether it is considered cheaper to pay high rates for insurance or to spend the large sum for protection. A third choice is also open, namely, to carry no insurance and to install no fire hydrants and to run the inevitable risk of losing the house by fire. Perhaps the decision is a mark of the type of man whose property is concerned.

*Rain water-supply.*

It will often happen that no pond or brook is available for a water-supply, and if water is obtained, it must come directly from the rain. Apparently, this is quite feasible, since an ordinary house has about 1000 square feet area on which rain water might be caught and carried to a tank. In the eastern part of the United States, the annual rainfall is, on the average, 3-3/4 vertical inches per month, or the volume of water from the roof will be 310 cubic feet. This is nearly 80 gallons a day, or enough for three or four [Pg 100] people. The rain from the house and barns might be combined, making perhaps 5000 square feet, and giving an ample volume of water for the needs of a dozen people.

In discussing the size of tank necessary to hold rain water for a family supply, it must be remembered that for many weeks at a time no rain occurs, and that a tank must be large enough to tide over these intervals of no rainfall. In the temperate zone there is no regularity in the monthly rates of rainfall. In the eastern part of the United States, the months of June and September are usually the months of least precipitation, although the general impression, perhaps, is that July and August have less rainfall than any other months. The truth is that, while wells and rivers are low in July and August, the actual rainfall for those months is not below the normal, and the low flows in the streams are caused by excessive evaporation and by the demands of growing crops. Although June and September have usually less rainfall than other months, in Boston the fall has been as high as 8.01 inches in June and 11.95 inches in September. Again, in Boston, typifying the eastern part of the United States, and taken because of the great length of rainfall statistics available there, the two months of highest rainfall on the average are March and August, and yet, in each month, in some particular year, the rainfall has been the lowest for any of the twelve months in the year.

As shown by statistics, the average rainfall in each month, taking a period of forty years or so, is practically constant for each month, and it is only the deviations from the average which would make trouble in a supply tank depending upon rainfall. Fortunately, statistics also [Pg 101] show that while a month whose average rate of rainfall is three inches may be as low as three tenths of an inch, it is not often that two months of minimum rainfall come together, and in looking over the rainfall statistics the writer finds that for any three consecutive months, including the minimum, the amount of rainfall is generally two thirds of the monthly average for that year; and this is stated in this way because it gives what seems to the writer a basis for determining a fair and reasonable capacity of a rain-water storage tank. It depends, one will notice, on the average annual rainfall; that is, on the depth to which the rainfall would reach in any year if none ran off. This varies from about ten inches in the southeastern part of the United States to one hundred inches in the extreme northwest, the average for the eastern part of the country being about forty-five inches, so that the monthly average is 3.75 inches.

*Computation for rain-water storage.*

With this for a basis, it may be determined how large a storage tank ought to be, assuming a family of five persons using water at the average rate of 25 gallons per head per day or 125 gallons each day. Doubling this amount to take care of emergencies and of the extra water used in hot weather, let us say that 250 gallons a day must be provided, or 7500 gallons a month. If we could be sure of starting at the beginning of any month with the tank full and that exactly thirty days would be the period of no rainfall, then a tank holding 7500 gallons would be the proper size. Unfortunately, with any month, as August, in which the rainfall may be practically zero, the preceding month may also have been so short of rain that the consumption was [Pg 102] equal to or even more than the rainfall, and the month of August would start with no rain in the tank.

But if we take a three-month period, those inequalities will be averaged and the supply will be, so far as one can foresee, ample in amount; that is, we shall take the supply required in three months, namely, 22,500 gallons, and subtract from it the amount of water furnished in the three months, which is presumably two thirds of the average rainfall on the area contributing to the tank. The normal rainfall in three months is three times 3-3/4 inches, or 11-1/4 vertical inches, and if this falls on a roof area of, say, 2000 square feet, the total amount of water is 1850 cubic feet or 13,875 gallons, and two thirds of this is 9250. The tank, then, must hold the difference between the 22,500 gallons and 9250, or 13,250 gallons, whereas a month's supply would be 7500 gallons. The actual tank, therefore, is made to hold a little less than two months' supply. Such a tank would be ten feet deep and fourteen feet square, a good deal larger tank, of course, than one ordinarily finds with a rain water-supply; but the estimate of the use of water has been high and a long period of rainfall has been assumed, so that there is little likelihood of a house with this provision being ever without water.

*Computation for storage reservoir on a brook.*

In determining the quantity of water that may be taken from a small stream the area of the watershed answers the same purpose as the area of the roof which delivers water into a tank, the only difference being that from the roof all the water is always delivered, except a small proportion that evaporates at the beginning of a rain in summer. From the surface of a watershed, on the contrary, [Pg 103] a large amount, and in some cases all of a stream, will be absorbed by the ground and by the vegetation and will never be delivered into the stream which drains an area. On large streams it is fair to assume that, on the average, only one half of the rainfall on the area will reach the stream, while with sandy soils this may be as small as 20 per cent. From December to May inclusive, when the ground is frozen, when there is no vegetation to absorb the water, and when evaporation is very light, practically all of the rainfall reaches the streams. From June to August, on the other hand, when the soil becomes rapidly parched, when vegetation is most active, and when evaporation is high, frequently no rainfall reaches the streams and the ground water sinks lower and lower, so that often streams themselves dry up. It is necessary, therefore, in providing for a definite quantity of water to be taken from a reservoir built on a small stream, to make the reservoir large enough to furnish water from June to September without being supplied with rain. This does not call for a very large dam or a very large storage, and three months' supply will usually be ample.

We have already estimated above that the quantity of water needed for three months will be 45,000 gallons, or about 6000 cubic feet. If the reservoir is built in a small gulley or ravine, its width may be twenty-five feet. If the length of the reservoir or pond formed by the dam is 240 feet, then the reservoir will furnish 6000 cubic feet for every foot of depth, and a reservoir of that size holding one foot of water will tide over a dry season.

Evaporation during these same three months will use up about a foot and a half in depth over whatever area the [Pg 104] reservoir covers, so that two and a half feet in depth must be provided above the lowest point to which it is desirable to draw off the water. It would be well to allow a depth of at least ten feet in order to avoid shallow, stagnant pools, and if this depth is provided, even more than the two-and-a-half foot depth mentioned might be withdrawn in extremely dry seasons, though perhaps at some reduction in the quality of the water.

*Deficiency from well supplies.*

A large number of water-supplies in the country, perhaps the largest number, at present comes from wells, either dug or drilled. It often happens that after plumbing fixtures have been installed with a pump to raise the water to the necessary elevated tank, the increased consumption causes the well to run dry for a number of weeks in the summer. The question then arises, Shall the well supply be supplemented or shall an entirely new supply be developed?

There are two methods of supplementing a dug well supply, and it may be of advantage to point them out. If the sand or gravel in which the water is carried is fine, it may be that the water will not at times of low water enter the well as fast as the pump takes it out. Such a well always has water in it in the morning, but a short pumping exhausts the supply. One remedy here is to provide a more easy path for the water, and that can be done by running out pipe drains in different directions. If there are any evidences that the underground water flows in any direction, then the drains should preferably run out at right angles to this direction, to intercept as much water as possible. The drains must be laid in trenches and be [Pg 105] surrounded with gravel, and of course the method is inapplicable if the well is more than about fifteen feet deep, because of the depth of trench involved.

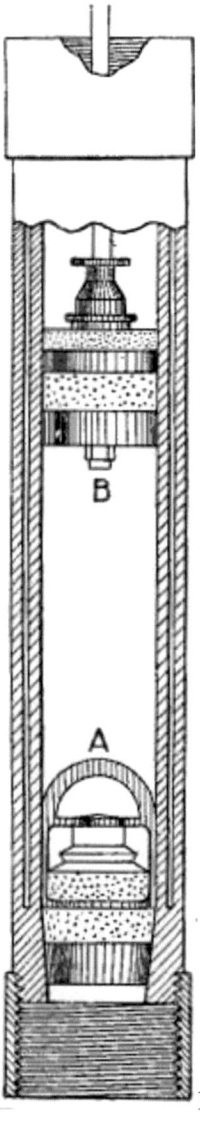

Fig. 22. — How a pump works.

Another remedy is to sink the well deeper, hoping to find a more porous stratum or to increase the head of water in the well. In one well, the writer remembers seeing two lengths of twenty-four-inch sewer pipe, that is, four feet, that had been sunk in the sandy bottom of the well by operating a posthole digger inside and standing on the top of the pipe to furnish the necessary weight for sinking.

Still another remedy is to drive pipe down in the bottom of the well, hoping to find artesian water which will rise into the well from some lower stratum. This method has been successfully employed in the village of Homer, New York, where the public supply formerly came from a dug well twenty feet in diameter. The supply becoming deficient, pipe wells were driven in the bottom and an excellent supply of water found fifty feet below the surface, the water rising up in the dug well to within eight feet of the surface of the ground.

If the well is a driven well and the water in the casing falls so low that the ordinary suction pump will no longer [Pg 106] draw, two remedies may be applied. A so-called deep-well pump may be used; that is, a pump which fits inside the piping and can be lowered down to the water level. The ability to bring up water then depends on the power to work the pump and on the presence of the water. Figure 22 shows the principle on which this pump works. At some point, it may be three or four hundred feet below the surface of the ground, a valve A opening upward is set in the well so that it is always submerged. Just above this is a second valve fastened to the lower end of the long pump rod which reaches up to the engine or windmill which operates the pump. At each up stroke water is lifted by the closed valve B and sucked through the open valve A. At each down stroke, the water is held by the closed valve A and forced up through the open valve B.

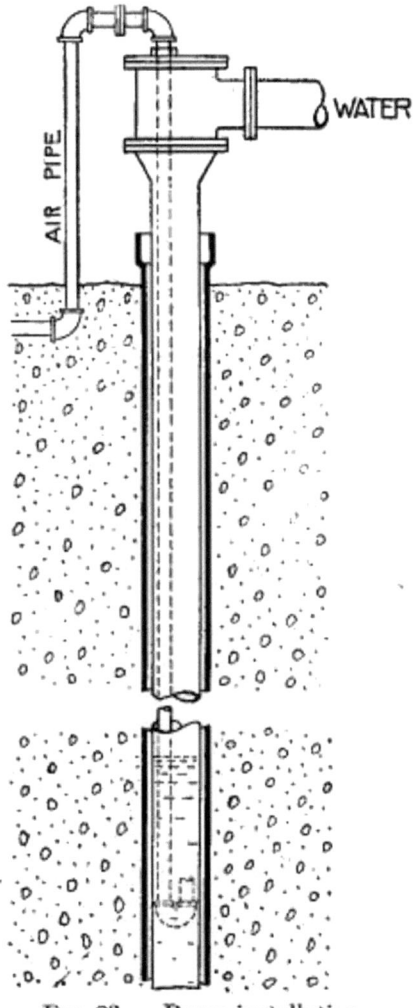

Fig. 23. — Pump installation.

Fig. 23. — Pump installation.

The other method of developing a greater quantity of [Pg 107] water from a deep well is to use air pressure to force the water either the entire distance to the tank or to a point where the suction of an ordinary pump can reach it, as indicated in Fig. 23. In this method an air blower is needed, and since this means an engine for operation, it is not generally feasible, but is suited to occasional needs, where an engine is already installed for other purposes and is therefore available.

The operation is very simple. An air pipe leads from a blower and delivers compressed air at the end of the air pipe, which must be below the level of the water in the well. The pressure of the air then causes the water to rise, the distance depending on the pressure at which the air is delivered.

[Pg 108]

**CHAPTER VI**

## *SOURCES OF WATER-SUPPLY*

Having arrived at the quantity of water necessary to supply the needs of the average household, we must next investigate the possible sources from which this quantity can be obtained. Before the advantages of running water in the house are understood, a well is the normal and usual method of securing water, although in a few cases progressive farmers have made use of spring water from the hillsides. It is rare, indeed, for surface water, so called, to be used for purposes of water-supply until after modern plumbing conveniences have been installed. Then the use of surface water becomes almost a necessity because of the large volume of water needed. The only drawback to its use is its questionable quality. Without modern plumbing, a well meets the requirements of family life, but does not answer the demands of convenience. With modern plumbing, a well is found to be pumped dry long before the domestic demands are satisfied. The result is an attempt to secure an unfailing supply, and for this a surface supply is sought.

Let us divide, then, the possible sources of water for domestic consumption into two groups, those found under [Pg 109] the surface of the soil and those found on or above the surface. In the first group will come wells and springs, and in the second group will come brooks, streams, and lakes.

*Underground waters.*

Springs result from a bursting out of underground waters from the confined space in which they have been stored or through which they have been running. Thus in Fig. 24 is seen how water falling on the pervious area *a-b* is received into the soil and gradually finds its way downward between impervious strata which may be clay or dense rock. At the point *B*, where the cover layer has, for any reason, been weakened, the pressure of the water forces its way upward and a spring is developed at the point *C*. Or, conditions may be as shown in Fig. 25, where the confined water, instead of being forced upward by pressure, flows slowly out from the side of a hill, making a spring at the point *D*, while the water enters the pervious stratum at the point *a-b* as before.

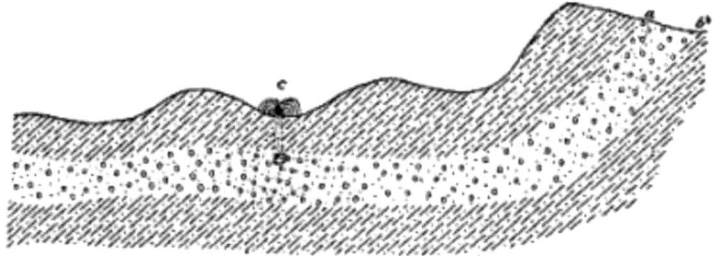

Fig. 24.—Diagram of a spring.

[Pg 110]

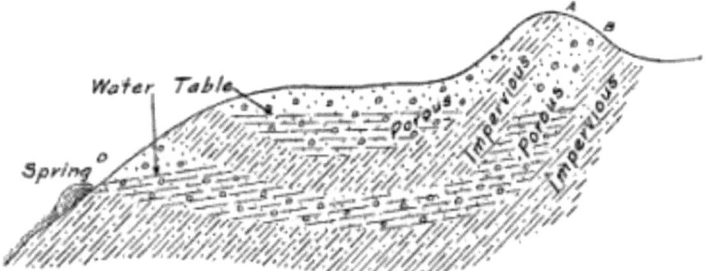

Fig. 25.—Water finding its way from a hillside.

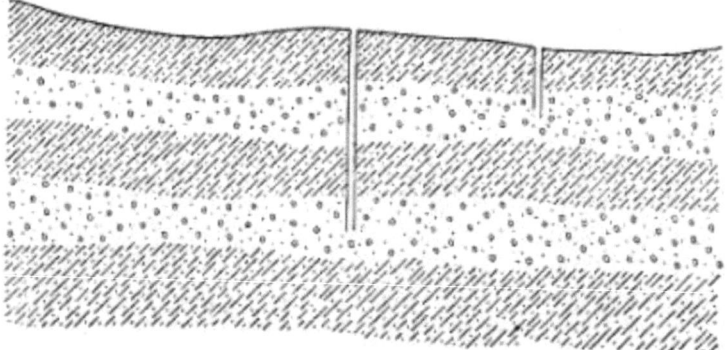

Fig. 26. — The sinking of wells.

If the water is held in the ground as in the first case, it is possible to develop the spring artificially; that is, to drill through or bore through the overlying impervious strata so as to allow the escape of the water. When this happens, the water bursts forth exactly as in a natural spring except that under some conditions the pressure may be sufficient to force the water rising in a pipe instead of through the ground to flow above the surface of the ground as a fountain or jet, making what is known as an [Pg 111] "artesian well." A true well, on the other hand, may be put down in the ground and through strata where springs could never develop; that is, where no pressure exists in such a way as to bring the water to the surface, as in Fig. 26. The well here is sunk until it reaches the water, and it is safe to say that one can always reach a layer of water in the ground by a well if the well is deep enough.

The flow of underground water is, however, always very uncertain and confusing, and even in localities where water would naturally be expected in quantity, as, for instance, in the bottom of a valley filled with glacial drift, much disappointment is often experienced because the expected water is not found. The city supply of Ithaca, New York, is a case in point. For six miles south of the lake there is a broad, almost level valley filled many hundred feet deep with glacial drift and presumably filled with water flowing at some unknown depth below the surface into the lake. When the city was recovering from the typhoid fever epidemic which, in 1903, committed such ravages, well water seemed to the panic-stricken citizens the only safe water. Geologists were called in, and they gravely asserted that the valley contained glacial drift to a great depth and that an ample supply of pure water could be counted on. It was known that water was met all through this valley at depths of from six to twelve feet and then that there would be found a layer of finely powdered silt to a depth of about one hundred feet, when another layer of water would be found, and that all the private wells reached this layer. When tested by the city, however, it was found that this water-bearing stratum was [Pg 112] of too fine material to yield its water freely, and the supply from the depth was altogether inadequate. In one section of the town large quantities of good water were found at a depth of about three hundred feet, and the city thought that other wells of the same depth should add to the quantity, but experiment showed that this three hundred-foot water was limited to one particular section, and after a considerable expenditure of money, an underground water-supply for the city was given up.

*Ordinary dug well.*

The ordinary well at a farmhouse is what is known as a shallow well or sometimes a "dug well," usually ten to twenty feet deep. This type does not usually pierce any impervious layer and thus reach a water-bearing stratum, otherwise inaccessible. The water is found almost at the surface, and the depth of the well is only that necessary to reach the first water layer. A very good example of this kind of well is to be found on the south shores of Long Island Sound, where a pipe can be driven into the sand at any point, and at a depth of a few feet an abundant and cheap supply of water may be secured. The amount of water that such a well can furnish depends upon the area from which the water comes and upon the size of the particles of sand or gravel through which the water has to percolate, it being evident that the finer the material, the more difficult for the water to penetrate.

The writer remembers superintending the digging of trenches in the streets of a city where the texture of the soil varied continually from clay to sand and even to gravel, all saturated with subsoil water into which wells could have been dug. It was very striking to see how the [Pg 113] coarseness of the material affected the quantity of water that had to be pumped from the trenches, — the finest sand requiring only one hand pump at a time, while the coarse gravel required either a dozen men or a steam pump to keep a short trench reasonably free from water. The same conditions exist when a well is in operation, modified by the fact that the coarse material yielding a larger supply will be most quickly exhausted unless the area drained is very large.

A shallow well is most uncertain as to its quantity and is likely to be of doubtful quality. There are, however, some examples of shallow well supplies which furnish large amounts of water; as, for instance, the one at Waltham, Massachusetts, or at Bath, New York, — the latter, a dug well some twenty feet in diameter and about twenty-eight feet deep, furnishing a constant supply of good water to a village of about 4000 people.

*Construction of dug wells.*

The construction of shallow wells requires little comment. Ordinarily, they are dug down to the water, or to such a depth below the level of the water as is convenient, by the use of an ordinary boat pump to keep down the water, and then are stoned up with a dry wall. Such a well for a single house requires an excavation of about eight feet diameter, with an inside dimension of about five feet. [Pg 114]

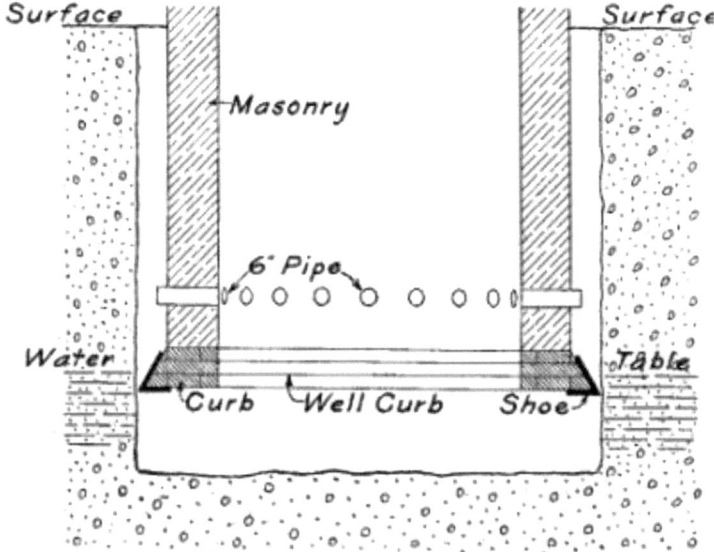

Fig. 27.—Mode of sinking a well.

If the soil at the bottom of the well is sandy, it is possible to take a barrel or a large sewer pipe and sink it into the bottom of the well in the water by taking out material from the inside and loading the outside to keep it pressed down into the sand. This same plan may be used to sink the whole body of the well wall, first supporting the lower course of masonry on a curb, so called (see Fig. 27). This curb is usually made of several thicknesses of two-inch plank well nailed together, the plank breaking joints in the three or four layers used. It is a good plan to have this shoe or curb extend outwardly beyond the walls of the well so that some clearance may be had, otherwise the dirt may press against the walls so hard as to hold it up and prevent its sinking. While this arrangement may be put down in water, it requires some sort of bucket which will dig automatically under water and has not been therefore a customary method [Pg 115] except for large excavations where machinery can be installed. There is no reason, however, why the method might not be used for a single house.

115

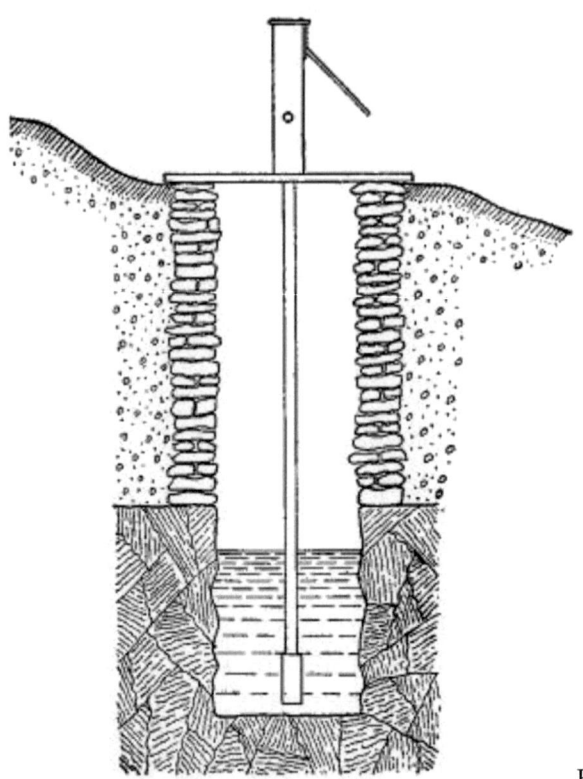

Fig. 28. — A well that will catch surface waste.

In whatever way the well is dug, one point in the construction that needs to be emphasized is that the wall should be well cemented together, beginning about six feet below the surface and reaching up to a point at least one foot above the surface. This is to prevent pollution from the surface gaining direct access to the well, and if [Pg 116] this cementing is well done for the distance named, it is not likely that any surface pollution in the vicinity of the well could ever damage the water. Figure 28 shows the section of a well where no such precautions have been taken, and it is evident that not only surface wash, but subsurface pollution may readily contaminate the water. Figure 29 (after Imbeaux), on the other hand, shows a shallow well properly protected by a good wall and water-tight cover.

Figure 30 shows a photograph also of this latter type of well. Even if a cesspool or privy is located dangerously near the well, in the second case the fact that the contaminating influence must pass downward through at least six feet of soil before it can enter the well is a guarantee that the danger is reduced to the smallest possible terms.

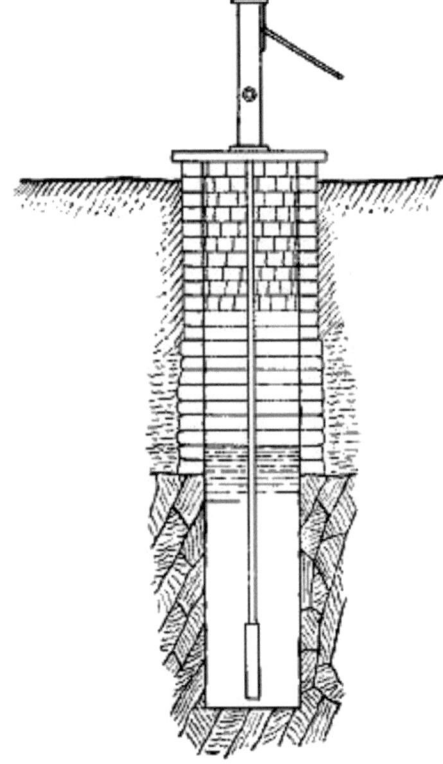

Fig. 29. — A well properly protected.

*Deep wells.*

Deep wells are of the same general character as shallow wells. Usually, the ground on which the rainfall [Pg 117] occurs is more distant, so that the source of the water is often unknown, and usually, also, the stratum from which the water comes is overlaid by an impervious one.

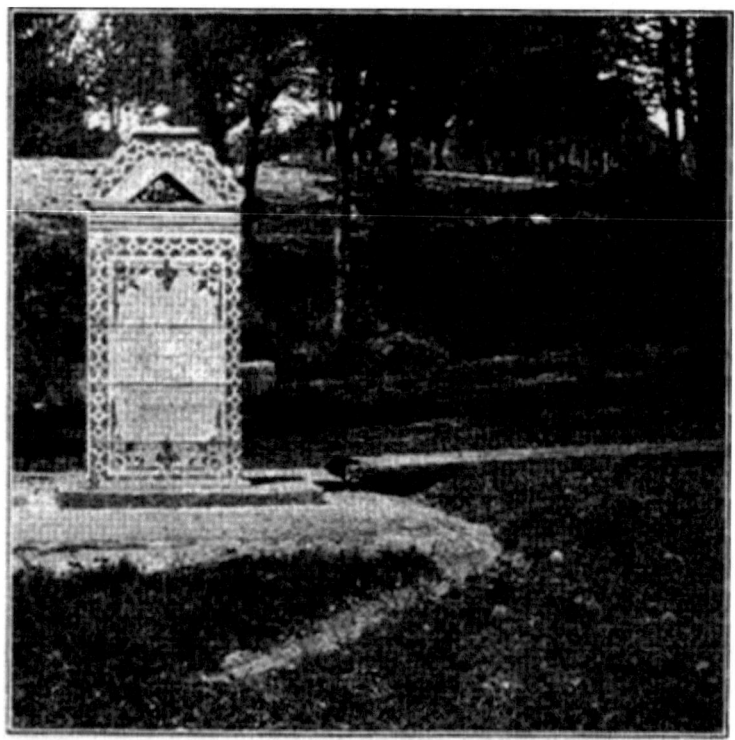

Fig. 30. — A properly protected well.

It often happens that there are several layers of water or of water-bearing strata alternating with more or less impervious strata, and that wells might be so dug as to take water from any one of them. Indeed, not infrequently in driving down a pipe to reach water, a fairly satisfactory [Pg 118] quantity is obtained at a certain level, and then, in order to increase the supply, the pipe is driven further, shutting off the first supply and reaching some other, less abundant.

Deep wells are reached usually by wrought-iron pipe driven into the ground. Sometimes this is done by taking a one-and-one-quarter inch pipe, with its lower end closed and pointed, and driving it with wooden mauls into the ground. When it has gone six or eight feet, it is pulled up, cleared from the earth, and replaced, to be driven six feet again.

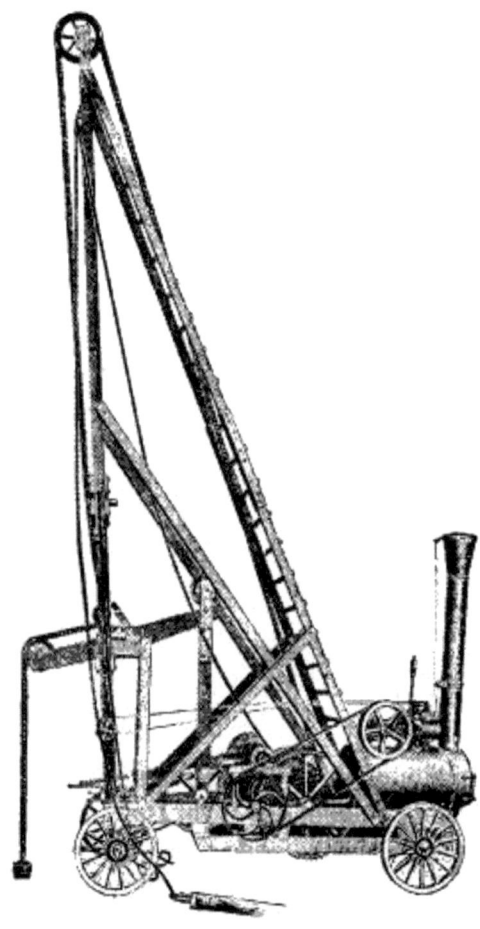

Fig. 31. — Well-drilling apparatus.

With ordinary soil, the pipe is easily withdrawn with a chain wrench, and two men will drive one hundred feet in a couple of days. When water is reached, a well point is put on through which water may percolate without carrying too much soil. This type of well is suitable for use in soft ground or sand, up to depths of about one hundred feet, and in places where the water is not abundant. It is most useful for testing the ground to see where water may be found and by pumping from such a well to see what quantity of water may be expected. This type is often [Pg 119] used as a shallow well, and the author has seen such wells driven only a dozen feet. Such a well has no protection against pollution, and an ordinary dug well is better for shallow depths. A driven well always has a disadvantage also from the ever present danger that the iron pipe will rust through at the top of the ground water and so admit to the well the most polluted part of the drainage.

For larger supplies and for greater depths, a machine like a pile-driver has to be used for forcing down the pipe. This is not usually removed, but driven down as far as possible, and when the limit of the machine has been reached, a smaller size is slipped down inside the driven pipe, to be in turn driven to refusal. In rock, that is, if the well has to penetrate a layer of rock, a drill is used that will work inside of the pipe last driven, and by alternately lifting and drop-ping the drill, and at the same time twisting it back and forth, a hole through rock may be made many hundred feet below the surface of the ground. Figure 31 shows a cut of a common type of well-drilling machine.

In some soils, not rock, it is necessary to keep the drill going in order to churn up or soften the earth so that the pipe may be low-ered. The churned-up soil is removed by a sand pump, which is a hollow tube with a flap valve at the lower end opening inwards and a hook on the upper end. By alternately drilling, pipe-driving, and pumping the wet material, length after length of pipe can be forced into the ground until water of a satisfactory quantity is reached. Very often a jet of water is used to wash out the dirt from the interi-or of the well instead of a sand [Pg 120] pump. As shown by Fig. 32 water under pressure is forced down the small pipe $A$ which runs to the bottom of the well. The large pipe $B$ can then, as the sand is loosened by the water, be driven down by the one thousand-pound hammer $M$. The water and sand together flow up in the space out-side the small pipe and inside the large pipe, overflowing through the waste pipe $W$. This type of well has been very largely used throughout New York State; on Long Island, in connection with the Brooklyn Water-supply; along the Erie Canal, in connection with the Barge Canal Work, and in New York City, in connection with building foundations.

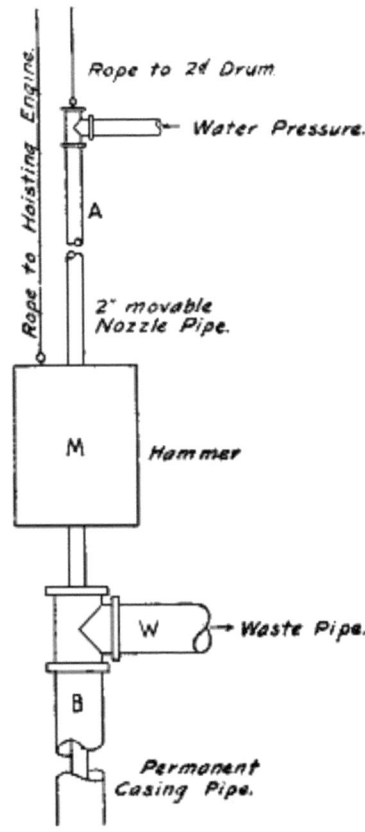

Fig. 32. — Sinking a well by means of a water-jet.

Sometimes, when a shallow dug well does not furnish the required quantity of water, the amount of water can be increased by driving pipe wells down into water strata below the one from which the dug well takes its supply, so that water will rise to the strata penetrated by the dug well. This has been done to increase the public supplies at Addison and Homer in New York State. Unfortunately, much uncertainty exists in [Pg 121] the matter of the yield of driven wells, and an individual undertakes a deep well usually with great reluctance on account of the expense involved and the uncertainty of successful results. In level ground, conditions are not likely to vary in the same valley, so that if one well is proved successful, the probabilities are that wells in the vicinity will be equally so, and yet, at some places, the contrary has proved to be true.

One may estimate the cost of putting down four-inch driven wells as approximately one dollar per foot besides the cost of the pipe, which will be about fifty cents per foot. The cost of one-and-one-half-inch pipe would be considerably less than fifty cents, the cost of driving varying not so much with the size of the pipe as with the soil conditions. The writer recently paid ninety dollars for driving two one-and-one-half-inch wells to a depth of about one hundred feet, the above cost including that of the pipe; the soil conditions, however, were very favorable. In Ithaca the cost of driving one-and-one-quarter-inch pipe is fifteen cents per lineal foot up to about fifty feet deep with the cost of the pipe fifteen cents per foot additional. Below fifty feet deep the cost increases, since the labor and time required for pulling up the pipe is largely increased, and at the same time the rate at which the pipe will drive is notably diminished.

The question of pumping from wells will be considered in a later chapter, together with methods of construction and operation.

*Springs.*

Springs should be the most natural method of securing water-supply for a detached house, since no expense is [Pg 122] involved except that of piping the water to the building. In Europe, spring water-supplies have been greatly developed in furnishing water for large cities. Vienna, for example, with its population of nearly two millions, obtains its water-supply from springs in the Alps mountains, and many smaller cities do likewise.

But in this country springs have been little used for water-supplies, partly because of the uncertain quantity furnished and partly because of difficulty in acquiring title to the water rights. If an individual, however, has on his farm, or within reach, a spring furnishing a continuous supply of water, it would seem quite absurd not to make use of such a Heaven-sent blessing. Care must be taken always that a spring is not contaminated by surface drainage, and for this reason, as with shallow wells, the wall surrounding the inclosed spring should be extended above the ground and made impervious to water for at least six feet below the surface. In some cases it may be wise to convert an open spring into an underground one, putting a roof over all and then covering with earth and sod. Figure 33 shows a type suggested by the French engineer, M. Imbeaux.

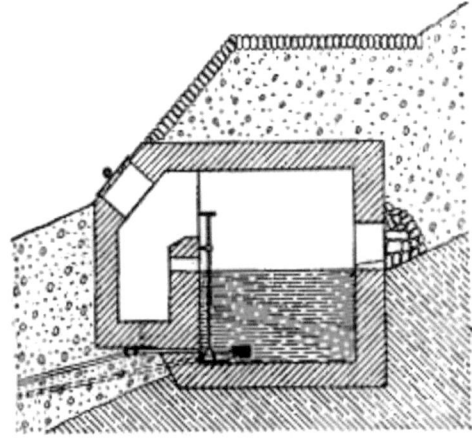

Fig. 33. — An inclosed spring.

[Pg 123]

Very often a larger supply from a spring may be obtained by collecting into one basin a number of separate and smaller springs. A swampy or boggy piece of ground is often the result of the existence of a number of springs, and if drains are laid to some convenient corner of the field, and a well dug there, into which the drains will discharge, not only will the swamp be drained, but an ample supply of water in this way be obtained. It would, of course, not be wise to have cows pasture in this part of the field, nor, even when the ground has been dried out, should this field be manured or cultivated. It should rather be fenced and left to grow up in underbrush, dedicated to the farm water-supply.

*Extensions of springs.*

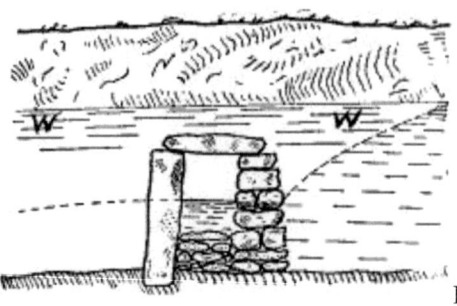

Fig. 34. — A spring extension.

Again, if the water comes from a stratum W-W, as shown in Fig. 34, a large additional yield can be obtained by extending the spring from the point where it breaks out along the edge of the water-bearing stratum on each side. This extension or gathering conduit can be made by building rough stone walls on each side of the ditch, covering with flat stones so as to form a pervious channel to intercept the water and lead it to the chamber from which the supply pipe to the house leads out. The ground-water level will then be altered as shown by the broken line in the draining. [Pg 124]

More simply it may be made by digging a trench along the hillside at the same level as the spring, or into the spring if necessary to find the water, and then laying draintile surrounded by coarse gravel or broken stone in the trench.

In the western part of the country much knowledge has been gained by investigating and experimenting on this kind of spring water development, only there the springs have been made artificially by digging down to meet the underground flow of water. For example, in the Arkansas River Valley, California, where it was suspected that water was flowing underground, a trench was dug transversely across the valley, and at a depth of six feet sufficient water was found to amount to 200,000 gallons per day for each one hundred feet of trench. On the South Platte River, near Denver, much the same thing has been done, and in a trench eighteen feet deep, water is collected at the rate of a million and a quarter gallons per day for each one hundred feet of trench. Other examples of the same sort might be given.

For a single house, the spring need usually only be extended by means of a short trench, and three-inch terra-cotta tile should be laid in the trench and surrounded by gravel and then covered over. The spring receiving water from these tiles should be inclosed, as will be described in a later chapter.

*Supply from brooks.*

Whenever a spring is not available and at the same time a supply of running water by gravity is determined on for a house, recourse is generally had to brooks which may find their way down the hillsides in the vicinity. In many [Pg 125] instances the water in such brooks is practically spring water and is the overflow of actual springs. Where the brook is not subject to contamination between the spring and the point at which the supply is taken, the latter is as truly spring water as the former, and if a long length of pipe is saved, there can be no objection to the brook supply. On the other hand, it is suggestive, at least, of misrepresentation for a summer hotel or boarding house to advertise that their water-supply comes from springs when really it comes from an open brook miles away from the spring which may be indeed the origin of the brook, but with so many intervening opportunities for contamination that the pure original source is unrecognizable.

There are two obvious drawbacks to the use of brooks: (1) that the quality of the water is, in many cases, objectionable, and (2) that brooks are very apt to dry up in summer on account of their limited watersheds. The discussion on the first point will be postponed to a later chapter, and we have now to consider the question of quantity only.

The wisest plan before deciding on a brook supply is to measure the volume of water which flows in the brook at the time when it is lowest, probably about the middle of August. The actual volume of water needed for the household is not large, although its required rate of flow may be high and, as already pointed out, a stream which furnishes water at the rate of one quart in five minutes is sufficient for a family of three persons, a rate which is almost a drop-by-drop supply. Such a stream would require a reservoir somewhere in order to supply the faucets at the proper rate, and for a single family a small cistern or [Pg 126] even a barrel sunk in the ground would be sufficient for this purpose. An objection to the utilization of so small a flow in connection with the smaller storage is that the temperature of the water in summer is so raised that vegetation and animal growths take place easily and freely, so that the taste and smell of such water is most disagreeable. These consequences can be avoided even with the low flow by increasing the storage, since the larger quantity of water has been found to resist the bad effects of the low flow and high temperature. Figure 35 shows a small reservoir actually in use to supply water for a single house.

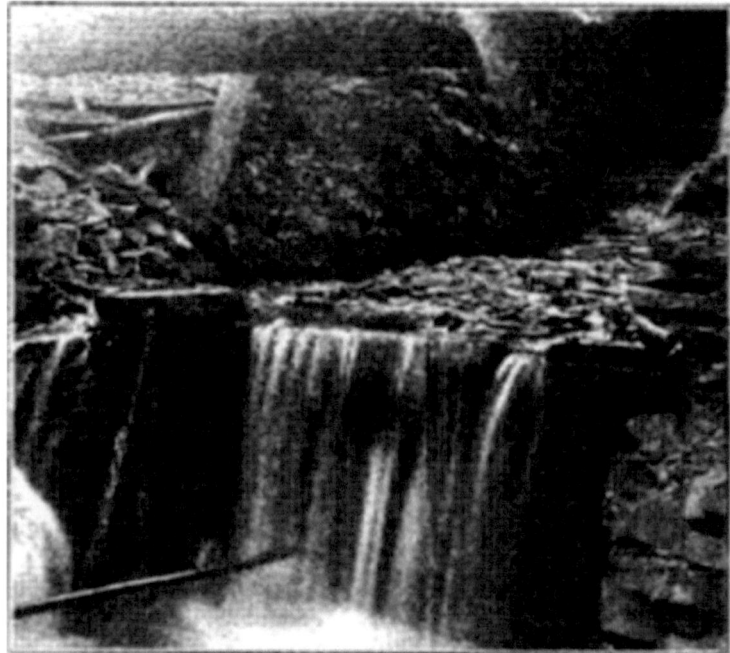

Fig. 35. — A reservoir for home use.

[Pg 127]

*Storage reservoirs.*

But even if the stream actually dries up for two or three months, it is still possible to use it for water-supply, provided a suitable location for a dam and pond can be found where storage, as described in the preceding chapter, can be secured. For this reason as well as for the greater benefit to the quality of the water, brooks flowing through rough, wooded, and uninhabited country are to be preferred as a source of water-supply to brooks flowing through flat agricultural land, and in many cases, where their flow is largely due to springs, the brooks themselves may compare favorably with springs in quality.

*Ponds or lakes.*

Water may be properly taken from ponds or lakes whenever the danger from pollution is negligible. No better source of supply can be imagined than a pond in the midst of woods, far away from human habitation, presumably furnishing an unlimited supply of pure soft water. Sometimes water from such ponds contains large amounts of vegetable matter, the result of decomposition of swampy or peaty material, as, for instance, from the ponds in the Dismal Swamp of Virginia, so that the water has a yellow, coffee-colored appearance. The appearance of such water is suspicious, but it need not be feared unless something more pernicious than the coloring matter is present.

As the country becomes more settled, ponds are more and more likely to become contaminated and hence unfit for a water-supply, and this possibility must be taken into account in planning for a water-supply. It would be most shortsighted to carry a long line of pipe from a house to a pond several miles away, only to have the pond made unfit [Pg 128] for use within a few years by the growth of the community around the pond. The possibility of coöperation ought not to be overlooked, however. It is quite possible that half a dozen householders might be so located with respect to each other and to a pond that an arrangement could be made whereby the owner of a small pond would agree to fence it around and dedicate it to the purposes of a water-supply, doing this as his share. The others might then well afford to pipe the water to one house after another, including that of the owner of the pond.

Water from a pond or lake has one great advantage over water from a brook, namely, that contaminating substances in the pond settle out, so that pond water, especially if the pond is deep, is always of much better quality than running water. For this same reason, water taken from a reservoir on a stream is much better water than that in the stream above the reservoir indicates, and pollution is much less to be feared where the reservoir exists.

*Pressure for water-supplies.*

The value of a high pressure in the water-pipes of a house has been much overestimated. For a number of years the water-supply in the writer's residence came from a tank in the attic, the pressure in the bath-room being not more than ten feet, and while the water flowing through a three fourths inch pipe was noticeably slow, it was not so slow as to discredit the supply.

A height or head of twenty feet above the highest fixture in the house would be better and ought to be secured whenever possible. This head is obtained by having the source of supply higher than the highest fixture, not merely the [Pg 129] twenty feet mentioned, but also an additional height necessary to offset the frictional losses caused by the running water. The loss from this source in case of fire supply has already been referred to, but for purely domestic supplies the loss is appreciable. The maximum rate as already indicated is not more than 7000 gallons per day, whereas the fire rate both for single houses and for a small hamlet is about a million gallons a day. For the lower rate, as well as for rates one half and twice this rate, the friction loss in vertical feet per 100 feet run in small pipes is shown in the following table: —

**Table X. Showing Loss of Head by Friction, for Different Quantities of Flow, and in Different Sizes of Pipes**

| Rate of Flow in Gallons Per Day | 1/2" Pipe | 5/8" Pipe | 3/4" Pipe | 1" Pipe | 1-1/4" Pipe |
|---|---|---|---|---|---|
| 3500 | 13.95 | 4.81 | 2.35 | 0.66 | 0.25 |
| 7000 | 47.17 | 17.30 | 7.45 | 2.04 | 0.74 |
| 14000 | 163.09 | 57.8 | 25.00 | 6.64 | 2.41 |

The table shows how much additional elevation is needed over the 20 feet already referred to. For example, suppose it is decided that a rate of 1 quart in 10 seconds is to be maintained from three faucets or a rate of 7000 gallons per day. Suppose that a pond 4000 feet away is found to be 50 feet above the highest faucet in the house, and it is a question what size pipe ought to be used. By the table a 1-inch pipe loses 2.6 feet per 100 feet or 104 feet in the 4000 feet, an impossible amount when only [Pg 130] 50 feet are available, although the size would be entirely proper if the difference of level was 124 feet or anything greater. A 1-1/4-inch pipe, however, loses only 0.74 foot in 100 or 39 feet per mile, so that the 1-1/4-inch pipe would be necessary, although that size would answer even if the pond were a mile and a quarter away.

When water from a well is pumped to an elevated tank there is the same necessity of providing about 20 feet difference in level between the tank and the highest fixture, but the length of pipe involved being small, the friction losses are not great. It should be noted even here that too small a pipe may reduce the pressure, a 1/2-inch pipe causing a loss of 47 feet in a 100-foot pipe line. If a tower is built by the side of the house, the distance down to the ground, across to the house, and up to the second floor would hardly be less than 50 feet, and this is a loss of 23-1/2 feet, which means that the tank would have to be set higher in the air by this amount. With a 3/4-inch pipe, it should go 3.7 feet, and with a 1-inch pipe but a foot higher than the level necessary to make the water flow out of the faucet at the rate already specified.

[Pg 131]

## CHAPTER VII

## *QUALITY OF WATER*

A pure water-supply has always been regarded as desirable and its value can hardly be overrated, from the standpoint of health, happiness, or economy. From the earliest history, no crime has been so despicable as that of deliberately poisoning a well from which the public supply was obtained, and in the past no charge more quickly could stir the populace to riot. In Strassburg in 1348 two thousand Jews were burned for this crime charged against them; and as late as 1832 the Parisian mob, frantic on account of the many deaths, insisted that the water-carriers who distributed water from the Seine, shockingly polluted with sewage as it was, had poisoned the water, and many of the carriers were murdered on this charge.

Yet no water, as used for drinking purposes, is absolutely pure, according to the standards of chemistry. Distilled water is the nearest approach to pure water obtainable, and it is said by physicians that such water is not desirable as a habitual and constant beverage. The human body requires certain mineral salts particularly for the bones and muscles, and while these salts are provided in a large measure by food, a number are also furnished [Pg 132] by drinking water. On the other hand, a wonderful natural process is accomplished by distilled or approximately pure water in that the water tends to dissolve, to add to itself, and to carry away whatever excess of solids may exist in the body. For certain kidney diseases, for example, pure water is prescribed, not merely as a means of preventing further accretions, but for the purpose of dissolving and removing the undesirable accumulations already existing.

Practically, considerable latitude is possible in the matter of the purity of drinking water, and no particular harm is to be apprehended by the constant use of either a water containing as little as ten parts per million of total solids or of water containing as much as three hundred parts per million of total solids. The human body, in this as in so many other ways, is so constituted as to be able to adjust itself to varying conditions of food, and, until an excessive amount of ingredients are absorbed, no great harm is done. There are, however, certain definite substances—animal, vegetable, and mineral—which, when found in water, are decidedly objectionable, and it is not the amount of foreign matter in a water-supply, but its character, which is of importance in a water to be used for drinking.

*Mineral matter in water.*

The mineral matter is the least objectionable as it is also the most common, since all water is forced to partake, more or less, of the nature of the rocks and soil over which it passes. Good waters contain from twenty to one hundred grains per gallon of mineral salts; that is, of various chemical substances which are able to be dissolved [Pg 133] by water. If the amount is much in excess of one hundred parts, the water is noticeably "hard," and this may increase to a point where the water cannot be used. For example, the writer once superintended the locating and drilling of a well which passed through a bed of sodium sulphate or gypsum, just before reaching the water, so that as the latter rose in the well it dissolved and carried with itself a large amount of this salt, so much that the water was useless. Water containing more than one hundred grains per gallon of such salts as magnesium sulphate or sodium phosphate is a mineral water rather than a good drinking water, and while an occasional glass may do no harm or may even have desirable medicinal effects, such a water is not fit for constant drinking.

It is worth noting that many attempts have been made to show the relative effect of various hard waters on the health. A French commissioner reported that apparently people in hard-water districts had a better physique than in soft-water districts. A Vienna commissioner also reported in favor of a moderately hard water for the same reason. It is to-day believed by many that children ought to have lime in water; that is, ought to drink hard water to prevent or ward off "rickets" or softening of the bones. An English commissioner, on the other hand, has concluded that, other things being equal, the rate of mortality is practically uninfluenced by the softness or hardness of the water-supply. This same commissioner has also shown that in the British Isles the tallest and most stalwart men were found in Cumberland and in the Scotch Highlands, where the water used is almost invariably very soft (Thresh's "Water-supplies"). [Pg 134]

It has been asserted that certain diseases, not necessarily causing death, are caused by hard water, as calculus, cancer, goiter, and cretinism; but, as already pointed out in Chapter II, no satisfactory proof has ever been established. One must conclude that within reasonable limits there is little to choose between a hard and soft water for drinking purposes, although a change from a soft water to a hard, or *vice versa*, usually produces temporary derangements.

*Loss of soap.*

For washing purposes the value of a soft water is more marked. When a hard water is used, a certain amount of soap is required to neutralize the hardness before the soap is effective, and this takes place at the rate of about 2 ounces of soap to 100 gallons of water for

131

each part of calcium carbonate per gallon, or about 3 ounces of soap to 10,000 gallons for each part per million increase in hardness.

The village of Canisteo, New York, has a hard spring water, the hardness being recorded by the State Department of Health as 162.8 parts calcium carbonate in a million parts of water. Clifton Springs water has a hardness of 208. Catskill, New York, which gets its water from a stream running down from the hillside, has a hardness of 22.1 or 140.7 parts less than Canisteo. Mr. G. C. Whipple says ("Value of Pure Water") he has found that 1 pound of soap is needed to soften 167 gallons of water when that water has a hardness of 20 parts per million, and that each additional part requires 200 pounds of soap to soften a million gallons. If Clifton Springs and Catskill should each use 100,000 gallons per day, the [Pg 135] additional cost of the hard water, at five cents a pound for soap, would be 20 × 140.7 × 0.05 = \$140.70, provided all the village water were neutralized with soap. Probably not over one fiftieth part of the water is so neutralized, so that the added cost of soap is actually about \$2.80 a day. Whipple expresses this cost as $H/100 = D$, where H is the hardness in parts per million and $D$ is the cost in cents for every 1000 gallons used for all purposes. Thus Canisteo water costs $162.8/100 = 1.6$ cents per 1000 gallons used, while Catskill costs only $22.1/100$ or 0.2 cent on account of soap.

This discussion is intended to suggest a comparison between a well of hard water and a surface supply of soft water, when both are available. It should arouse an interest in securing a soft water as well as a clear water, and the advantages of the softer water, in so far as soap consumption alone is concerned, are seen to be not inconsiderable.

*Vegetable pollution.*

The vegetable and animal matter is organic in its origin and nature, and their effect on water may be taken up together.

Vegetable pollution is generally the result of decayed leaves, roots, bark, and such other vegetable tissue as would be likely to be found where the water-supply flows through a swamp or accumulates in hollows and depressions. This sort of water is likely to have a brownish or yellowish brown color, to have a slightly sweetish taste, and to [Pg 136] be soft, that is, free from mineral solids. Usually such water can be used for drinking purposes without serious consequences. Æsthetically, it is objectionable because of its color, and the city of Boston has expended many thousands dollars in building channels around swamps and in providing artificial outlets for swamps, so that the color of the water collected on the watershed shall not show the color induced thereby. Water from the Dismal Swamp of Virginia is so discolored as to look like coffee, and yet, in the vicinity, it is much prized for drinking, and formerly great pains were taken to fill casks with this water when in preparation for a long sea voyage.

Such matter always has a marked influence on a chemical analysis of the water, shows large amounts of nitrogenous matter, and apparently indicates a polluted supply; but, if the reason for this apparent pollution lies in the presence of a swamp, no danger to health therefrom is to be apprehended. Such water also is less subject to decay or putrefaction, and if a water-supply for a house is to be taken from a small pond, a gathering ground containing swamps is likely to furnish a more satisfactory water, color alone excepted, than one free from such swamps.

*Pollution of water by animals.*

Animal pollution usually comes from the presence on the watershed of domestic animals, that is, cows, sheep, and horses, or from manure spread on fields draining into the brook, or from barns or barnyards close by the water. It is the presence of this sort of pollution that furnishes the other kind of organic matter not to be distinguished by chemical analysis from the organic matter just referred to, but vastly more objectionable. [Pg 137]

Drainage from houses and barns is responsible for the same kind of animal pollution, and while it is difficult to prove by statistics that such pollution is always dangerous to health, it is sufficiently repulsive from an æsthetic standpoint to be done away with whenever possible. Such pollution applies only to surface water, such as brooks or lakes, and the best method of detecting and evaluating this pollution is to make a careful inspection of the watershed.

If it is proposed to use the water from a certain stream for drinking purposes, the first step should be to examine carefully the area draining into the stream, to detect, if possible, all opportunities for animal wastes to find their way directly into the stream and to note whether fields sloping rapidly to the streams are manured; to see whether the stream flows through pasture land in which cows are kept, and especially to note whether houses with their accompanying outbuildings are near enough the brook so that water may at any time wash impurities down into the stream. Whenever a brook flows through woodland free from all animal pollution and not subject to pollution before entering the wood, the water is probably as pure as that in any spring or well.

On the contrary, when the water in a brook flows through a meadow used for pasture or through gullies, the sides of which are manured, or in the vicinity of houses and barns, the water is probably unfit for drinking purposes. This can be realized by standing at the edge of a barnyard and watching the rain falling first on the roof of the barn, then in larger quantities from the eaves on to the manure pile into the yard below, then accumulating in [Pg 138] pools of reddish black concentrated liquid, until the volume is sufficient to form small rills which gradually assemble into a fair-sized stream. Similarly, the pig-pen drainage is washed out from under or even through the building, and, after combining with the barnyard drain, is carried into the stream near by. The very idea of drinking such filth is nauseating in the extreme. It is common for small slaughter-houses to be built on the side of a stream, so that the offal, carrion, and refuse of the place may be carried off without effort on the part of the owner, and there are a number of such places where brooks, used as places of deposit for slaughter-house refuse, discharge directly into the reservoirs of water works.

But this sort of animal refuse is not the most serious pollution. The leachings and washings from privies and cesspools, carrying, as they do, germs of contagious diseases, are most to be dreaded, and when a privy (with no vault underneath) is built on the side of a steep ravine and is so located that the natural drainage of the sidehill on which it is built cannot help but run around and through the building, then the pollution of the stream in the gulley is not only direct and inevitable, but of a deadly sort (see Fig. 36). Fortunately, the germs thus carried into the stream suffer the vicissitudes of all life exposed to the attacks of hostile forces.

At the time of freshets the streams carry mud in abundance, which mud is continually settling out of the water as opportunity offers, and with this settlement of mud there occurs also the settlement of the germs. Also the pathogenic or disease-producing germs are usually weaker and more susceptible than the putrefactive and other [Pg 139] organisms which are found in the water in great abundance after any rain storm, and which tend to inhibit or destroy the pathogenic germs. But some will survive, and, with favoring conditions, may pass through the water-pipe to the house, causing sickness, if not death.

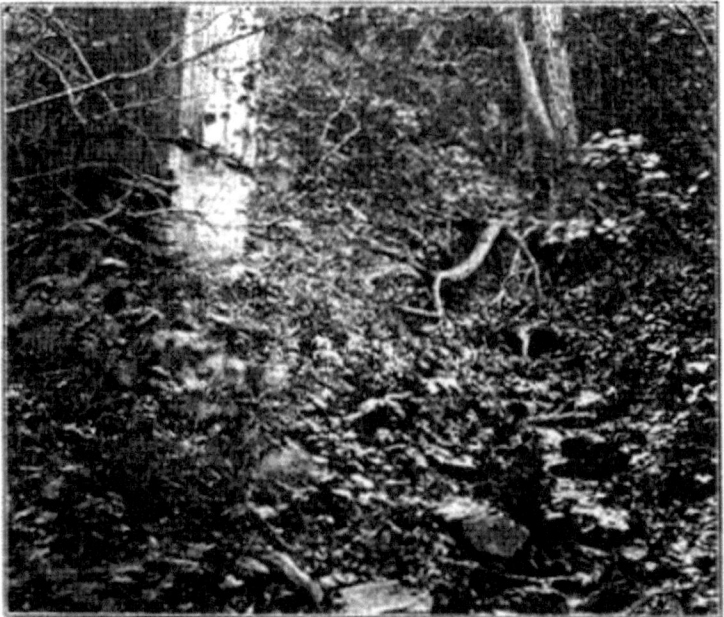

Fig. 36.—Stream draining a privy.

Any inspection of the watershed, therefore, should look to the elimination of the dangers above described, and to the location of barns and barnyards, pig-pens and poultry yards, privies and cesspools, so that no direct drainage into the stream shall be possible. [Pg 140]

It is out of the question for any surface water-supply to be pure, since the mere fact of the passage of water over the soil inevitably results in the collection of organic matter; and it is no exaggeration to say that the time will inevitably come in this country, as it has already in Germany, when no surface supply will be considered satisfactory unless the water is filtered. The only alternative is water gathered from areas that are owned by the individual and on which, therefore, all dwellings may be prohibited, all cultivated land avoided, and where the primeval forest may be restored, making the watershed equal to that from which forest streams emerge.

But usually, in the case of a single house, it will not be possible entirely to eliminate the dangers of surface pollution, although an inspection will show the dangers, and possibly some of them may be avoided. Certainly any direct drainage into the streams should be cut out, as well as the drainage from barnyards in the immediate vicinity of the point where the water is taken out. Just what percentage of pollution may be eliminated in this way it is impossible to determine, but it is not too much to say that no brook or pond should be used for a water-supply of a house unless *every known pollution* of an organic nature has been removed. Under the most favorable circumstances there will be enough accidental contamination to make the water at times dangerous, and no added risks ought to be assumed.

In looking over a watershed the possibility of sewage entering the stream is, of all pollutions, the most to be avoided. To adequately investigate the quality of a stream, the inspector must satisfy himself as to the point [Pg 141] of discharge of the sewer of every house on the watershed, and this must be done personally, without apparently reflecting on the statements of the owner of the house. If any such points of discharge are found, the sewage should be either diverted into some other watershed, or spread out over the ground away from the stream, or purified by some artificial treatment before discharge, or else the creek water cannot be used.

The next point to be noted in the source of the water-supply is the presence and location of privies. These nuisances should be as far back from the banks of the streams as possible to eliminate all danger since the surface of the ground always slopes toward some stream, and pollution may be carried for considerable distances over or through the soil. Water-tight boxes can be provided so that no possible pollution of the surface-wash can occur, and if periodically the contents of these boxes be hauled away and buried, the privy loses its dangerous character. The city of Syracuse has installed on the watershed of Skaneateles Lake a most admirable system of collection of privy wastes, and the lake water is thoroughly protected, although there are several hundred privies on the watershed.

Cesspools, in general, are not dangerous if they are located fifty feet or more from the stream and if no overflow occurs.

Barnyards ought not to drain directly into streams, but when, as in so many cases, the stream flows through the barnyard, the only remedy is to move either the stream or the barnyard, and it is difficult to persuade even a well-disposed neighbor to do either. It is sometimes [Pg 142] possible to appeal to his sense of right; but, too often, the neighbor feels that it is his land, his barn, his drain, even his brook, and he will do whatever he pleases with them, whether the water further down stream is to be used for drinking purposes or not. The question resolves itself into an inspection of the watershed and a determination of the existing conditions. If those are tolerable, the water may be used. If evident contamination is present, the water must usually be given up, and some other source of supply sought.

*Well water.*

The pollution of wells, if it exists at all, is usually very pronounced, and it is probably safe to say that, except where buildings, drains, or cesspools have been crowded too close to wells, or where some manifest and gross cause of pollution exists, a well water is safe to drink.

To protect properly a well from gross pollution, two precautions should be observed. The wall of the well should be built up in water-tight masonry, so that surface wash cannot enter the well except at a depth of at least six feet, and second, this water-tight masonry should be carried above the surface of the ground at least six inches and the well then covered with a water-tight floor so that no foreign matter can drop through the floor into the well or can be washed in by the waste water from the pump (see Figs. 28, 29, 30). If these precautions are taken, it is safe to say that nine tenths of the pollution occurring in isolated wells would be stopped.

Besides the above, a well may be polluted by a stream of underground water washing the contaminating matter through the soil. Experiments have been made to show [Pg 143] this very plainly. A large number of bacteria were placed six feet below the surface just in the top of the underground stream of water. Within a week they were found in considerable numbers in the water of the soil one hundred feet distant, but when the same number of bacteria were placed in the soil four feet below the surface above the level of the ground water, none of them found their way into the water of the soil. This experiment shows the folly of building a cesspool in the vicinity of a well when they both go down to the same water level, since the contents of the cesspool will be carried into the well if the underground stream flows in the proper direction. A shallow cesspool, however, would not be open to the same objection.

It is always difficult to detect the direction or flow of underground water, and various technical and delicate methods have been selected to make this determination. A very simple test, however, is to dig a hole at the point where pollution is suspected, carrying the hole down to where ground water is reached, and then to throw a gallon of kerosene oil into the hole, and if the ground-water flow is toward the well, the presence of kerosene in the well water will make the fact known. This would not, however, prove that the actual contamination would produce disease, since a liquid like kerosene can find its way through the pores of the soil to much greater distances than bacteria can be carried. But, to be on the safe side, water from such a well should not be used.

To make sure of the quality of the water proposed for a water-supply, it is wise to have such water examined by a chemist. The chemist will make certain determinations [Pg 144] of ammonia and other chemical combinations, and will report his findings with an interpretation or explanation of the result. What he finds is not the presence or absence of disease or disease germs, but substances that suggest or involve the presence of organic pollution. A test is made for the number of bacteria, and a well of spring water which contains more than about fifty in a cubic centimeter is a suspicious water. Surface water, on the other hand, may contain two or three hundred without being necessarily bad, the types of bacteria being harmless. Generally, a chemist will also determine the presence of the colon bacillus which is found in the intestinal tract of man or warm-blooded animals. Wherever this is found, in even such a small quantity as one cubic centimeter of water or less, there is strong presumption that the water has been polluted by human wastes and is therefore not fit to drink.

*Dangers of polluted water.*

Since no evidence of the danger of drinking polluted water can be so graphically expressed as by a direct reference to epidemics caused by the unwise use of such water, it will not be out of place to refer briefly to some of the instances in which a direct connection has been traced between a specific pollution of a certain water and disease or death resulting from it.

Although, as has already been explained, an infected water causes various kinds of intestinal disorders, particularly among children, the most characteristic evidence of pollution occurs when the noxious material comes directly from a typhoid fever patient, so that this same disease can be recognized as transmitted to another individual [Pg 145] or family. This transmission of typhoid fever, while in some cases very plainly due to other agencies than water, as, for example, milk, oysters, and flies, yet, by far the largest proportion of the transmitted cases comes through the agency of polluted drinking water, and there are many examples both of contaminated wells and streams which emphasize this possibility beyond all question.

Two historic investigations of epidemics which have thoroughly convinced sanitarians that typhoid fever is a communicable disease and that water is the vehicle for its transmission may be briefly cited.

In 1879 Dr. Thorne reported an epidemic in the town of Caterham, England, which he had investigated, and disclosed the following facts: The population of the village was 5800. The first case of fever appeared on January 19. Others followed in rapid succession, until the number reached 352, of whom in due time 21 died.

The possibility of infection was carefully looked into. The influence of sewer air was ruled out because there were no sewers. The milk supply was proved unobjectionable. No theory of personal or secondary infection could account for the widespread prevalence, particularly as only one isolated case had occurred during the preceding year, and this had been imported.

Of the first 47 persons attacked, 45 lived in houses supplied with the public water-supply, and the other two were during the day in houses supplied with public water. Further, in the Caterham Asylum, with nearly 2000 patients, not a single case appeared, their water coming from driven wells. Investigation of the water-supply [Pg 146] showed the undoubted cause of the epidemic. The public water-supply was derived from three deep wells, connected by tunnels in the chalk. In one of these tunnels, from January 5 to the end of the month, a laborer worked, who, though unattended by a physician, was evidently suffering from mild typhoid fever, the symptoms of the disease being carefully detailed by Dr. Thorne. The laborer at the time of his going to work had a severe diarrhœa, and while in the tunnel was obliged to make use of the bucket, in which the excavated chalk was hauled to the top. He admitted that at times the bucket, in being hauled up, would oscillate in such a way as to spill part of its contents and thereby pollute the water of the well below. Two weeks from this accidental pollution the epidemic began, and there can be little doubt of the relation of this mild case of typhoid to the epidemic which followed.

A second illustration may be cited at Butler, Pennsylvania, which occurred in 1903. The water-supply of Butler, a borough of 16,000 people, comes from a reservoir on the creek which flows through the phase. On account of the gross pollution of the water at the pumping-station, a long supply pipe has been laid from the reservoir directly to the pumps. The water also was filtered through a filter of the mechanical type. Through some accident the filter was thrown out of service for eleven days, between October 20 and 31, 1903, and unfortunately, on account of the failure of the reservoir dam, the water was at that time being taken directly from the creek at the pump well, and had been since August 27. Only ten days after the filter was shut down, the epidemic broke out in all parts of the [Pg 147] town. Between November 10 and December 19 there were 1270 cases and 56 deaths. In the subsequent investigation it developed that not only was the stream generally polluted by the sewage at various points above the intake, but that there had been several cases of typhoid fever on the watershed, some on a brook that enters the creek within one hundred feet of the filter plant. As at Caterham, the inference is patent that the introduction of some specific infection into the drinking water was the direct cause of the general epidemic.

The occasional outbreaks of typhoid fever which occur in single families are not so easy to explain, particularly since the small number of persons affected does not usually call for a widespread interest on the part of those experienced in such epidemics. In the Twenty-seventh Annual Report of the New York State Department of Health, the following description of an outbreak in a small hamlet, where the cause seems to have been the use of a pond for a wash tub by some Italian laborers, thereby transmitting the disease germs from their clothes to the water afterwards used in a creamery, is given. The diagram, Fig. 37, shows that the creamery secured its water for the purpose of washing cans from a small pond by means of a gravity pipe line. The foreman of the creamery, who boarded at the residence marked *A*, first contracted typhoid fever. A week later an employee at the creamery also contracted the fever, the residence of the latter being marked *B* on the diagram. About six weeks later the railroad station agent, living at the point marked *C*, contracted the fever, and two weeks later his wife was attacked with the same disease. The residences at [Pg 148] *B* and *C* are only about three hundred feet apart, both families taking their water-supplies from a spring between the two, but nearer *B*. During the summer previous to this outbreak a gang of Italian laborers, engaged in double-tracking the Central New England Railroad, were housed in box cars standing on one track of the railroad. One of the members of the gang was reported to have been taken ill with a fever and was at once removed, it was supposed, to a hospital in New York. It was the practice of the Italian laborers to bathe and wash their clothes in the upper of the two ponds from which water is supplied to the creamery by the pipe line. All the persons who contracted the fever were supplied with milk from the creamery. The foreman, who was the first to contract the fever, used water from the creamery and from the well at the house where he boarded. The other families, as already mentioned, used water from the spring. The conclusions, therefore, are that the creamery in some way became infected with typhoid fever, probably through the water-supply from the pond, and that the first two cases were due directly to this cause; that the station agent and his wife contracted the fever because of the infection of the spring, either from some small stream which is the outlet of the ponds or from some infection due to the illness of the owner of the house *B* near by. The report concludes as follows: "The use of water for creamery purposes from a pond exposed to such unwarranted and unchecked pollution as is shown here, or the permitted abuse of a water-supply for a creamery, appears little less than criminal negligence on the part of those responsible for the management of the creamery."

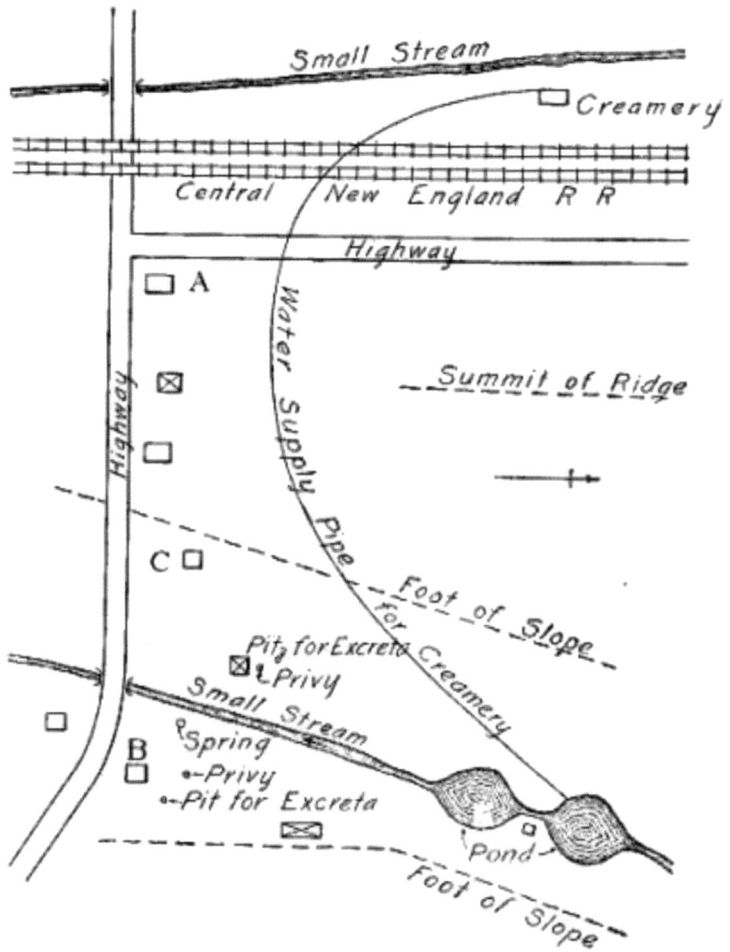

Fig. 37.—Contamination of a creamery from the water-supply.

[Pg 149]

Another report in this volume of the New York State Department of Health illustrates very well how a spring or well may be contaminated, and is taken from a report on an outbreak at Kerhonkson, Ulster County. The report reads as follows: "The village of Kerhonkson is built mainly on the side of a mountain of solid rock covered by a thin top soil of variable depth. Owing to its rocky nature, only one or two wells exist throughout the whole place; such a thing as a drilled well has never been seriously considered. [Pg 150]

"The inhabitants obtain their drinking water from a well on the property adjacent to and above the present school building, and known as the "Brown" well, and from a clear spring at the bottom of the hill in the rear of the village store and known all over the region as the Loundsbury spring.

"The school building is an old-fashioned two-story ramshackle affair with overhanging eaves, especially designed to obstruct light and darken the upper schoolroom. The building is in the center of a pine grove 250 × 150 feet in size, which also obstructs the light and tends to dampen the building. At the extreme ends of this school lot are two privies for the boys and girls, built on loose stone foundations, innocent of mortar or cement, which allows the water in heavy storms to wash out the fecal contents of from nearly a hundred pupils down upon the habitations below. Were the wells existing in the village as carelessly constructed as the Brown well and the various privy vaults which I have inspected, the loss of life from typhoid fever would be terrible indeed.

"Obtaining the names of all the patients who had suffered from this disease, I found that all but three were Kerhonkson public school pupils, and all had drunk the water of the before-mentioned well on the Brown property. [Pg 151] Two out of these three cases were mothers of pupils who had been stricken with the fever and who had nursed the children through their long and exhausting illnesses and afterward had been attacked by the disease themselves, while the third and remaining case was a puzzler. This boy had never been a pupil of the school in question, nor had he partaken of any of the water of the suspected well. He was a pupil of another school entirely and lived in an adjoining village a considerable distance away. A special visit to him, however, developed the fact that some time before his illness he had come to the village store in Kerhonkson to purchase goods and had drunk water from the Loundsbury spring.

"Two years ago two cases died of typhoid fever on the property on which the Brown well is situated. Their stools were treated with lime and buried on the hill behind the house. Three cases of the same fever have occurred in the same house this season. The well in question is laid up with stone and cement and was supposed to be tight and impervious to surface water contamination. Investigation, however, proved that there were openings in the stone work in the side toward the privy. On examining the privy it was found that the foundation was composed of loose stones without cement or mortar that would readily allow the fecal contents to be washed down toward the well, the privy being about three feet higher than the well, the natural descent of the land being about one foot in twenty-five, the distance between privy and well being only about eighty feet. Another factor favoring the well contamination from this privy is that any filth washed downward from the privy toward the well would be stopped by the wall [Pg 152] of the house proper and carried directly toward the well which lies close to the southeast corner of the house. Thus all of the conditions point to privy contamination of this well which should be at once cemented up on the inside, thoroughly cleansed and purified, before its use should be permitted, while all the privies in question should be provided with vaults of brick eight inches thick with eight-inch brick floors all laid with cement, and their inside surfaces lined with cement at least one inch thick, to prevent any further possible contamination."

In view of the imminent danger always possible wherever human wastes are directly discharged into streams, whether from privies or sewers, it is obvious that water so contaminated should never on any account be used as drinking water. It does not follow, because a stream so contaminated has been used for months or years without producing any evidence of disease, that the water is safe. Unless an excessive amount of organic matter is so transmitted, no evidence will be found that such pollution has existed through any outbreak of disease. But if once the discharges become affected through a person having typhoid fever, then the result of the infection is apparent immediately. If, therefore, an inspection of the stream above the point where it is proposed to take the water-supply shows the existence of privies, as shown by Fig. 36, the water should not be used for domestic supply, although a number of individuals may have been using the water for years without bad effects. It is a case in which prevention is much wiser than cure, and while economy and convenience may indicate such a polluted stream to be a desirable source of supply, a proper regard for health conditions will rule it out absolutely.

[Pg 153]

## CHAPTER VIII

# *WATER-WORKS CONSTRUCTION*

Construction methods and practices which lend themselves to the development of the water-supply for an individual house may be divided into three parts, namely:—

(1) Construction at the point of collection, whether this point be a well, spring, brook, or reservoir;

(2) The pipe line leading from the collection point to the buildings;

(3) Constructions involved in the house, other than the plumbing fixtures.

Taking up these different points in order, we may note at the outset that it is possible to employ either very simple or very complicated construction.

*Methods of collection of water.*

The common method is to lay a galvanized iron pipe in a ditch as far as a spring and there to protect the end of the pipe with a sieve or a grating and to leave it exposed in the water with no efforts expended on the spring itself. In a brook with waterfalls or with good slope, it is not uncommon to project a large pipe or a wooden trough into the stream at the top of a waterfall and so carry a certain amount of the water into a tub or basins from which the [Pg 154] small pipe leads to the house. On the shores of a lake or pond the galvanized iron pipe is laid out on the bottom of the lake with the end protected by a strainer.

In all these cases the simplest method is the best, provided the supply of water is not needed in the winter; but such simple methods as just described fail when frost locks up the surface flow of the stream. Then the pipe throughout its entire length must be in a trench below the frost line at the entrance to the spring as elsewhere. To permit this, the spring must also be deep, or else so inclosed that the pipe leading into the spring can be covered by earth banked up against it. Not long ago the writer saw a pipe taking water from a small lake recently improved by a stone wall. Instead of conveying the water-pipe down under the wall the unwise stone mason had built the wall around the pipe and the pipe line was frozen up through the entire winter following.

Such simple methods also fail when the supply of water is not adequate, since, in order to secure a large quantity from a stream whose flow is periodic and irregular, some storage must be provided, and storage usually requires more or less elaborate construction work at the reservoir. Another reason for more elaborate construction at a spring is to prevent surface contamination, and it is always desirable to roof over a spring in order to protect it from surface flows. The writer has seen, as an example of objectionable construction, a spring in the bottom of a ravine or gully down which, in time of rain, torrents of water passed, although in a dry season the spring was the only sign of water in the vicinity. It could not but happen that this torrent of water, which carried all kinds of pollution from [Pg 155] the road above, practically washed through the spring, destroying its good quality. In such a case, another channel for the gulley water ought to have been made, or else the spring dug out and roofed over, so that the torrential water could pass above it.

In other cases, the spring is found at the lowest point in a general depression, so that, while no stream passes through the spring, the spring is a catch-all for the surface drainage in the vicinity. In such cases the water should be protected by a bank of earth around the spring, behind which the drainage should be led off through a special pipe line if necessary.

*Spring reservoirs.*

In protecting the spring and in building up around it in order to put it underground, concrete is the most suitable material, although a large sewer pipe or a heavy cask or barrel will answer the purpose. It is usually sufficient to dig out the spring to a depth of four or five feet, and with a pump it is possible to keep the water down, so that the concrete walls may be laid. In building these walls, it is important to notice from which side the spring water comes, and on that side holes should be left in the wall. These openings may properly be connected with agricultural tile drains laid out from the spring in different directions, serving both to drain the ground and to add volume to the spring. It is often possible instead of pumping out water during construction to drain a spring temporarily, in places where the ground slopes rapidly, by carrying out a drainpipe from the lowest level; this drain is to be later stopped up.

The size of this spring reservoir depends on the average [Pg 156] rate of flow of the spring and on the quantity of water used. If there is always an overflow from the spring, that is, if it always at all times of the year furnishes more water than is required by the house at that time of day when the greatest demand is made, then a two-foot sewer pipe is just as good as a concrete chamber ten feet square. But if at times the spring is low, so that the flow during the night must be saved to compensate for the excess consumption during the day, or if the rate at which the water is drawn at certain hours is greater than the average rate at which the spring flows, then storage must be allowed for in preparing the spring to act as a reservoir.

We have already estimated that a family of ten persons might use five hundred gallons of water a day, and the most exacting conditions would never require the spring to hold more than one day's supply. This would mean a chamber four feet deep and in area four by five feet. If the average supply of the spring is less than the average consumption of the family, then the spring must become a storage basin for the purpose of carrying water enough over the dry season, and the capacity of the basin must be computed from the number of days' storage required. It may not be out of place to suggest again the possibility of increasing the yield of the spring by laying draintile in a ditch running along the permeable stratum. These pipes may run fifty or one hundred feet each way from the main spring, so long as they continue to find ground water.

The walls of such a spring reservoir as here suggested for depths of six to eight feet need not be more than nine inches thick, whether built of brick or concrete. For [Pg 157] greater depths the thickness should be increased to twelve inches.

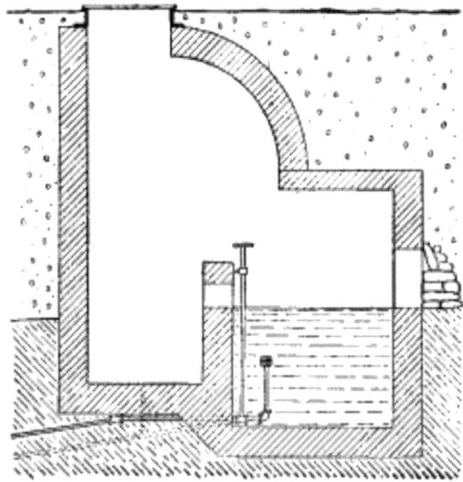

Fig. 38. — A protected spring-chamber.

The roof of the spring-chamber may be of plank, but this is temporary and undesirable. It is far better, for all spans up to ten feet, to make the roof a flat slab of concrete six inches thick, imbedding in the concrete in the bottom of the mass some one-half-inch iron rods, spaced about a foot apart each way and extending well into the side walls. The size of these rods should increase with the size of the chamber, making them three-quarter-inch rods up to a nine-foot span, and one-inch rods up to a twelve-foot span. There should be some way of getting into the spring, preferably by an opening in one corner so arranged as to carry the side walls of the opening or manhole up above the ground, where it may be protected with an iron cover locked fast (see Fig. 38, after Imbeaux). Besides the outlet pipe from the spring, which will naturally pass through the side walls about halfway between top and bottom in order to get the best water, there should be a drainpipe from the lowest part of the inclosure, the valve of which can be reached through a valve box coming to the surface. In the figure [Pg 158] the drainpipe is shown by the dotted line, and the twofold chamber is for the purpose of allowing an examination of the spring to be made at any time.

The concrete used in this work should be of good quality, one part of cement to five parts of gravel or to four parts of stone and two parts of sand. A concrete bottom, although sometimes used, is not necessary. The position of the drain, of the house pipe, and of the several collection pipes must not be overlooked when the wall is being built, since it is much easier to leave a hole than to dig through the concrete afterwards.

*Stream supplies.*

If the volume of a stream is more than enough for the maximum consumption, nothing is needed but to carry the intake pipe from the shore out under water and protect the end with a strainer. In this case, however, the stream may freeze down to the level of the strainer and even around the strainer, so that the supply of water in winter would be cut off. To avoid this possibility the intake pipe ought to be in a pool of water so deep that it never freezes, and this means sometimes creating a pool for this very purpose. If storage is to be provided, a reservoir must be built, and this intake pipe would naturally be placed at least two feet below the surface of the water.

*Dams.*

If the stream is not deep, or if there is not a pool of satisfactory depth, or if the minimum flow of the stream is not adequate for the maximum needs of the consumers, a dam across the stream becomes a necessity. There are two or three types of dams suitable for a reservoir on a small stream, and they may be described briefly. [Pg 159]

A dirt dam is not generally desirable, since in most cases the dam must also be used as a waste weir; that is, the freshets must run over the dam. This means that unless the crest of the dam is protected with timber or masonry the dam will be washed out; as happened, indeed, in the terrible flood at Johnstown, Pennsylvania, several years ago. If it is possible to carry the overflow water of the stream away in some other channel than over the dam, then a dirt dam is not objectionable, although always a dirt dam is best with a masonry core. A very good dam can be made by driving three-inch tongue-and-grooved planking tight together across a gulley and then filling in on each side so that the slope on each face is at least two feet horizontal for every foot in height. This last requirement means that if the dam is ten feet high, the width of the dam at the base shall be at least forty-five feet, the other five feet being required to give the proper thickness to the dam at the top.

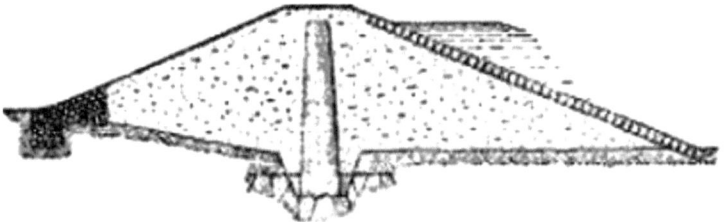

Fig. 39.—Concrete core in a dam.

In the second type of dam this central timber core is replaced with a thin wall of concrete as shown in Fig. 39, from six to twelve inches thick, sufficing to prevent small animals burrowing through the dam and at the same time to make the dam more nearly water-tight. Sometimes stone masonry is used, building a light wall to serve as the true dam, and then holding up this light wall with earth-filling on each side. If neither plank, [Pg 160] stone, nor concrete can be used, the central core is made of the best earth available, a mixture of clay and sand preferably, and special pains are taken in the building to have this mixture well rammed and compacted.

The writer has recently heard of a dam on a small stream being made by the continual dumping of field stone from the farm into the brook at a certain definite place. This stone, of course, assumed a slope at each side and settled in place from year to year as the dam grew. The mud and silt of the stream filled up the holes between the stones, so that the dam was finally practically water-tight. This made a cheap construction and had the additional value of serving to use up stones from the fields. It was necessary, since the spring floods poured over the top of this dam, to protect the top stones, and a plank crest was put on, merely to keep the dam from being washed away.

The third type of dam is entirely of concrete or stone masonry, concrete to-day being preferable because more likely to be water-tight. The problem with a concrete dam is to get a foundation such that the impounded water will not leak out under the dam, imperiling the very existence of it. The ideal foundation, of course, is rock,

151

and in a great many locations can be found in the small gulleys where the limestone and shale peculiar to this region will answer as well as more solid rock for dams not more than ten feet high; but with gravel banks on the sides or with soft sandy bottom, or where the clay soil becomes saturated with water at times, the gulley offers great difficulties for the construction of a dam. It will be wise, under such conditions, to carry a cut-off wall, not necessarily more than twelve inches thick, well into the bank, that is, about ten [Pg 161] feet on each side, and under the dam this cut-off wall ought to go down until it reaches another stratum of sand or clay or rock. This cut-off wall, then, surrounding the main dam, shuts off the leakage, and the dam itself can be built without danger of undermining. In many large dams this cut-off wall is carried down more than a hundred feet, especially where the depth of water behind the dam is great. For small dams, a row of plank driven down behind a timber sill across and in the bed of the stream will often be sufficient.

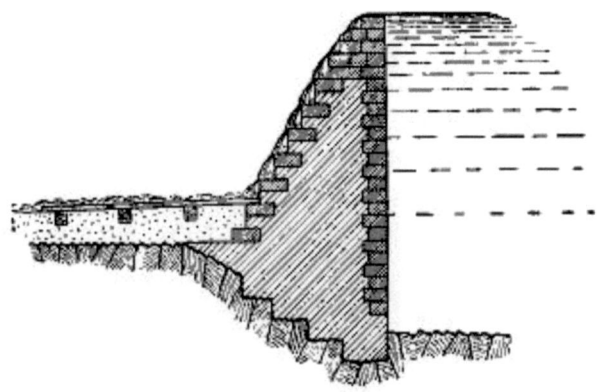

Fig. 40. —

Section of a flood dam.

The cross section of the main dam, in cases where flood water in the spring runs over the dam, should be such that the bottom thickness is about one half the height, and Fig. 40 (after Wegman) shows a suitable cross-section of a dam ten feet high. Figure 41 (after Wegman) shows a cross-section intended to carry the water over the dam, especially in times of flood, without danger of erosion.

Sometimes, in a narrow gorge with rock sides, it is possible to save masonry by building the dam in the form [Pg 162] of an arch upstream, the resistance to the force of the water being then furnished by the abutment action of the rock sides, instead of by the weight of the dam, as in ordinary construction. For a dam ten feet high, the necessary thickness of the curved dam would probably not be more than twelve inches, while the ordinary gravity dam would be three or four feet thick. The workmanship on the former, however, must be of a very superior order.

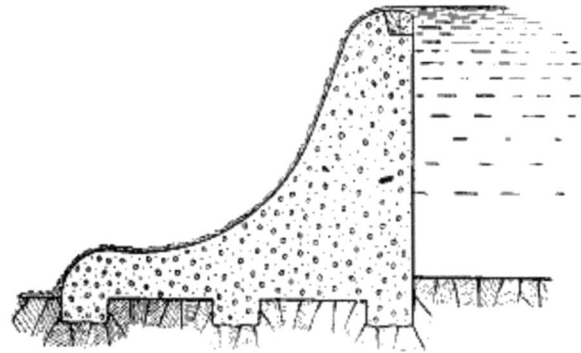

Fig. 41. —

Section of a flood dam.

It is never desirable to allow the water flowing over the dam to fall directly on the ground in front, since the falling water will rapidly carry away this soil and undermine the front of the dam. For this reason, the lower section of the dam is made curved, as shown in Fig. 41, giving the water a horizontal direction as it leaves the dam instead of a vertical. A plank floor is often added to carry even further from the dam any possible erosion (Fig. 40). Where it can be done, it is a good plan to provide a small body of still water below the dam, so that the force of the falling water may be distributed through the water on to the soil below. [Pg 163]

There are other forms of dams often used. For example, brush dams, formerly common, are made by cutting off the tops of trees and dropping them in place and loading them with stones so as to make a mass of interwoven branches. These branches hold together particles of earth which are dumped in and form a dam.

Another dam that has been much used in rural communities is the old-fashioned crib dam, where logs are piled up crib fashion, held together at the corners by iron pins, a bottom spiked on, and the crib then filled with stone, a succession of these cribs across the stream forming the dam. Dirt is filled in on each side of this crib work, and, in some cases, cross timbers are set in, and both sides of the dam covered with tongue-and-grooved planking. But such dams are not permanent, and their construction involves an expense nearly equal to that of a permanent structure, and consequently they are not to be recommended.

*Waste weirs.*

When the dam is made of earth with or without a core wall and when no opportunity exists for carrying the waste water around the dam, a waste weir of masonry through the dam must be provided, so that freshets may be carried off without destroying or washing out the earth work.

The size of this weir is a matter of considerable concern, since its ability to carry off the high water is fundamental. The capacity of such waste weirs depends on the volume of flood-water, and this, in turn, depends on the area of the watershed. This volume cannot be predicted with any absolute certainty, but, in general, it may be said that [Pg 164] the maximum run-off in the eastern part of the United States, from small areas not exceeding twenty-five square miles, will be about one hundred cubic feet per second per square mile, so that the freshet flow for a watershed of twelve square miles would be twelve hundred cubic feet per second. Ordinarily, the height of the weir is taken to be from two to four feet and the length made sufficient to care for the volume of discharge.

If the depth of water flowing over the weir is taken at one foot, the length of weir in feet necessary to carry the flood flow may be computed by multiplying the number of square miles of watershed by thirty. Then an area of twelve square miles would need a length of waste channel of three hundred sixty feet; in most cases, for small dams, longer than the dam itself.

If the depth be taken at two feet, then the number of square miles of watershed must be multiplied by ten to get the length of weir, so that a shed of twelve square miles would mean a weir one hundred twenty feet long.

The factor for a depth of three feet on the weir is six, making for the same area the length of weir seventy-two feet, and for four feet depth the factor is four. There is no more important part of the construction of a dam than that involved by a proper design of a waste weir, since a failure either to provide proper area or to so build as to withstand the erosive action of the running water will inevitably wash away the dam.

When the valley is narrow and the watershed large, the waste weir will occupy the entire width of the dam, and then it becomes necessary to construct the dam in masonry. On the other hand, when the watershed is small and the [Pg 165] width of the valley great, then it is proper to make the waste weir only a certain portion of the entire width of the dam, making the rest of the dam either masonry or earth, as may be convenient.

*Gate house.*

In connection with a reservoir and at the back of the dam at the bottom of the bank, it is convenient to have what is called, in larger installations, a "gate house"; that is, a masonry or wooden manhole through which the water-pipe leading out from the reservoir passes and in which a gate is placed to shut off the water. In larger installations, it is usually possible to admit water at this point from different levels of the reservoir into the water-pipe, so as always to get the best quality of water, but for a small plant that is not necessary. A gate or valve, however, should always be provided, and while this may be on the bank of the pond with the intake pipe extending twenty or thirty feet into the pond, the valve should not be omitted. The end of the pipe extending into the pond should be placed about two feet above the bottom of the pond, instead of resting in the mud, in order to get a better quality of water.

*Pipe lines.*

In bringing the water from the spring or pond to the house, some kind of a pipe line must be provided. Such a pipe line is made of various materials; hollow wooden logs, vitrified tile, cast-iron pipe, wrought-iron pipe, and lead pipe having all been used. The last-named pipe is now too expensive for use in any great lengths. Hollow wooden pipes are employed occasionally, but, except in unusual localities, they also are more expensive than other [Pg 166] forms, and are short lived on account of their tendency to decay. Cast-iron pipe, commonly used for municipal water-supplies, is not made in small sizes and may be excluded from the possibilities for an individual house. There remains only tile and wrought-iron pipe. Under certain conditions, the use of tile pipe is to be recommended, since it may be installed even in large sizes at a comparatively low cost, the objection to it being that it is very difficult to make the joints water-tight, and practically impossible when the pressure is greater than ten feet. It is more difficult to make joints in a pipe line of small diameter water-tight than in a pipe line of larger diameter, because the space for the cement in the former is so small. The writer has tried both four-inch and six-inch pipe, and while the four-inch line can be laid with tight joints, it requires much more careful and conscientious effort on the part of the workman than with six-inch pipe. The joints must be thoroughly filled with cement, not very wet, so that it can be rammed or packed with a thin stick into every part of the joint. Merely plastering the cement over the surface of the joint will always result in a leaking joint.

It often happens that a water-supply coming from a distance of a mile or so runs at first nearly level, so that, except for surface pollution, the water might be carried in an open ditch. An open ditch is, however, far better replaced by vitrified tile, six inches in diameter, which entirely prevents surface pollution, and which costs only about ten cents a running foot. When the slope of the ground exceeds the natural fall of the water, so that a pressure inside the pipe is created, iron pipe must be used. If vitrified [Pg 167] pipe is used, the joints must be made with the greatest care, and every precaution taken to prevent leakage. Figure 42 shows a section of a joint in tile pipe.

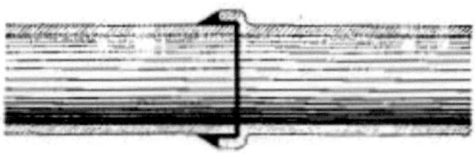

Fig. 42. — A joint in tile pipe.

In using iron pipe large enough to furnish the amount of water required, due regard must be paid to friction in the pipe. In flowing through a pipe of small size, water loses a great deal of head by friction. This friction between the sides of the pipe and the water, which must be duly considered in a pipe of small size, increases very rapidly as the velocity of the flow increases. It is always a great temptation to use a small pipe, since the cost of the pipe increases rapidly as the diameter increases, but it is penny wise and pound foolish to lay a line of pipe several thousand feet long to furnish water to a house and find when completed that the amount of water furnished by the pipe is on account of friction only a small dribble. In a previous chapter we estimated that the flow of water, in order to furnish three faucets at a reasonable rate, ought to be at least two thousand gallons a day or about one and a half gallons a minute, and the effect of a reduced size of pipe on the head necessary to carry a definite amount of water was shown.

The cost of cast-iron pipe should not be more than thirty cents per running foot for four-inch pipe and fifty cents per running foot for six-inch pipe. To this must be added the cost of about seven pounds or ten pounds respectively of lead for each joint and the cost of all the labor [Pg 168] involved. The price of terra-cotta pipe is much less, as already indicated, so that it is quite worth while to expend some additional effort on making the tile pipe joints water-tight, if it allows the cheaper pipe to be substituted for the more expensive iron pipe.

*Pumping.*

Although the present methods of securing water for isolated farm buildings will not corroborate the statement it is safe to say that the proper method of obtaining a water-supply is always to make use of a pond or stream at such an elevation that water will flow to the house by gravity, provided this is possible. Only when the conditions are such that a gravity supply is impossible and water from a well or stream at some lower elevation becomes inevitable is pumping properly resorted to.

The advantage of a gravity supply is twofold. First, the daily charges for maintenance are practically nothing, so that when once the intake and the pipe line have been installed, there will be no additional charges. When pumping is resorted to, on the other hand, there must be a daily expenditure which, even if small, in the course of a year amounts to the interest on a large sum of money. For example, suppose that the cost for supplies for a small pumping engine was only ten cents per day, not counting in the cost of labor. This would amount to $36.50 a year, which at 5 per cent is the interest on $730. It would be $200 cheaper, therefore, to borrow $500, at 5 per cent, to pay for a gravity supply rather than to pay $30 for a pump which costs ten cents a day to run. This same reasoning may be applied to the cost of different kinds of pumps. One pump may cost $200 more than [Pg 169] another, but the saving in fuel and repairs may be sufficient to more than justify this additional cost.

Second, a gravity supply is to be preferred because of its greater reliability. It is hardly possible to imagine any excuse for a gravity supply failing to deliver its predetermined quantity of water regularly day after day. A pumping plant, on the other hand, both breaks down and wears out. Valves are continually requiring to be repacked, nuts drop off and have to be replaced, pieces of the machinery break and require repairs, so that with the best machinery it is almost inevitable that for many days in the year the water-supply is interrupted by some failure of the machinery. In planning water works for cities, an engineer weighs and estimates the value of a continuous service, and even if the gravity supply costs somewhat more than the pumping system, it is in many cases adopted because the greater cost is supposed to be compensated for by the greater reliability of the supply.

*Windmills.*

Perhaps the cheapest source of power for pumping water is a windmill, and in many cases it proves entirely serviceable. It has two drawbacks which are self-evident. Unless the wind blows, the mill will not work, and, unfortunately, at those times of the year when a large supply of water is most to be desired, that is, during the hot summer months, the wind is particularly light. It is necessary, therefore, when using wind as a source of power, to provide large storage which will tide over the intervals between the times of pumping. Again, the wind may blow frequently enough, but may be so light as not to turn the large vanes necessary to pump rapidly and easily the [Pg 170] large amount of water needed. Nothing less than a twelve-foot mill ought to be erected, and, to be efficient, the wind must blow at the rate of twelve to sixteen miles an hour.

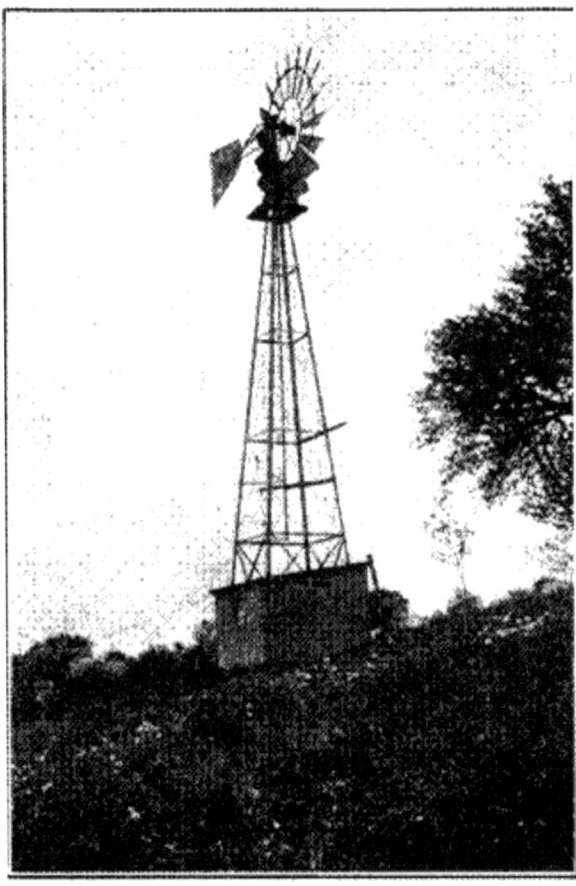

Fig. 43. —
Windmill and water tank.

A windmill of the best design is made entirely of steel with small angle irons for posts for the tower, and with [Pg 171] the mill itself made of galvanized iron. It requires a good foundation and must be well anchored to the masonry piers by strong bolts set well down into the masonry. If the mill is set directly over the well and the storage tank supported on the tower, a very compact arrangement is accomplished and the danger from frost is the only difficulty to be apprehended. However, the tank is often placed in the attic, some distance from the well, to which it is connected by suitable piping.

The location of the windmill requires careful consideration in order that it may receive the prevailing winds in their full force and at the same time be properly located with reference to the well. It must be remembered that the surface of the wheel is exposed to the full fury of a storm, and both the wheel and the tower must be strong enough to withstand such storms. Figure 43 shows windmill and water tank in the vicinity of Ithaca, New York.

*Hydraulic rams.*

A hydraulic ram is the cheapest method of pumping water, provided that the necessary flow with a sufficient head to do the work is available. It requires about seven times as much water to flow through the ram and be wasted as is pumped, so that if it is desired to pump five hundred gallons a day, the stream must flow at the rate of about thirty-five hundred gallons per day to lift the necessary water.

The two disadvantages of a ram are, first, that a fall of water is not always obtainable or that the stream flow is not always sufficient, and second, that the action of the ram is subject to interruptions on account of the accumulation of air in summer and on account of the formation [Pg 172] of ice in winter. In fact, in winter it is necessary to keep a small fire going in the house where the ram is at work in order that this interruption may not take place. Its great advantage is that it requires no attendance, no expense for maintenance, and practically nothing for repairs. It operates continuously when once started, and, except for the occasional interruption on account of air-lock, is always on duty.

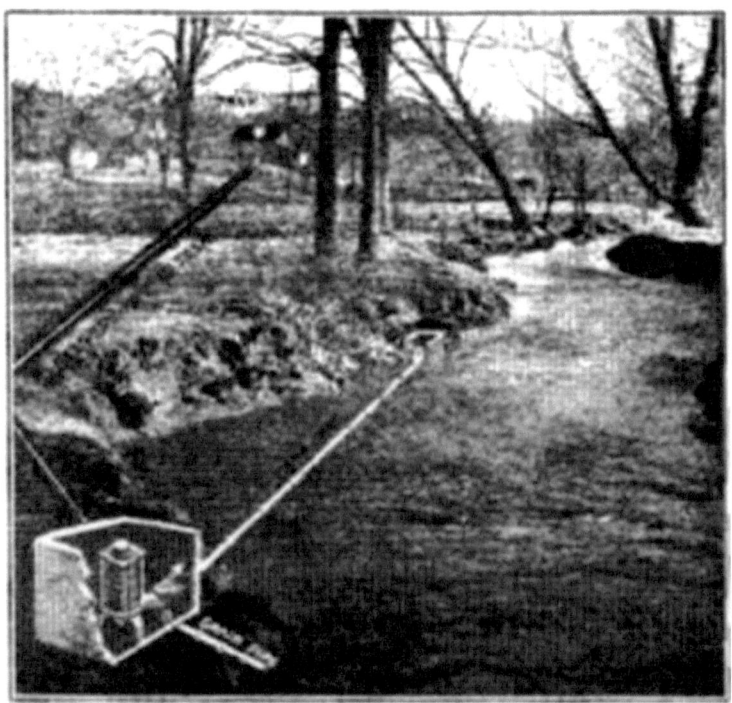
Fig. 44. — Installation of ram.

Usually the water is led from above the dam or waterfall [Pg 173] in a pipe to the ram and flows away after passing through the ram, back into the stream. The water pumped is generally taken from the same stream and is a part of the water used to operate the ram. This is not necessary, however, and double-acting rams are manufactured which will pump a supply of water from a source entirely different from that which operates the ram. The following table from the Rife Hydraulic Engine Manufacturing Co. gives the dimensions and approximate costs of rams suitable for pumping against a head not greater than about thirty feet for each foot of fall available in the drive pipe: —

## TABLE XI

| mensions | |
|---|---|

| Height | Length | Width | Size of Drive-pipe | Size of Delivery-pipe | Gallons per Minute required to operate Engine | Least Feet of Fall Recommended | Weight | Price Single-action |
|---|---|---|---|---|---|---|---|---|
| ' 1" | 3' 2" | 1' 8" | 1-1/4" | 3/4" | 2-1/2 to 6 | 3 | 150 | $ 50 |
| ' 1" | 3' 4" | 1' 8" | 1-1/2" | 3/4" | 6 to 12 | 3 | 175 | 55 |
| ' 3" | 3' 8" | 1' 9" | 2" | 1" | 8 to 18 | 2 | 225 | 60 |
| ' 3" | 3' 9" | 1' 9" | 2-1/2" | 1" | 11 to 24 | 2 | 250 | 66 |
| ' 7" | 3' 10" | 1' 10" | 3" | 1-1/4" | 15 to 35 | 2 | 275 | 75 |
| ' 3" | 4' 4" | 2' 0" | 4" | 2" | 30 to 75 | 2 | 600 | 150 |
| ' 4" | 8' 4" | 2' 8" | 8" | 4" | 150 to 350 | 2 | 2200 | 525 |
| ' 9" | 8' 4" | 2' 8" | 12" | 5" | 375 to 700 | 2 | 3000 | 750 |
| ' 9" | 8' 4" | 2' 8" | 2-12" | 6" | 750 to 1400 | 2 | 6000 | 150 |

If the length of the discharge pipe is more than a hundred feet, the effect of friction is to reduce the amount of water pumped, but rams will operate successfully against a head of three or four hundred feet. The writer remembers an installation in the northern part of New York State, where two large hydraulic rams furnish the water-supply supply for an entire village, pumping every day several hundred thousand gallons. Figure 44 shows an installation by the Power Specialty Co. of New York, using the fall of some rapids in a brook to pump water into a tank in the attic of a house. [Pg 174]

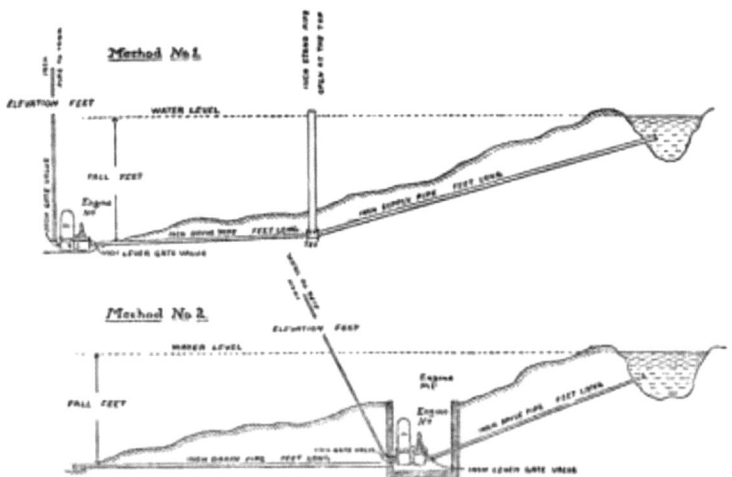

Fig. 45. — Means of securing fall for hydraulic ram.

[Pg 175]

In Fig. 45 are shown two methods of securing a fall for hydraulic rams, recommended by the Niagara Hydraulic Engine Co. The first method shows no drain pipe, but a long drive pipe; while the second method puts the ram in an intermediate position, with considerable lengths of each.

There are other methods of utilizing the fall of a stream, but usually they involve a greater outlay for the construction of a dam and other appurtenances. An old-fashioned bucket water wheel may be used, which, though not efficient, utilizes the power of the stream. The wheel may be belted or geared to a pump directly or may drive a dynamo, the power of which may in turn be transmitted to the pump. The objection to such construction usually is that during the summer the small streams which could be made of service at slight expense run dry or nearly so, while the expense of damming and utilizing a large stream where the water-supply is always sufficient is too great for a single house.

*Hot-air engines.*

The simplest kind of a pump worked mechanically is the Rider-Ericsson hot-air engine (see Fig. 46), which is made to go by the expansive force of hot air. The fuel used may be wood, coal, kerosene oil, gasolene, or gas, the [Pg 176] amount used being very moderate and the daily expense of maintenance very small.

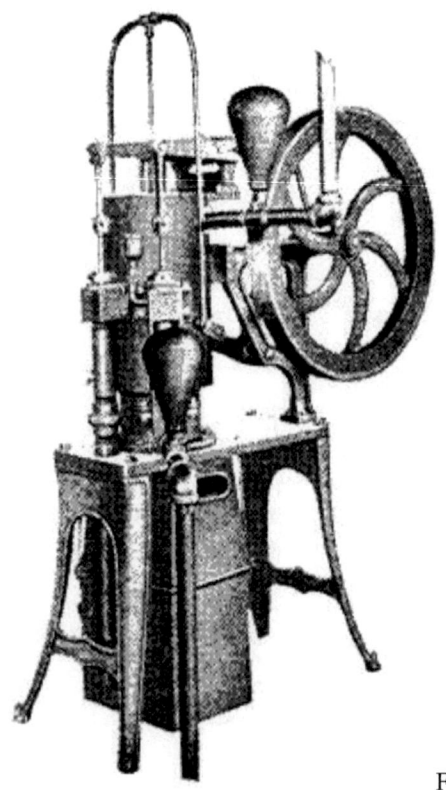

Fig. 46. — A hot-air engine.

For a number of years the writer used one of these machines to pump water from a tank in his cellar to a tank in the attic, so that running water could be had throughout the house. With an engine and pump costing $100, it was necessary to pump twice a week for about an hour to supply the attic tank and to furnish the necessary water for the family. The following table shows the dimensions, the capacity, and the fuel consumption of the different styles of pumps made by this company: —

**TABLE XII**

| Size of Cylinder | Suction and Discharge Pipe | Capacity Per Hour | Cu. Ft. of Gas | Kerosene Per Hour | Anthracite Coal Per Hour | Price |
|---|---|---|---|---|---|---|
| 5" | 3/4" | 150 gal. | 12 | 1 qt. | 4 lb. | $ 90 |
| 6" | 1" | 300 gal. | 16 | 2 qt. | 4 lb. | 130 |
| 8" | 1-1/4" | 500 gal. | 20 | 2 qt. | 5 lb. | 160 |
| 10" | 1-1/2" | 1000 gal. | 50 | 3 qt. | 6 lb. | 240 |

[Pg 177]

*Gas engines for pumping.*

During the last few years, on account of the great demand for gas engines for power boats and automobiles, the efficiency and reliability of these engines depending upon the explosive power of the mixture of gas and air has greatly increased. To-day, probably no better device for furnishing a satisfactory source of power in small quantities at a reasonable cost can be found. One engine might readily be used in several capacities, pumping water during the day or at intervals during the day when not needed for running feed cutters; and possibly running a dynamo for electric lights at night. It would be easy to arrange the gas engine so that a shift of a belt would transfer the power of the engine from a dynamo to a pump or to other machinery. In this case the pump is entirely distinct and separate from the engine, and while the gas engine may be directly connected with the pump and bolted to the same bed plate, if the engine is to be used for other purposes than pumping, an intermediate and changeable belt is desirable.

The term "gas engine" is properly restricted to engines literally consuming gas, either illuminating gas or natural gas; but the term is also applied to engines using gasolene as a fuel. The same principle is used in the construction of oil engines where kerosene oil is the fuel instead of gasolene, and it is probable that the latter engines are safer; that is, less subject to dangerous explosion than the former. Whichever fuel is used, the engine may be had in sizes ranging from one half to twenty horsepower and are very satisfactory to use. Any ordinary, intelligent laborer with a little instruction can start and operate them, [Pg 178] and except for occasional interruptions they may be depended upon to work regularly. The cost of operation with different fuels may be estimated from the following table, which also shows the cost when coal is used as in an ordinary steam plant, the data being furnished by the Otto Gas Engine Works: —

**TABLE XIII**

| Fuel | Price of Fuel | Fuel Consumption Per Brake H.-P. 10 Hours | Cost of Fuel Per Brake H.-P. 10 Hours |
|---|---|---|---|
| Gasolene | 10c per gal. | 1.25 gal. | 12.5c |
| Illuminating gas | $1.00 per 1000 cu. ft. | 180 cu. ft. | 18c |
| Natural gas | 25c per 1000 cu. ft. | 130 to 160 cu. ft. | 3.25 to 4c |
| Producer gas, anthracite pea coal | $4.00 per ton | 15 lb. | 2.67c |
| Producer gas, charcoal | $10.00 per ton | 12 lb. | 5.35c |
| Bituminous coal, ordinary steam engine | $3.00 per ton | 80 to 100 lb. | 10.7 to 13.4c |

A photograph of a small (2 H.P.) gas engine made by the Foos Gas Engine Co. with pump complete is shown in Fig. 47. This pump will lift forty gallons of water per minute, with a suction lift up to twenty-five feet, to a height of about seventy-five feet above the pump. The pump gear can be thrown out of connection with the [Pg

179] engine, so that the latter can be used for other purposes where power is desired.

*Steam pumps.*

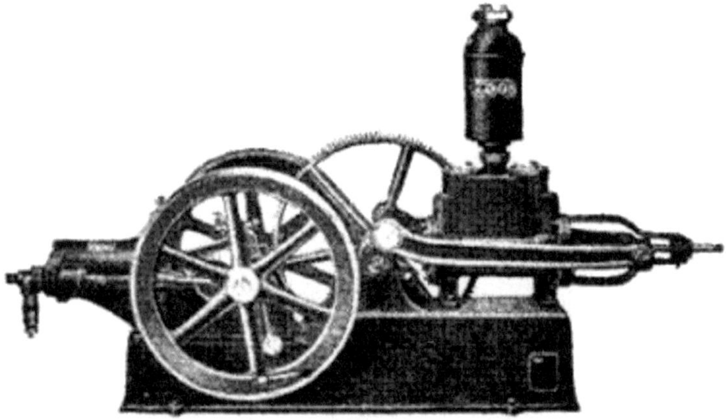

Fig. 47. — A gas engine.

The use of a steam pump would probably not be considered for a single house unless a small boiler was already installed for other purposes. Not infrequently a boiler is found in connection with a dairy for the purpose of furnishing steam and hot water for washing and sterilizing bottles and cans. Where silage is stored in quantity, a steam boiler and engine are often employed for the heavy work of cutting up fodder. In both these cases it may be a simple matter to connect a small duplex pump with the installed boiler, as is done frequently in creameries, for the sake of pumping the necessary water-supply for the house. Whenever extensive improvements are contemplated, it is well worth while to consider the possibilities of one boiler operating the different kinds of machinery referred to. In Fig. 48 is shown a small pump, made by The Goulds Manufacturing Co., capable of lifting forty-eight gallons of water per minute against a head of a hundred feet. The diameter of piston is four inches and the length of stroke is six inches. It is operated by a belt from a steam engine used for other purposes as well. [Pg 180]

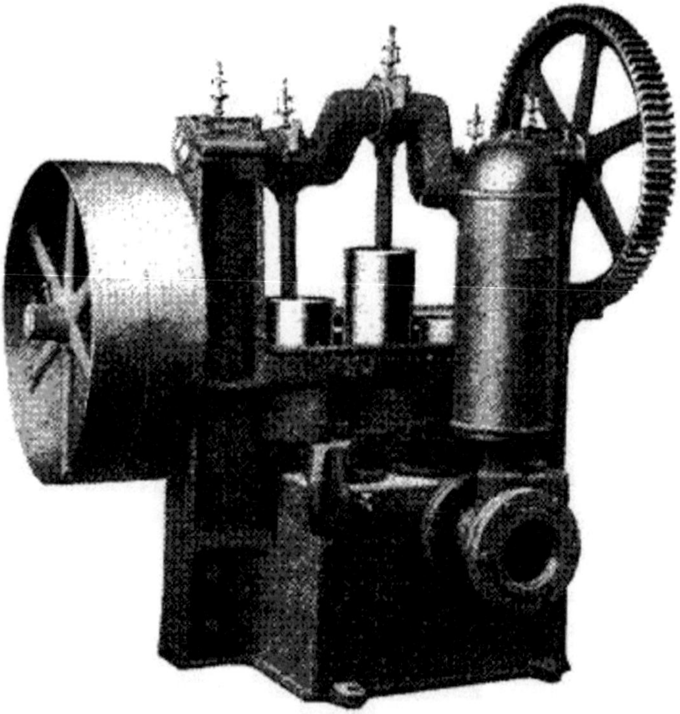

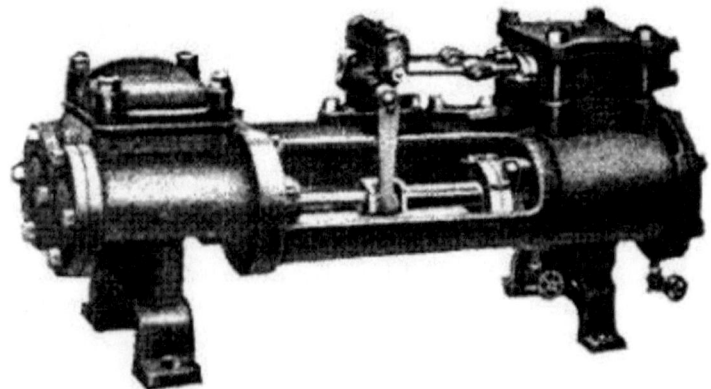

Fig. 48.—Pump operated by belt.

Fig. 49.—Duplex pump, operated directly by steam.

[Pg 181]

**TABLE XIV**

| ...er ...r | Length of Stroke | Gallons per Revo-lution | Revolutions per Minute | Gallons per Minute | Size of Pipes for Short Lengths To be increased as Length Increases | | | |
|---|---|---|---|---|---|---|---|---|
| | | | | | Steam Pipe | Exhaust Pipe | Suction Pipe | Delivery Pipe |
| | 3 | 0.019 | 80 | 1.5 | 3/8 | 1/2 | 1-1/4 | 1 |
| | 3 | 0.033 | 80 | 2.6 | 3/8 | 1/2 | 1-1/4 | 1 |
| | 4 | 0.044 | 75 | 3.6 | 1/2 | 3/4 | 2 | 1-1/2 |
| | 4 | 0.064 | 75 | 4.8 | 1/2 | 3/4 | 2 | 1-1/2 |
| | 5 | 0.08 | 70 | 5.6 | 3/4 | 1-1/4 | 1-1/2 | 1 |
| | 5 | 0.18 | 70 | 12.7 | 3/4 | 1-1/4 | 1-1/2 | 1 |
| | 6 | 0.22 | 65 | 14.0 | 1 | 1-1/4 | 1-1/2 | 1 |
| | 6 | 0.29 | 65 | 19.0 | 1 | 1-1/4 | 1-1/2 | 1 |
| | 6 | 0.38 | 65 | 25.0 | 1 | 1-1/4 | 1-1/2 | 1 |
| | 6 | 0.38 | 65 | 25.0 | 1-1/2 | 2 | 4 | 3 |
| | 6 | 0.48 | 65 | 31.0 | 1 | 1-1/4 | 1-1/2 | 1 |
| | 6 | 0.048 | 65 | 31.0 | 1-1/2 | 2 | 4 | 3 |
| | 6 | 0.056 | 65 | 36.0 | 1-1/2 | 2 | 4 | 3 |
| | 6 | 0.056 | 65 | 36.0 | 1-1/2 | 2 | 4 | 3 |
| | 6 | 0.079 | 65 | 51.0 | 1-1/2 | 2 | 4 | 3 |

[Pg 182]

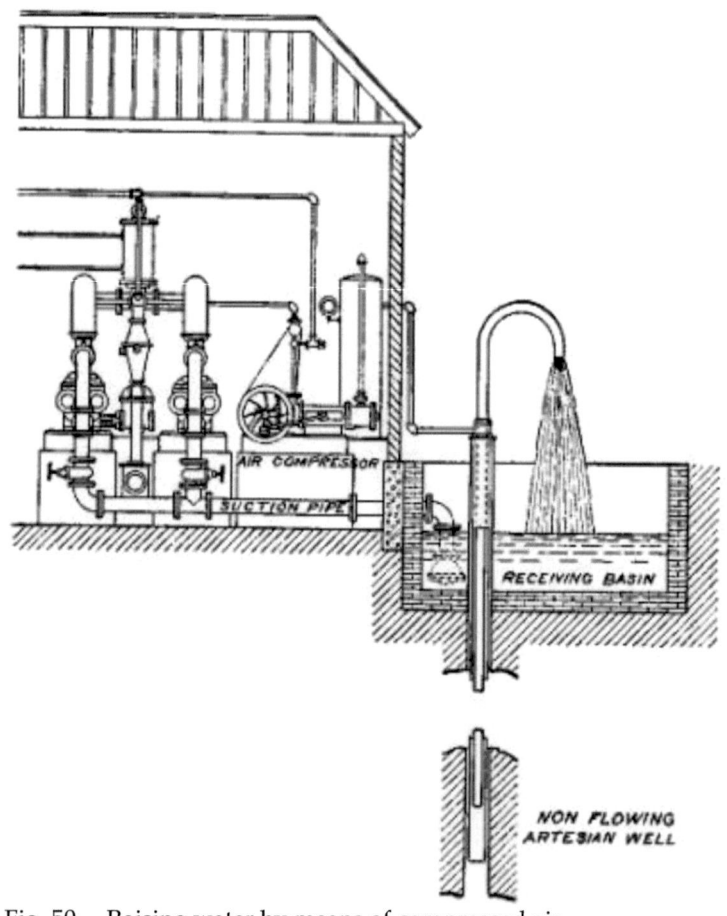

Fig. 50.—Raising water by means of compressed air.

Figure 49 shows a cut of a small duplex Worthington pump which operates by steam, not requiring any intermediate engine. To show the variety of pumps made and the way in which the proportions vary with the capacity [Pg 183] of the pumps, the preceding table is given of pumps of small capacity designed to work with low steam pressure.

*Air lifts for water.*

Compressed air is also a source of power for raising water from a deep well; but it is neither economical in first cost of apparatus nor in operation. The principle is shown by the diagram of Fig. 23, and explains without words how air pressure may be carried down into the well through one pipe and thereby force the water of the well up into another pipe far above its natural level. The machinery needed involves an engine or motor and an air compressor, the latter taking the place of the ordinary pump. It has the single advantage that it avoids the maintenance of valves and similar deep-well machinery at a great distance below the ground, the air pump not requiring any mechanism in the well.

In Fig. 50 is shown a plant installed by the Knowles Pump Co. for a hotel where the air compressor furnished compressed air to raise the water from the deep well into a tank, whence a steam pump lifts the water to a reservoir, not shown.

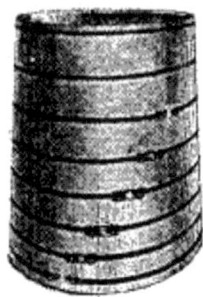

Fig. 51. — Wooden tank.

*Water tanks.*

The standard form of wooden tank in which water may be stored and from which it may be delivered to the house fixtures is pictured in Fig. 51. Figure 52 shows a galvanized iron tank for the same purpose. The tables appended, taken from catalogues of firms building such tanks, show [Pg 184] the dimensions, weights, and costs of the two kinds of tanks.

**TABLE XV. Dimensions and List Prices of Water Tanks.**

**Wooden Stave Tanks**

| th e, | Dia. Bottom, Feet | Capacity, Gallons | No. of Hoops | Price Galv. Hoops, Extra | 1-1/2 In. Cypress | | 2-In. Cypress | | 2-In. Pin |
|---|---|---|---|---|---|---|---|---|---|
| | | | | | Weight Lb. | Price | Weight Lb. | Price | Weight Lb. |
| | 3 | 66 | 2 | $ .30 | 105 | $ 9.30 | 127 | $12.00 | 110 |
| | 3 | 108 | 3 | .40 | 146 | 12.00 | 182 | 15.00 | 157 |
| | 4 | 125 | 2 | .35 | 150 | 14.30 | 186 | 17.50 | 160 |
| | 4 | 283 | 4 | .65 | 260 | 21.00 | 321 | 26.00 | 277 |
| | 5 | 207 | 2 | .45 | 190 | 19.80 | 240 | 24.00 | 207 |
| 2 | 5 | 272 | 3 | .65 | 247 | 21.30 | 305 | 26.00 | 263 |
| | 5 | 337 | 3 | .65 | 267 | 22.80 | 332 | 28.00 | 287 |
| | 5 | 467 | 4 | .85 | 342 | 25.80 | 425 | 32.50 | 367 |
| | 5 | 597 | 4 | 1.00 | 409 | 28.90 | 508 | 37.00 | 438 |
| | 5-1/2 | 252 | 2 | .50 | 233 | 22.50 | 317 | 27.50 | 251 |
| 2 | 5-1/2 | 312 | 3 | .75 | 275 | 24.00 | 341 | 31.70 | 294 |
| | 6 | 304 | 2 | .50 | 265 | 23.50 | 331 | 28.00 | 284 |
| 2 | 6 | 400 | 3 | .75 | 310 | 26.30 | 387 | 31.00 | 334 |
| | 6 | 688 | 4 | 1.25 | 443 | 31.80 | 546 | 41.00 | 473 |
| | 6 | 880 | 4 | 1.40 | 520 | 36.90 | 645 | 48.00 | 557 |
| | 6 | 1072 | 5 | 1.60 | 600 | 42.00 | 744 | 55.00 | 642 |
| 2 | 7 | 550 | 3 | .85 | 381 | 29.00 | 475 | 38.00 | 409 |
| | 7 | 1210 | 4 | 1.60 | 630 | 45.00 | 780 | 58.00 | 675 |

| 7 | 1474 | 5 | 2.00 | 738 | 51.50 | 910 | 66.00 | 789 | 5... |
|---|---|---|---|---|---|---|---|---|---|
| 7 | 1738 | 6 | 2.35 | 829 | 58.00 | 1028 | 74.00 | 889 | 6... |
| 8 | 551 | 2 | .80 | 408 | 31.00 | 506 | 40.00 | 436 | 3... |
| 8 | 725 | 3 | 1.20 | 472 | 35.00 | 587 | 45.00 | 507 | 3... |
| 8 | 1943 | 5 | 2.60 | 880 | 61.00 | 1083 | 78.00 | 938 | 6... |
| 8 | 2639 | 7 | 3.50 | 1113 | 76.00 | 1363 | 97.00 | 1193 | 8... |
| 9 | 3825 | 8 | 5.20 | | | 1770 | 124.40 | 1539 | 1... |
| 10 | 3093 | 5 | 4.30 | | | 1458 | 107.00 | 1266 | 9... |
| 10 | 4200 | 7 | 6.20 | | | 1867 | 131.00 | 1630 | 1... |
| 10 | 5308 | 9 | 8.10 | | | 2277 | 155.00 | 1994 | 1... |
| 10 | 6516 | 11 | 10.00 | | | 2653 | 179.00 | 2323 | 1... |
| 12 | 4494 | 5 | 6.30 | | | 1930 | 138.00 | 1685 | 1... |
| 12 | 7714 | 9 | 11.35 | | | 2910 | 200.00 | 2555 | 1... |
| 12 | 9324 | 11 | 14.00 | | | 3393 | 231.00 | 2984 | 2... |

[Pg 185]

**GALVANIZED IRON TANKS**

| No. | Height Ft. | Diameter Ft. | Capacity Bbl. | Weight Lb. | Price |
|---|---|---|---|---|---|
| 150 | 5 | 8 | 60 | 475 | $ 47.50 |
| 151 | 6 | 6 | 41 | 340 | 35.00 |
| 152 | 6 | 8 | 72 | 530 | 52.50 |
| 153 | 8 | 6 | 54 | 430 | 43.00 |
| 154 | 8 | 8 | 96 | 640 | 65.00 |
| 155 | 8 | 10 | 150 | 875 | 85.00 |

| 156 | 10 | 8 | 120 | 750 | 73.00 |
| 157 | 10 | 10 | 180 | 970 | 95.00 |
| 158 | 10 | 12 | 270 | 1400 | 128.00 |
| 159 | 12 | 12 | 324 | 1600 | 150.00 |

There are many combinations and forms of these structures, and a detailed description of their characteristic construction and cost would occupy too much space for this present work. By referring to the pages of any agricultural, architectural, or engineering magazine, advertisements may be found of firms who build such towers and who may be depended upon for satisfactory work.

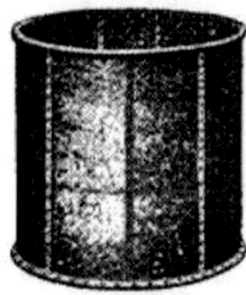

Fig. 52. — Iron tank.

If the tank is to be placed inside a building, it may be built of steel or of wood, although a lining of lead, copper, or galvanized iron is of advantage in the latter case. If the tank is out of doors, protection against frost must be carefully attended to, both to prevent an ice cap forming in the [Pg 186] tank — the cause of many failures of tanks — and to prevent standing water in the connecting pipes being frozen. If the tank is to be placed inside the building, care must be taken to have it water-tight and to have the supports of the tank ample for the excessive weight which will be thereby imposed. Wooden tanks are likely to rot, and if left standing empty, become leaky. They are, therefore, less worth while than iron tanks.

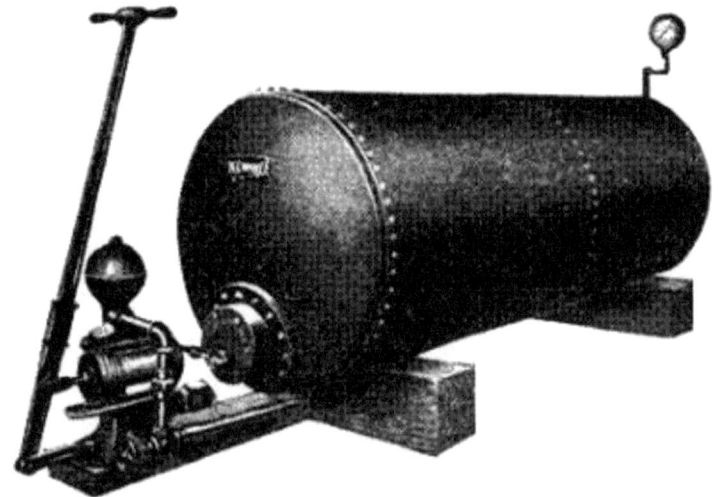

Fig. 53.—Hand pump applied to air-tank.

*Pressure tanks.*

A simple and very satisfactory method of storing water, and at the same time making provision for pumping water, is to place in the cellar or in a special excavation outside the cellar a pressure tank similar in shape to an ordinary horizontal boiler. The water in this tank is forced up into the house through the agency of compressed air, pumped [Pg 187] in above the water, either by hand or by machinery, and in some cases automatically regulated so that the air pressure in the tank remains constant, no matter whether the tank contains much or little water. The village supply of Babylon, Long Island, is on this principle, the tanks there being eight feet in diameter and one hundred feet long,—much larger, of course, than is needed for a single house.

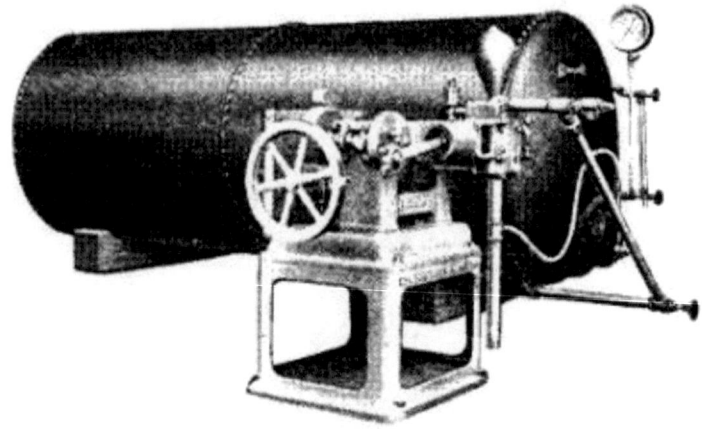

Fig. 54.—Engine applied to air-tank.

The accompanying diagram and figures show the method of installing this system, which is known generally as the Kewanee system, although a number of other firms than the Kewanee Water Supply Co. are prepared to furnish the outfit necessary. [Pg 188]

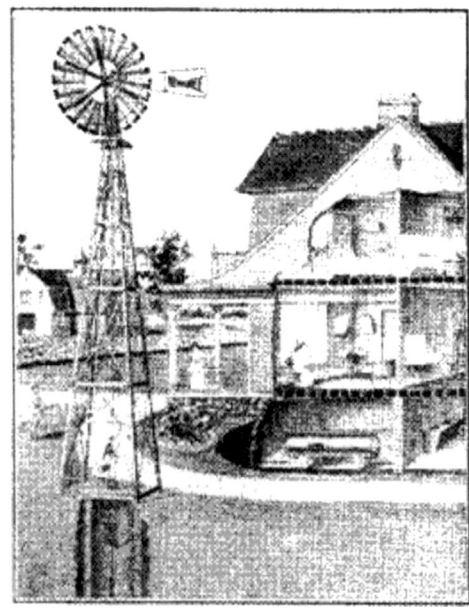
Fig. 55.—Windmill connection with tank.

How the air-tank may be used in connection with a hand force pump is shown in Fig. 53. The water is pumped from a well into the tank, usually in the cellar, whence it flows by the pressure in the tank to all parts of the house. Figure 54 shows the tank with a gas engine and a power pump substituted for the hand pump. Figure 55 shows the using of a windmill in connection with the tank and also shows the relation of the tank to the fixtures in the rest of the house.

[Pg 189]

## CHAPTER IX

## *PLUMBING*

A generous supply of water for a house brings with it desires for the conveniences necessary to its enjoyment. As soon as running water is established in a house, the kitchen sink fails conspicuously to fulfill all requirements, and a wash-tub seems a sorry substitute for a modern bath-room. A single pipe supplying cold water only, no matter how pure the water or how satisfactory in the summer, does not afford the constant convenience which an unlimited supply of both cold and hot water offers, and the introduction of running water is usually followed by an addition to the kitchen stove whereby running hot water may be obtained as well as running cold water. The next step is the equipment of a bath-room, affording suitable bathing facilities and doing away with the out-of-door privy.

*Installation of the plumbing.*

These things are reckoned as luxuries, not among the necessities of life, and it must be understood at the outset that such conveniences cost money, both for original installation and for maintenance; the water-back in the stove will become filled up with lime if the water is hard, the boiler will become corroded and have to be replaced, the [Pg 190] plumbing fixtures will certainly get out of repair and need attention, and there will be, year by year, a small but continuous outlay.

Again, it is idle to propose installing plumbing fixtures unless the house is properly heated in winter time, and this calls for a furnace for at least a portion of the house. Usually the kitchen is kept warm enough through the winter nights, so that running water may be put in the kitchen without danger from frost; although the writer knows of a house where it is the task of the housewife each winter night to shut off all water in the cellar and to clean out the trap in the sink drain in order to prevent freezing in both the supply pipe and drainpipe. Usually a water-pipe may be carried through the cellar without danger of freezing, but in most farmhouses heated by stoves, except in the kitchen and sitting room, water-pipes would, the first cold night, probably freeze and burst.

Various makeshifts have been employed to secure the convenience of a bath-room without adding to the expense by installing a furnace. In one house the bath-room was placed in an alcove off from the kitchen, with open space above the dividing partition, so that the kitchen heat kept the bath-room warm. This is not an ideal location for a bath-room, but, in this case, it avoided the necessity for an additional stove or furnace. In another house the bath-room was placed above the kitchen, with a large register in the floor of the former, so that the kitchen heat kept the room warm; and in still another case the bath-room was over the sitting room, and a large pipe carried the heat from the stove below into the room above. The stovepipe also went through the bath-room and [Pg 191] helped to provide warmth. It is better, all things considered, to defer the installation of a bath-room until a furnace can be provided, since then there is no danger of frozen water-pipes at intermediate points where the cold reaches the pipes. A full list of fixtures and piping required is as follows:—

1st. A tank in the attic to store water in case the main pipe-flow or pump-capacity is small. This tank, of course, is not needed if the direct supply from the source is at all times adequate for the full demand.

2d. A main supply pipe from the outside source or from the attic tank connecting with and supplying the kitchen sink, the hot-water boiler through the kitchen stove, the laundry tubs, the bath-tub, the wash-basin, and the water-closet tank. It is wise, in order to save expense, to have all these fixtures as close together as possible; as, for instance, the laundry tub in the basement directly under the kitchen sink and the bath-room fixtures directly over the kitchen sink.

3d. A hot-water pipe leading out of the hot-water boiler to the kitchen sink, to the laundry tubs, and to the bath-tub. Although not essential, it is desirable to carry the hot-water pipe back to the bottom of the hot-water boiler, so that the circulation of hot water is maintained. This will avoid the necessity of wasting water and waiting until the water runs hot from the hot-water faucet whenever hot water is desired.

4th. The necessary fixtures, such as faucets, sinks, tubs, wash-basins, kitchen boiler, water-back for the stove, water-closet, tank, and fixtures. These may be now taken up in order and described more in detail. [Pg 192]

*Supply tank.*

The attic tank may be of wood or iron, and its capacity should be equal to the daily consumption of water. Its purpose, as already indicated, is to equalize the varying rates of consumption from hour to hour and between day and night. The minimum size of this tank would be such that the flow during the night would just fill the tank with an amount of water just sufficient for the day's needs. Of course, the additional supply entering the tank during the day would reduce the size somewhat, but the basis for computation given is not unreasonable.

Several accessories must be provided for such a tank. An overflow is essential, and this is best accomplished by carrying a *pipe out through a hole in the roof*. This must be ample in size, provided with a screen at the inside end, and be examined frequently to make sure that the overflow remains open. A light flap valve to keep out the cold in winter is also a desirable feature for the overflow pipe. The tank must be water-tight, and while it is possible to make a wooden tank water-tight, it is wiser to line a wooden tank with lead or sheet iron. The latter can be painted at intervals, so that it will not rust, and is safer than wood alone to prevent leakage.

Care must be taken to give sufficient strength to the wooden tank; it should never be made of less than two-inch stuff, and should not depend upon nails or screws alone for holding the sides together. Figure 56 shows a suitable way to put together such a tank. Certain firms that make windmills and agricultural implements generally can furnish wrought-iron tanks, warranted to be water-tight, of suitable size to go in an attic. Such a tank, as [Pg 193] we have already said, should hold about five hundred gallons and should therefore be a cube four feet on a side or its equivalent. It needs to be very carefully placed in the house, or else its weight will cause the attic floor to sag. A tank of the size named will weigh a little more than two tons, and such a weight, unless special precautions are taken, cannot be placed in the middle of an attic floor without causing serious settlement, if not actual breaking through, of the floor.

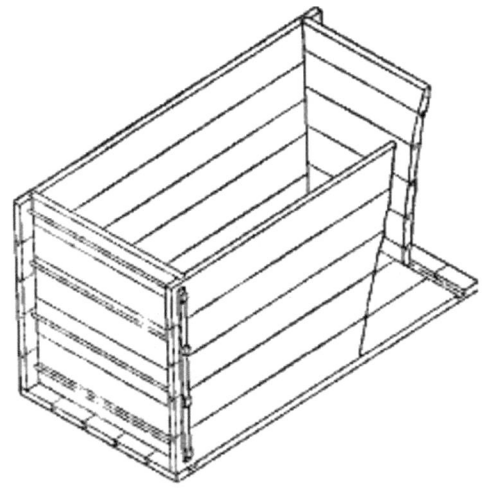

Fig. 56.—Construction of a wooden tank.

A good way of placing such a tank is to nail the floor joists onto the bottom of the rafters, so that a truss is formed, and the box or tank is properly supported on the floor and also hung from the rafters by iron straps bolted both to tank and rafters. If possible, this tank should be placed directly over a partition carried through to the cellar, in which case no settlement is possible.

*Main supply pipe.*

The main supply pipe, except when pressure is very great, is most satisfactory when made of three-quarter-inch galvanized iron pipe. Even with a high pressure, half-inch pipe is unsatisfactory because of the great velocity with which the water comes from the faucets and [Pg 194] because the high pressure causes the packing in the faucets to wear out rapidly. This three-quarter-inch pipe should have a stop-and-waste, as it is called, just inside the cellar wall, so that if the house is not occupied at any time, the valve may be shut and the water in the pipes drawn off, to prevent possible freezing. The pipe should never be carried directly in front of a window or along the sill of the building unless protected by some kind of wrapping. The laterals and the different fixtures are taken off from this main supply pipe as it rises through the house, and the pipe is capped at the top.

*Hot-water circulation.*

To provide hot water, a branch must be taken off at the level of the kitchen stove and run into the hot-water boiler at or near the bottom. The circulation in the tank and through the house is then provided for by a separate circuit running from the bottom of the hot-water tank to the water-back and back into the tank at a point about halfway up. The house circuit is then run from the top of the boiler around through the house, and if a return pipe is provided, it comes back and enters at the bottom. This hot-water pipe is also of galvanized iron and should be of the same size as the main supply pipe (see Fig. 57). [Pg 195]

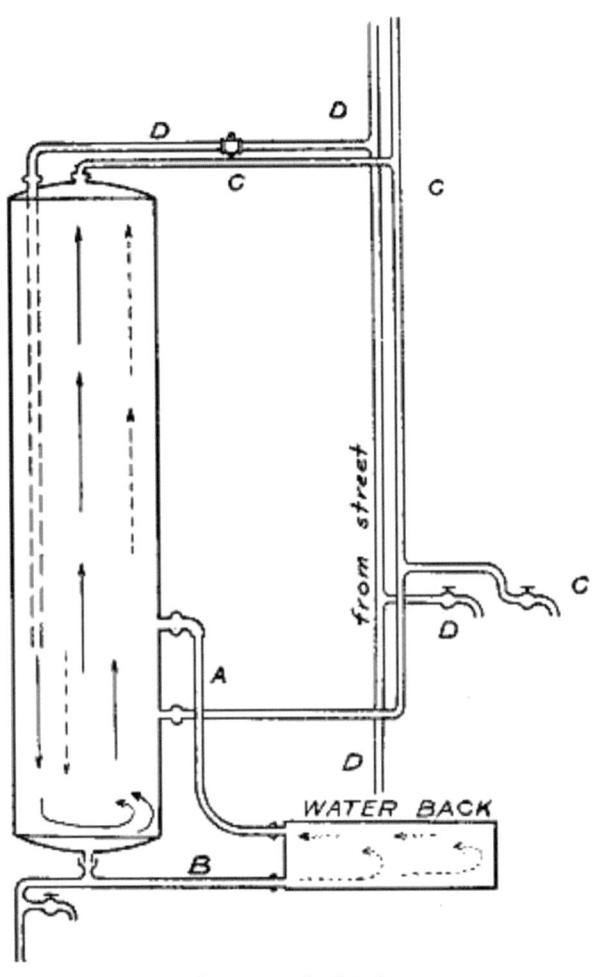

Fig. 57. — Hot-water attachment to the kitchen stove.

The fixtures may be as elaborate as the purse and taste will allow, but some general instruction may not be out of place. There are many types of faucets, all good, and differing from each other only in some minor detail of construction. Experience with the so-called self-closing faucets or bibbs has not been entirely satisfactory, since, with high pressure, the packing very quickly wears out. Similarly, experience with those faucets that open and shut by a single turn of a handle shows that frequent renewals of packing are necessary. The simplest, most reliable, and the easiest faucets to repair are those in which the valve is screwed down onto the valve seat, which is a plane, and where the water-tightness is made by the [Pg 196] insertion of a rubber or leather washer that can always be cut out with a knife from a piece of old belting or harness. The faucets may be nickeled or left plain brass, and the advantage of the added expense of nickel is in the appearance alone. If the faucets themselves are nickel, then the piping also should be nickel; that is, brass nickel-plated. Galvanized iron piping and brass faucets do not, to be sure, have the same satisfactory appearance as highly finished nickeled faucets, but the one is quite as serviceable as the other.

*Kitchen sinks.*

In providing a sink for the kitchen, choice lies between plain iron and enameled iron. For special work, sinks have been made of galvanized iron, of copper, slate, soapstone, and of real porcelain. There is hardly any limit to the cost of a porcelain sink, and while an enameled iron sink with fittings costs from $30 to $60, a cast-iron sink of the same size will cost only $3 or $4. A good quality of white enameled iron sink, of size suitable for a kitchen, with white enameled back and a drainboard on the side, costing $30, is very attractive as an ornament, but it serves no more useful purpose than a $3 sink and a fifty-cent drainboard. Figure 58 shows an enameled iron sink, containing sink, drainboard, and back all in one piece. This is pure white, and when fitted with nickel faucets makes a very attractive fitting.

*Laundry tubs.*

If running water is to be put in a house, stationary tubs for the laundry, into which water runs by a faucet and which can be emptied by pulling a plug, are certainly worth their cost over movable wooden tubs in the labor saved. [Pg 197] Stationary tubs may be made of wood, of enameled iron, or of slate.

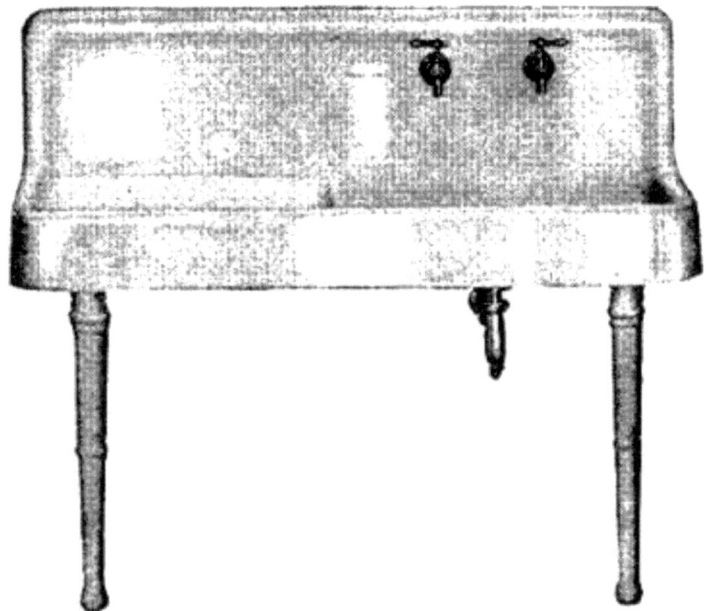

Fig. 58. — Enameled iron sink.

Wooden tubs are not as desirable as the others because in the course of time they absorb a certain amount of organic matter and have a persistent odor. They are, however, very inexpensive, a man of ordinary ability being able to build them himself at the cost of the wood only. Enameled iron tubs of ordinary size cost, with the fixtures, from $20 to $40 apiece, and a set of three slate tubs costs $25. To these figures must be added the expense of the piping to bring both hot and cold water to [Pg 198] the tubs, together with the two faucets and the drainpipe connections necessary. Figure 59 shows three white enameled iron laundry tubs costing about $75 installed.

*Hot-water boiler.*

The kitchen boiler is to-day almost always made of galvanized iron and is placed on its own stand, usually back of the kitchen stove, although it may stand in an adjoining room, — the bath-room, for instance, — and aid in keeping that room warm. Such a tank costs about $12, to which must be added the necessary piping, and it is always desirable to put a stop-cock on the cold-water supply entering the tank. Then if the tank bursts, the cold water may be shut off without doing harm.

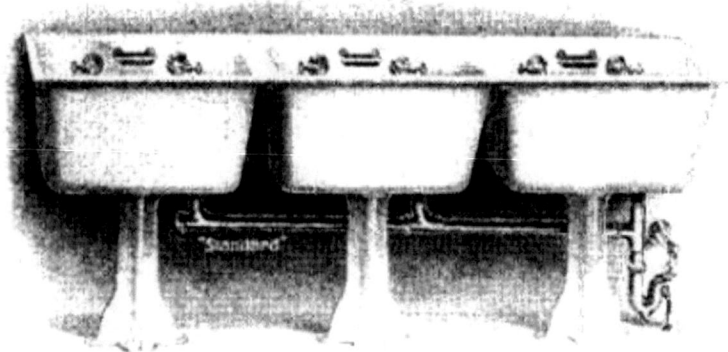

Fig. 59. — Enameled laundry tubs.

A drainpipe from the bottom of the tank is also desirable to draw off the accumulations of sediment. [Pg 199]

*Water-back, wash-basin, bath-tub.*

The water-back is merely a hollow box made to fit the front of the fire box in the stove, usually shaped so as to replace the front fire brick. The cold water comes in at the bottom of the box, is heated by contact with the fire, and the hot water goes out through the other pipe into the boiler.

The wash-basin in the bath-room is either marble, enameled iron, or porcelain. The marble basins with a slab can be had for about $7.50, while the enameled iron basins cost from $6 to $40. To this must be added the cost of faucets and piping, together with the drain and the trap that belongs with the drain. The enameled iron basins which are being used to-day more than ever before have proved very satisfactory, have but little weight, can be fastened to the wall without difficulty, and take up less room than the old marble basin. A fancy porcelain basin costs about $75, and is no better for practical use than either of the others.

Much the same kind of material may be used for bath-tubs, although warning ought to be given to avoid the use of the old-fashioned tin-lined bath-tub. This lining will easily rust or corrode, is very difficult to keep clean, and while the first cost is less than the enameled iron tub, it has no other advantage. An enameled iron tub five and a half feet long will cost from $20 to $100 without fixtures.

*Cost of plumbing installation.*

A fair estimate of the cost of the plumbing in a house, including all the fixtures mentioned except the tank in the attic, including also the plumber's bill, is $150. This [Pg 200] requires very careful buying, and implies an entire absence of brass or nickel-plated piping. If a high grade of fixtures, including nickel fittings and nickel piping, wherever it shows, is used, the cost of the fixtures alone, not including labor or piping other than mentioned, will be from $150 up.

*House drainage.*

The term "plumbing" is generally used to include both the water-supply in the house, with all the fixtures pertaining thereto, and the carrying of the waste water to a point outside the house; it remains, therefore, to discuss the waste pipes connected with the plumbing fixtures.

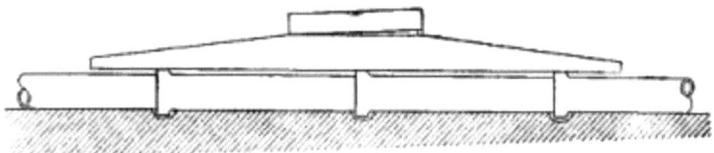

Fig. 60.—Leveling the drain.

The house-drain, or the pipe which carries the wastes from the house to the point of final disposal, is generally made of vitrified tile, and in ordinary practice is five inches inside diameter. The lower end of this drain discharges into a cesspool, or settling tank, or into a stream, as local conditions permit. This house-drain should be carefully laid in a straight line, both horizontally and vertically, for two reasons. In the first place, the velocity of flow in a straight pipe will be greater, and therefore the danger of stoppage will be decreased, and in the next place, if a stoppage does occur in the pipe, it can be cleaned out better [Pg 201] if the pipe is straight than if it is laid with numerous bends. Such a pipe should have a grade of at least one quarter inch to a foot, and this is conveniently given by tacking a little piece of wood one half inch thick on one end of a two-foot carpenter's level and then setting the pipe so that with this piece of wood resting on the pipe at one end and the end of the level itself on the pipe at its other end, the bubble will be in the middle. Figure 60 shows the carpenter's level in position on a level board, which rests on the hubs of three pipes. The joints of this pipe should be made with Portland cement mixed with an equal part of sand, and the space at the joint completely filled. When nearing the house, it is very desirable that a manhole should be built so that if a stoppage occurs, it may be cleaned out without taking up the pipe. In city houses a running trap is always inserted just outside the house with a fresh-air inlet on the house side of the trap, as shown in Fig. 61. But for a single house this is not necessary, and it is wiser to omit the running trap.

The soil-pipe begins at the trap or at the cellar wall and runs up through the roof of the house, so that any gas in the drain or soil-pipe may escape at such a height as not to be objectionable. Through the cellar wall and up through the house the soil-pipe should be of cast-iron, which comes in six-foot lengths for this special purpose. Y's are provided by which the fixtures are connected to the soil-pipe, and the top of the pipe is covered with a zinc netting to keep out leaves and birds. This soil-pipe weighs about ten pounds per foot and is almost always four inches inside diameter. The length necessary is easily computed, since it runs from the outside cellar wall to the point where the [Pg 202] vertical line of pipe rises and from that point in the cellar extends to the roof. Such a pipe may be estimated at two cents a pound with something additional for the Y's.

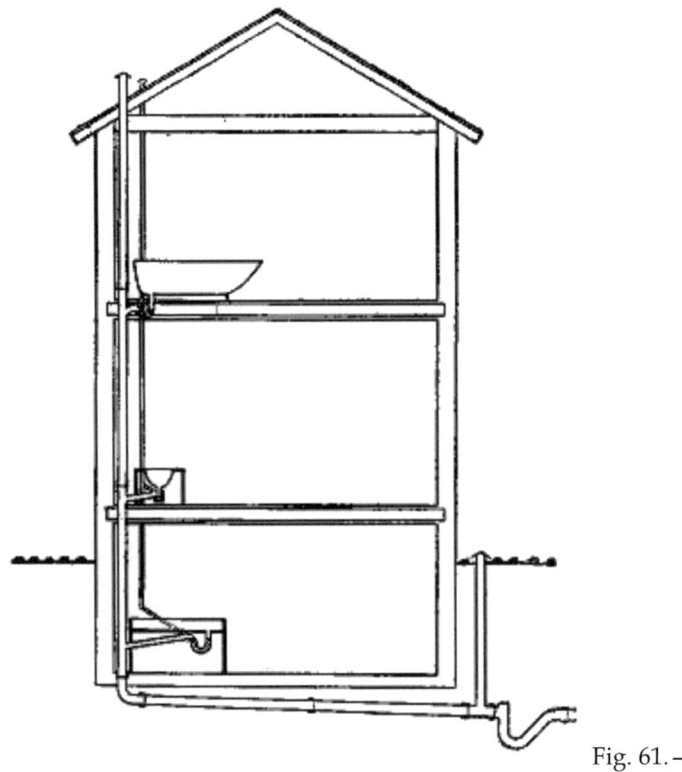

Fig. 61.—
Water-supply installation.

The soil-pipe must be well supported along the cellar wall on brackets or hung from the floor joists by short pieces of chain or band iron. Special care must be taken to support the pipe at the elbow, where it turns upward, since a length of thirty feet of this pipe, weighing three hundred pounds, has to be provided for. It is a good practice to [Pg 203] build a brick pier from the cellar bottom up to and around the elbow to support it firmly in the masonry.

The joints in this drainpipe should be made with lead, ramming some oakum into the joints first and then pouring in enough lead melted to the right degree to provide an inch depth of joint. After the lead cools, it must be expanded or calked by driving the calking tool hard against it.

To prevent rain finding its way between the soil-pipe and the roof, a piece of lead is generally wrapped around the soil-pipe for a distance of twelve inches or so above the roof, and then a flat piece of lead extending out under the shingles is slipped over and soldered fast to the other lead piece.

The fixtures are connected to the iron pipe usually by lead pipe, the lead pipe being first wiped onto a brass ferrule, the ferrule being leaded into the Y branch. These Y branches are usually two inches in diameter and the lead pipe usually one and one quarter inches. Between the soil-pipe and the fixtures a trap must be provided with a water-seal of about an inch.

*Trap-vents.*

In city plumbing it is customary to vent traps; that is, to carry another system of pipes from the top of the trap nearest the fixture up to and through the roof. On most roofs, where modern plumbing has been installed, are seen two pipes projecting, one the soil-pipe and the other the vent-pipe, indicating the location of a bath-room below (see Fig. 61). In a single house, however, and particularly in view of experiments made recently on the subject of trap siphonage, these trap-vents seem hardly necessary. [Pg 204] They were formerly insisted upon because of the feeling that by the passage of a large amount of water down the soil-pipe, sufficient suction might be induced to draw out the water from some small trap on the way, thereby opening a passage for sewer gas into the room. Experiments have shown that it is practically impossible to draw off the water from a trap in this way, and that the system of vent-pipes does little more than add to the cost.

The traps themselves, however, are essential, and great care should be taken to see that each trap is in place and has a seal of the depth already mentioned. The best trap to use in any fixture is the simplest, and a plain S trap answers every purpose. It is always wise to have a clean-out at the bottom of the trap; that is, a small opening which can be closed with a screw plug, so that when the trap becomes clogged, it can be easily opened and cleaned (see Fig. 62).

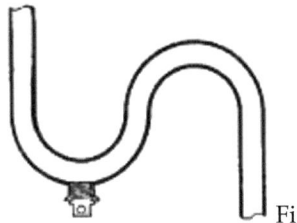 Fig. 62. — A trap.

*Water-closets.*

A great many kinds of water-closets have been made and used, with various degrees of success. The old-fashioned pan-closet becomes easily clogged, allows matter to decompose in the receptacle under the valve, and, in spite of its being cheaper, should not be used. The long-hopper closet is also objectionable, for the same reason. A recent bulletin of the Maine State Board of Health, which gives the relative merits of the different forms now available, very directly and briefly, is here repeated: —

"The choice of a water-closet should be made from those [Pg 205] which have the bowl and trap all in one piece, which are simple in construction, are self-cleansing, and have a safe water-seal. None should be considered except the short-hopper, the washout, the washdown, the syphonic, and the syphon-jet closets.

"Short-hopper closets not many years ago were considered desirable, but other styles costing but little more are better.

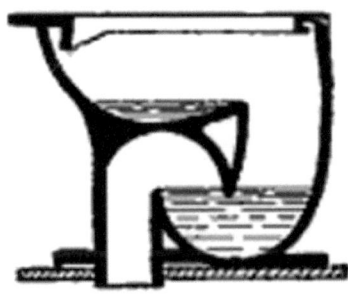 Fig. 63. — Washout water-closet.

"The washout closet (Fig. 63) has too shallow a pool of water to receive the soil, and the trap below and the portion above the trap do not receive a sufficient scouring from the flush.

191

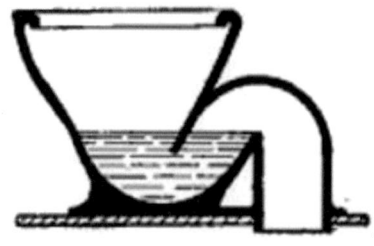

Fig. 64. — Washdown water-closet.

"The washdown closet (Fig. 64) is an improvement over the washout. Having a deep basin, a deep water-seal, smaller surfaces uncovered by water, and a more efficient scouring action, it is more cleanly. The washdown closet is really an improved short hopper.

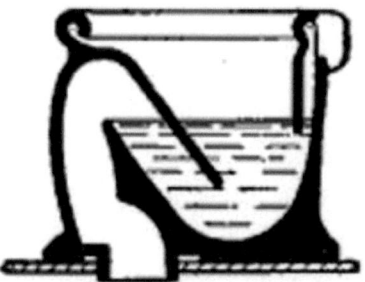

Fig. 65. — Syphonic closet.

"Of late years the principle of syphonic action has been applied to the washdown closet. Figure 65 shows the outline of a syphonic closet. It will be seen that the basin, as in the washdown closet, has considerable depth and holds a considerable quantity of water; but it differs in having a more contracted outlet. When the closet is flushed, the filling of this outlet forms a syphon, and then the pressure [Pg 206] of the air upon the surface of the water in the basin drives the water into the soil-pipe with much force. At the breaking of the syphon, enough water is left in the trap to preserve the seal.

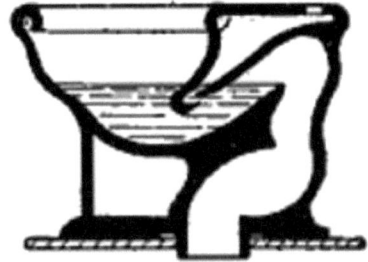

Fig. 66.—Syphon-jet closet.

"In the syphon-jet closet (Fig. 66) there is added to the mechanism of the syphon closet a jet of water which helps to drive the contents of the bowl more rapidly into the outlet. These two closets, syphon and the syphon-jet, are preferable to those of any other style. Among other advantages they are more nearly noiseless than any other kinds.

"Recapitulating, it may be said, while the short-hopper and the washout closets may not deserve absolute condemnation, the advantages of the washdown, syphon, and the syphon-jet closets are so much greater that they should be chosen in all new work."

Properly to flush out the closet, a water-pipe connection must be made from the supply main. It would be quite possible to connect directly to the closet rim where the flush enters, but there are two objections urged against this. Sometimes, when the pressure is low and water is being drawn in the kitchen, if a faucet in the bath-room is opened, not only will no water come, but air is drawn into the pipe by the force of the running water below. A direct connection with a water-closet, it is conceivable, might allow filth to be drawn up into the water-pipe under certain conditions. The other objection is that the small pipe generally used in a house does not deliver water fast enough for effective flushing. [Pg 207]

It is common, therefore, to put in, just back of or above the closet, a small copper-lined wooden tank which holds about three gallons and which can be discharged rapidly through a one-and-a-quarter-inch pipe. This tank with fittings costs about $10, and in a great many cases is probably unnecessary. It has the advantage, however, of allowing a small flow to enter the tank whenever emptied, to be automatically shut off by a float valve when filled. If the house has a tank supply or if the pressure is strong enough to insure a positive flow at all times, there can be no objection in a single family, where the flushing action will be insisted on by the mistress of the house in the interests of cleanliness, to making a direct connection between the closet and the house supply pipe. An automatic shut-off bibb would then be used on the water-pipe, allowing the water to flow freely as long as the bibb was opened, but closing automatically when released.

[Pg 208]

## CHAPTER X

## *SEWAGE DISPOSAL*

The subject of sewage disposal for a single house in the country does not at all present the elaborate problem that is suggested when the disposal of sewage of a city is under discussion. In the first place, the amount of sewage to be dealt with is moderate in quantity; and in the second place the area available on which the sewage may be treated is in almost all cases more than ample for the purpose. Nor is there the complication that arises with city sewage, due to the admixture of manufacturing wastes. The material to be handled is entirely domestic sewage and varies only according to the amount of water used in the house, making the sewage of greater or less strength according as less or more water is used. Sewage from a single house differs only in one respect disadvantageously from city sewage, namely, in the fact that the sewage, not having to pass through a long length of pipe, comes to the place of disposal in what is known as a fresh condition; that is, no organic changes have taken place in the material of which the sewage is composed.

*Definition of sewage.*

The great bulk of sewage is water, and, in quantity, the amount of sewage to be cared for is about equal to the [Pg 209] amount of water consumed in the household, although this will depend somewhat on the habits of the family. If, for example, part of the water-supply is used for an ornamental fountain in the front yard, or if in the summer time a large amount of water is used for sprinkling the lawns, that water is not converted into sewage, and the amount of the latter is thereby diminished; but, ordinarily, it is safe to say that the quantity of water supplied to the house and the quantity of sewage taken away from the house is identical, and since it is much easier to measure the water-supply than the sewage flow, the former is taken as the quantity of sewage to be treated.

In the course of its passage through the house, however, the water has added to it a certain amount of polluting substances, largely derived from the kitchen sink, where dirt from vegetables and particles of vegetable material, together with more or less soap, are carried by the waste water from the sink into the drain. In the bathroom, also, some small amount of organic matter is added to the water, but the proportion of such matter to the total volume of water used is very small, probably not exceeding one tenth of one per cent. This small proportion is nevertheless sufficient to become very objectionable if allowed to decompose, and the problem of sewage disposal for a single house is to drain away the water, leaving behind the solids so disposed that they shall not subsequently cause offense by their putrefaction.

The process of decay is normal for all organic matter and is due to the agency of certain bacteria whose duty it is, providentially, to eliminate from the surface of the earth organic matter which otherwise would remain useless, [Pg 210] if not destructive, to man. It is impossible to leave any vegetable or animal matter exposed to the air without this process of decay at once setting in. Apples left in the orchard at the end of the season inevitably are reduced and disappear in a short time. Dead animals, whether large or small, in the same way succumb to the same process of nature, and it has been pointed out that, unless this provision did exist, the accumulation of such organic wastes since the settlement of this country would be so great as to make the country uninhabitable. Fortunately, however, this inevitable process breaks down the structure of all organic material, partly converting fiber and pulp into gas, partly liquefying the material and converting the remainder into inorganic matter which is of vast importance as food for plant life. A cycle is thus formed which may be best illustrated in the case of cows which feed on the herbage of a meadow, the manure from the cows furnishing food for the grass which otherwise would soon exhaust the nutriment of the soil.

*Stream pollution.*

The first fundamental principle of sewage disposal, therefore, is to distribute the organic matter in the sewage so that these beneficent bacteria may most rapidly and thoroughly accomplish their purpose. During the last fifty years, a great deal of study has been expended on this problem, and while it has not as yet been entirely solved, certain essential features have been well established.

The most important factor promoting the activity of these agents of decay is the presence of air, since in many ways it has been proved that without air their action is impossible. Thus it has been shown that discharging [Pg 211] sewage into a stream, whether the stream be a slow and sluggish one or whether it be a mountain stream churned into foam by repeated waterfalls, has little other power to act on organic matter than to hold it for transportation down stream, or to allow it to settle in slower reaches until mud banks have been accumulated which will be washed out again at the first freshet. Experiments have shown that the agencies to which certain diseases are attributed, commonly known as pathogenic bacteria, are frequently, if not always, found in sewage, and that when these bacteria are discharged into streams they may be carried with the stream hundreds of miles and retain all their power for evil, in case the water is used for drinking purposes. No right-minded person to-day will so abuse the rights of his fellow-citizens as deliberately to pour into a stream such unmistakable poison as sewage has proved itself to be. The fact is so well known that it is not worth while pointing out examples. It is enough to say that some of the worst epidemics of typhoid fever which this country has known have been traced to the agency of drinking water, polluted miles away by a relatively small amount of sewage.

In a number of states, laws have been passed which expressly prohibit the discharge of sewage, even from a single house, into a stream of any sort, even though the stream is on the land of the man thus discharging sewage and where it would appear as if he alone might control the uses of that stream. Unfortunately, the machinery of the law does not always operate to detect and punish the breakers of the law, but any law which, as in this case, has so positive a reason for its existence, and violation of which [Pg 212] is so certain to bring disaster on persons drinking the water of the stream below the point where the sewage is discharged, any law which appeals for its enforcement so directly to the common sense and right feeling of all intelligent people, seems hardly to need legal machinery for its enforcement. It must depend, as indeed all laws must depend, upon the intelligent support of the community, and surely no law would commend itself more urgently than this one forbidding the pollution of drinking water.

In spite of the fact that the lack of air in the water will prevent bacterial action, there are, nevertheless, many cases where the discharge of sewage into a stream may be permitted as being the best solution of the disposal problem, provided always that the stream is not used and is not likely to be used for drinking water. Such cases occur where the stream is relatively large and where the level of the stream is fairly regular, so that there is no likelihood of the deposit of organic matter on the banks during the falling of the stream level. Examples of this sort might be cited in the vicinity of the Mohawk or Hudson River, or in the vicinity of any of the larger rivers of any populous state, since although the water of the Mohawk is used by the city of Albany for drinking purposes, yet the amount of organic matter which inevitably finds its way into such rivers precludes its use for drinking without filtration. Into the Hudson below Albany there can hardly be any question of the propriety of discharging sewage from a single house.

Again, houses in the vicinity of large bodies of still water may without question be allowed to discharge into those [Pg 213] lakes. For example, houses in the vicinity of Lake Ontario or Lake Michigan, or even of much smaller lakes, should not contribute any offensive pollution to the waters of the lake. In New York State, some of the smaller lakes are used as water-supplies for cities, as, for example, Owasco Lake for the city of Auburn and Skaneateles Lake for the city of Syracuse, and, acting under the statutes, special laws have been passed by the State Department of Health, forbidding any discharge of any kind of household wastes into these lakes. The same is done in other states. Here, again, it is a question of the drinking supply which is being considered, and not a question of the possibility of any nuisance being committed.

*Treatment of sewage on land.*

If no stream suitable for the reception of sewage is available, then the sewage must in some way be treated on land before it passes into the nearest watercourse. For the second fundamental principle about the treatment of sewage is that of all places the action of putrefactive bacteria is most energetic in the surface soil and that it is there that the organic matter of sewage can be most rapidly accomplished. Experiments already referred to have shown not only this, but also that their activity is most noticeable in the surface layers of the soil and that their action continues for scarcely two feet downward, and it is customary to assume that the largest amount of work done is accomplished in the top twelve inches. Further than this, it has been established that in order to persuade the bacteria involved to do their work as promptly as possible, the application of sewage to any particular locality should be made intermittent; that is, that a resting [Pg 214] period should be given to the bacteria between successive applications of sewage.

For example, one can recall without difficulty the conditions on the ground at the back of the house where the kitchen sink-drain commonly discharges. At the beginning of summer perhaps a rank growth of grass starts up vigorously in the vicinity, and the path of the surface drain can be traced by the heavy vegetation along the line of the drain. If the slope of the surface away from the house is considerable, no other effect may be noticed through the season, since the surface slope carries away the sewage, spreading it out over the ground so that the soil really has a chance to breathe between successive doses. But if the ground is flat, it will be remembered that before many weeks the sewage ceases to sink into it; the ground becomes "sewage-sick," as they say in England, and a thick, dark-colored pool of sewage gradually forms, which smells abominably. If a piece of hose a dozen feet long had been attached to the end of the drain and each day shifted in position so that no particular spot received the infiltration two days in succession, it is probable that no such pondage of sewage would occur, but that the mere intermittency of the application thereby secured would permit the successful disposal of this sink waste throughout the season.

The same effect is to be noted in some cesspools where, because of the great depth to which they are dug and because no overflow into the surface layers of the soil is provided, the pores of the ground around the cesspool become clogged and choked, and the cesspool becomes filled with a thick, viscous, dark-colored, objectionable-looking, and evil-smelling liquid. [Pg 215]

The three principles which will avoid these conditions are, as already stated, plenty of air, presence of bacteria normally found in the surface layers of the soil, and intermittency of application.

In order to secure the operation of these three principles in the application of sewage onto land, the sewage must be made to pass either over the surface of the land in its natural condition in such a way that the sewage may sink into the soil and be absorbed and at the same time give up its manurial elements to whatever vegetation the soil produces; or, as a modification of this principle, the sewage may be required to pass through an artificial bed of coarse material by which the rate of treatment may be considerably increased. In the latter case, although probably the greater part of the action of the bacteria takes place in the top twelve inches, it is customary to make the beds about three feet thick, chiefly in order to prevent uneven discharge of the sewage through the bed. Finally, wherever, for æsthetic reasons, it is desirable that the sewage should not be in evidence, either before passing through the natural soil or exposed in an artificial bed, the practice may be resorted to of distributing the sewage through agricultural tile drain laid about twelve inches below the surface. In this way, the sewage is scattered through the top soil, where bacteria are most active, without being apparent, and a front lawn thus treated would not give any indication of its use.

Taking up now in order these three methods of treatment, we may consider some of the details of construction. In spreading the sewage over the lawn or in distributing it on the surface, due regard must be paid to the kind of soil. Clay soils and peaty soils are useless for the purpose [Pg 216] of sewage disposal unless as the result of continuous cultivation a few inches of top soil may have accumulated on the clay. This top soil is adapted to sewage purification, provided the quantity applied is not excessive.

*Surface application on land.*

Two methods of operation may be pointed out. The sewage (and this is the simplest method of disposal possible) may be brought to the upper edge of a small piece of ground, usually sowed to grass, and allowed merely to run out over the surface of the ground. There should be, however, some method of alternating plots of ground, one with another, so that the sewage is turned from one to the other every day. Each plot will then have one day's application of sewage and one day's rest, and this would complete the disposal, were it not for the interference of rain and cold. The winter season practically puts a stop to this method of treatment, and rainy weather reduces the power of the soil to absorb sewage. For these two reasons, it is desirable to have one plot in reserve, or three in all, and the area of each plot should be based on the amount of sewage contributed. For a family of ten persons using twenty-five gallons of water per day the total area provided should be one tenth of one acre, or an area seventy feet square divided into three plots. Figure 67 shows six beds arranged to care for the sewage of a public institution in Massachusetts. As a guide to the amount of land needed, it will be safe to provide at the rate of one acre for each forty persons where the soil is a well-worked loam but underlaid with clay. The effect of this irrigation on the grass will be to induce a heavy, rank growth which must be kept down by repeated cutting or by constant grazing. Both [Pg 217] methods are practiced in England, and it may be said in passing that no injury to stock from the feeding of such sewage-grown grass has been recorded. The grass cut from such areas (and the cutting is done every two weeks through the whole summer) is packed into silos and fed to cattle through the winter with advantage. Or, if grazing is resorted to to keep the grass down, the herd is alternated with the sewage from one field to the other, so that the bed which has received sewage one week is used for pasture the next week, and the number of head which can thus be fed is astonishing. In order to secure an even flow of sewage over such grass land as is here contemplated, there must be a gentle slope to the field, and the ditch or drain bringing the sewage to the field should run along its upper side. Openings from the drain, controlled by simple stop planks, are provided at intervals of about ten feet, and no attention is needed further than the opening and closing of these admission gates.

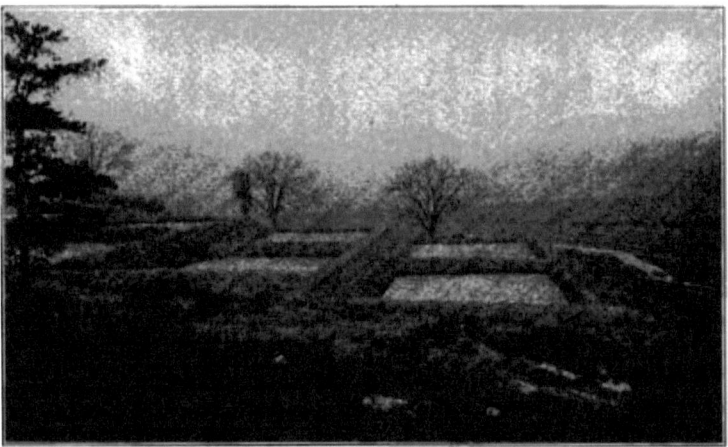

Fig. 67.—Sewage beds.

[Pg 218]

Another method of applying sewage to the surface of the ground is to lead it in channels between narrow beds on which vegetables have grown. These beds are made about eight feet wide with two rows of root crops, such as turnips or beets, set back about two feet from the edge. The beds are made by properly plowing, the channels between the beds being back-furrowed. Here, again, the principle of intermittent application is essential, and the area to be provided is the same as already given for the surface irrigation. Three beds should be provided, as before; but, in general, no provision need be made for carrying off the sewage at the lower end of the beds, since it may be safely assumed that all of the sewage will be absorbed [Pg 219] by the soil. Of course, a sandy soil will absorb more water than a clay soil, and if the soil is entirely clay, it is not suitable for such treatment. Sewage passed over the surface of clay soil, however, will, in the course of a few months, so modify the clay as to convert it into a loam, and in this way increase its absorptive power.

When possible, it is desirable to have a plot of plowed ground over which the sewage may pass before reaching the beds, so that the grosser impurities may be left behind and harrowed in or plowed under. If proper regard is paid to intermittent application, no danger from odors need be feared, and the repeated plowing in will increase immensely the fertility of the soil. Nor need one be afraid that all of the manurial elements will be left behind on this plowed ground. About two thirds of the organic matter in sewage is in solution, and this will be carried onto the beds just as if passage over the plowed ground had not occurred.

*Artificial sewage beds.*

In order to secure a higher rate of discharge of sewage through the soil it is best to arrange an artificial bed which shall be made of coarse, sandy material which will allow a rate of at least 10 times that already given. The best material out of which to make such an artificial bed is a coarse sand; that is, a sand whose particles will not pass through a sieve which has 60 meshes to the inch and which would pass through a sieve of 10 meshes to the inch. Such an ideal sand will purify sewage at the rate of 50,000 gallons per acre per day, or an acre will take care of the sewage of at least 1000 persons. This means that it is necessary to provide about 50 square feet for each person [Pg 220] in the family, or a family of 10 persons could have all the sewage taken care of on an area 25 feet square. The same principle of intermittency of application, however, must be observed by dividing the bed into three parts, so that the sewage may be alternated from one bed to another. Practice has indicated that it is better to shift from bed to bed about once a week and to deliver the sewage onto each bed intermittently; that is, to discharge a bucketful at a time with short intervals between, rather than to allow a small stream to flow continuously onto a bed. Such a bed should be about 3 feet deep, as already stated, and preferably should have light concrete side walls and bottom, as shown in the sketch (Fig. 68). Ordinarily, the surface of the sand will be level, and the dose of sewage applied to the bed will cover it a fraction of an inch deep, and in the course of an hour or so will disappear into the sand and reappear in the underdrains as clear water.

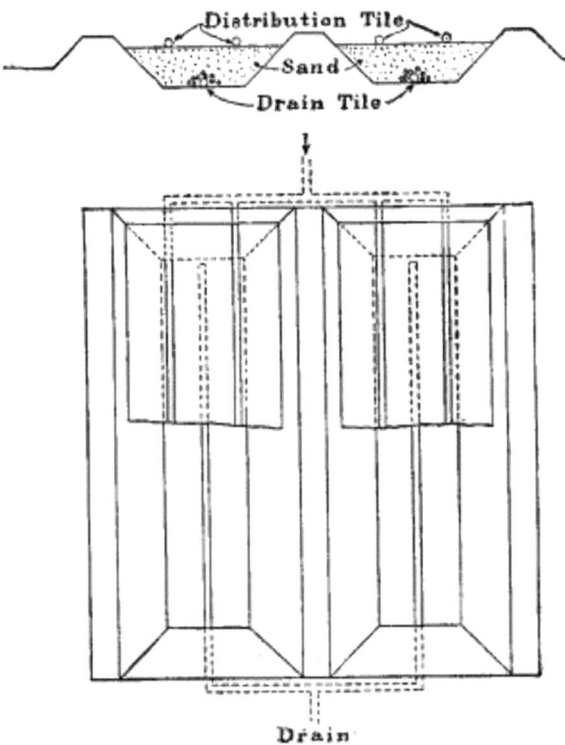

Fig. 68.—

Sewage beds.

[Pg 221]

In cold weather a thin sheet of sewage spread out over the surface of the sand would freeze before penetrating the bed; therefore, in the winter time, it is usual to furrow the beds; that is, dig furrows across the beds 2 or 3 inches wide at the bottom and about 10 inches deep, so that in the bottom of these furrows the sewage may be, partly at least, protected against frost. It has been found that, if sewage is discharged intermittently,—that is, in bucketfuls into such furrows,—the beds open and allow the filtration of the sewage. To be sure, the purification effected in cold weather is not quite that accomplished in warm weather, but the results are sufficiently satisfactory, and no nuisance ensues.

*Subsurface tile disposal.*

The other method of distributing sewage over land is by means of draintile placed in shallow trenches, so that the sewage may leach out into the soil through the open joints of the pipe. These draintiles receive the sewage intermittently, and by the constant rush of water are presumably filled throughout their length. The sewage then gradually works out of the joints into the surrounding soil, and the pipes are empty and ready to receive another dose when next delivered. [Pg 222]

Two essential points must be considered in the successful operation of such a plant: the grade of the tile and the length of the tile.

The grade of the tile must be properly adjusted to the porosity of the soil; that is, in open, porous, and gravelly soils a grade must be steeper than in loamy and dense soils. The reason is manifest. In a gravel soil, the sewage is at first rapidly absorbed, so that as the sewage goes down the pipe line the first joints take up the water and deliver it to the soil, where it disappears, and probably no flow reaches the end of the line at all. This means that the soil surrounding the first joints does the work which the entire pipe line was intended to do and thus becomes overworked. When overworked, the soil always refuses to do anything, so that when the succeeding joints take up the sewage and in their turn become overworked, the line is useless. If, on the other hand, the grade had been steep enough to carry the sewage down the pipe line gradually so as to secure a uniform distribution, then the same or approximately the same amount of sewage would be taken out of the pipe at each joint, securing a long life for the system. In loamy soil, on the contrary, there is not the same absorption at the joints, and so on a steep grade there is the tendency for all the sewage to follow down the pipe line to the lower end and there escape to clog the soil and thus spoil the system. As a general average, it may be said that the proper grade for such a subsurface distribution pipe line in a fairly good sandy loam should be 5 inches in 100 feet; less than this as the loam becomes clay and more as the loam becomes gravel.

The other essential point for the successful operation [Pg 223] of this method of distribution is to provide a proper length of pipe for the number of persons contributing sewage. The soil itself will absorb about the same amount as when the sewage is spread over the surface, so that a family of ten persons would require, as before, an area about 70 feet square. The pipe lines may be laid in different sections, provided the different lines of pipe are not nearer together than 10 feet. On an area 70 feet square there would be, therefore, 7 lines of pipe each 70 feet long, or 490 lineal feet of pipe in all, or 49 feet per person. The writer generally allows 40 feet in well-cultivated soil as a reasonable length of pipe for each person in the family. If the soil is sandy, this may be reduced one half, but need not be increased under any conditions, since a soil requiring a greater length of pipe than 40 feet per person would be so dense as to be unfit for use. To properly arrange the lines of pipe on a sloping ground requires careful study of the inclination of the ground and of the relation of direction of lines of pipe to slope. Usually the slope of the ground is greater than the 5 inches per 100 feet just referred to, but by laying out the lines of pipe across the slope instead of with it any grade desired may be obtained. Nor is it necessary that these lines of draintile be run in straight lines; they may very properly follow the curving slope, the proper grade being always carefully maintained. [Pg 224]

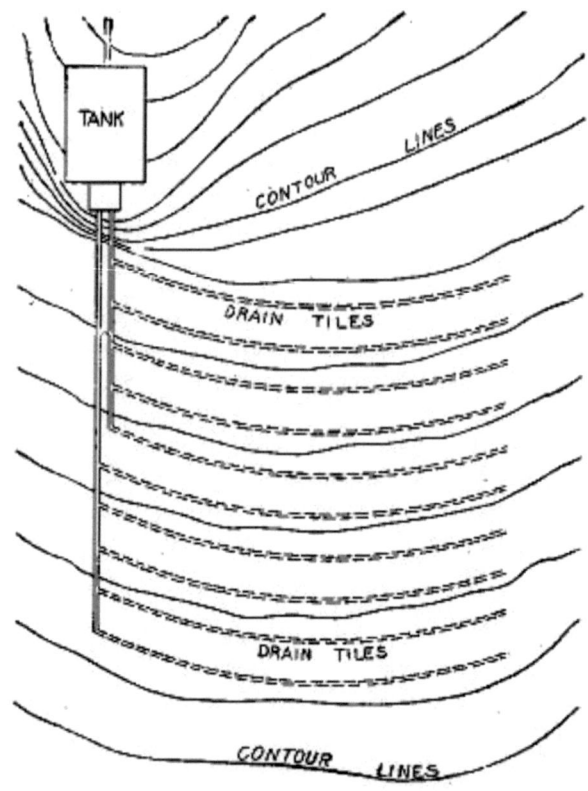

Fig. 69. —
Plan of subsurface irrigation field.

Common agricultural tiles three inches in diameter and costing about two cents per running foot are suitable material for these distribution lines. The sewage enters these distribution lines from a larger pipe, usually six inches in diameter, and a difficult adjustment is presented that each branch tile line shall receive its own proportionate share of the sewage. If only one line of tile is provided, say 200 feet long for 5 members in the family, then all the sewage goes into that line with no question of distribution arising, but if a number of short parallel lines must be used, as shown in the sketch (Fig. 69), the difficulty of subdividing the sewage properly among the different branch lines becomes very great. For that reason the writer prefers to use not more than two lines, with the [Pg

225] possibility of delivering the sewage alternately in the one and the other. In this way, the bed not receiving sewage is resting, while the other bed is acting, and also the outlet for the sewage is always definitely known. And particularly in the case of these subsurface tile, the necessity for the intermittent dosing is apparent, since with small, constant trickling discharges the difficulty of distribution through the long length of tile is gradually increased, and usually saturation of the soil occurs from joint to joint, as already described. Therefore it becomes most necessary, in this case, for the best results on the soil not merely to alternate the beds receiving sewage, but also to effect the intermittent discharge onto the beds or through the pipes although the sewage itself may flow very uniformly in volume.

*Automatic syphon.*

This intermittent discharge is accomplished by constructing on the pipe line from the house and before it reaches the beds an "automatic syphon," as it is called, the operation of which may be described as follows: As the sewage enters the tank containing the syphon and rises outside the syphon-bell, air is compressed between the water surface inside the bell and the water left inside the syphon-leg. With greater and greater height of water outside, this compression inside becomes greater and forces the water in the syphon-leg lower and lower. Finally, the water sinks so low as to allow the compressed air to escape suddenly around this bend, instantly relieving the compression, and the water outside rushing in to fill up the space occupied by the air starts the syphon (see Fig. 70). [Pg 226]

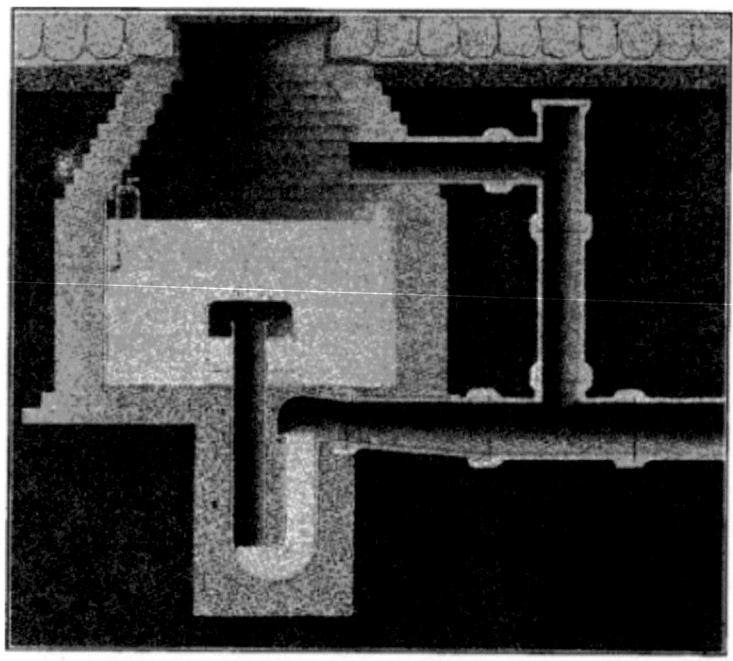

Fig. 70.—Section of "Miller" syphon.

This syphon, in size suitable for a single house, costs about $12 delivered, and will always be available to secure an intermittent dosing of the bed or pipe line. Usually the chamber in which this syphon is placed holds about one hour's flow, so that it may be estimated that this syphon will discharge on the bed every sixty minutes. The exact interval of time is not essential nor, perhaps, important, although it may be noted that the coarser the material,— that is, the nearer uniform all the sand particles are to the largest size passing the ten-mesh size,—the smaller must be the dose applied, but the more frequently [Pg 227] must the application be made. This has been very thoroughly studied in Massachusetts, and the views of experts on this subject may be found in the report of that Board.

Such an intermittent discharge may be made and often is made by a hand valve leading out from this chamber in institutions or in private houses where some one constantly is available for the purpose. Thus it becomes the duty of the man in charge every hour or perhaps three times a day to pull the valve and allow the sewage to discharge (see Fig. 71). An overflow pipe should always be provided, so that if he forgets to pull the valve, the sewage will still find its way into the system rather than out on the ground.

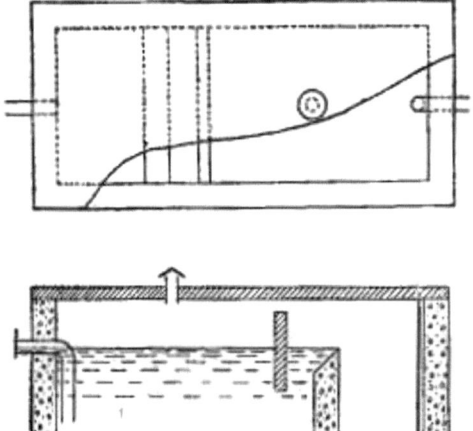

Fig. 71.—Plan and section of a septic tank with valve.

*Sedimentation.*

As a matter of economy of operation, it has been found desirable to take out from the sewage before the treatment already described as much of the solid matter as may be reasonably done, and for this purpose sedimentation is made use of. Most of the solids in sewage are slightly heavier than water, so that if they be allowed to stand in the water for a short length of [Pg 228] time, they will settle to the bottom of the tank and allow the liquid above to pass on, considerably clarified. It has been found worth while to do this, since all three processes described are interfered with if the solids taken out by sedimentation are allowed to be deposited either upon the surface of the ground, giving rise to odors as well as to objectionable appearances, or onto the surface of the sand beds, which they clog up, or in the three-inch tile drain, which may be filled in a short time.

It has been further found by experience that if these sedimentation tanks are made large, really larger than necessary for sedimentation, in some way a large proportion of the matter accumulating in the tank will disappear, so that the amount of sediment to be taken out of the tank is not as large as might be expected. In fact it is usual for such tanks to run one or two years without cleaning, although the amount of solids shown by chemical analysis to have been removed from the sewage would fill the tank twice over.

It has been found that a tank, in order to do successful work in separating solids and in eliminating as much as possible of the sediment, needs to be of a capacity to equal about one day's flow of the sewage, and this is a good basis for computation. Here, again, the fact that the sewage from a single house is considerably fresher than the sewage from a city must be remembered, since, while many cities build tanks holding only one third or one fourth of their daily flow with good results, in the case of a single house this is not possible, and the tanks, if built at all, ought to hold at least the full day's flow. Ten persons, at 25 gallons each, furnish 250 gallons per day or 33 cubic [Pg 229] feet. The tank, then, must be large enough to hold this volume, and suitable proportions generally require that the tank be at least 5 times as long as wide. A certain allowance must always be made for deposit in the bottom and for the accumulation of scum on the top, so that an extra foot or more of depth is desirable. The tank, then, to furnish the required 33 feet, might be made 3 feet wide, 3 feet deep, and 5 feet long, and probably in no case would a tank much smaller than this be used.

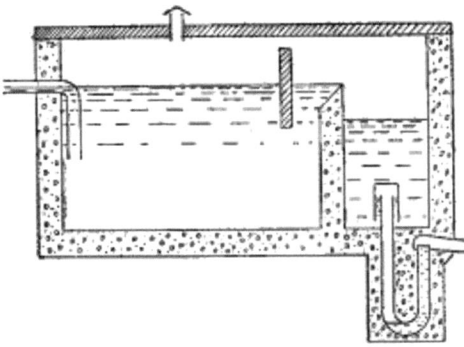

Fig 72.—Section of a septic tank with syphon chamber.

There are two or three details of tank construction which may be suggested, although almost any kind of tank will answer the purpose. It is desirable in order that the surface scum may not be disturbed, and in order that the inflowing sewage may distribute itself as uniformly as possible across the tank, to attach an elbow to the entering pipe so that the sewage enters about halfway between the top and bottom of the tank (see Fig. 72). Similarly, at the outlet or weir an elbow should be provided because it is not desirable to allow the floating matter of the surface to be carried onto the bed, and a pipe taking off liquid, open halfway between top and bottom, will carry away but little of either the surface scum or bottom sediment. Such a tank must be built of concrete or masonry or timber, although the latter is not [Pg 230] to be recommended because of its short life. The walls of an ordinary tank may be built 6 inches thick at the top and 12 inches to 18 inches thick at the bottom, the latter being necessary if the depth is over 8 feet. The tank should have 6 inches of concrete on the bottom, and the roof may be made of flagstone or of concrete slabs in which some wire mesh has been buried.

It is not necessary to ventilate this tank, although it is desirable to have perhaps a foot of air-space between the water level and the roof of the tank. During the first few months of its operation such a tank is very likely to smell badly, and, if ventilators are provided, the presence of the tank will be well known by the odors sent off. After the tank has been in operation two or three months these odors gradually disappear, due presumably to the fact that the surface of the water in the tank has become coated with a thick blanket through which odors cannot penetrate. On the other hand, there have been a few cases recorded where the production of gas in a septic tank was so great that an explosion occurred, tearing off the roof and otherwise doing considerable damage.

The full plant, therefore, will consist of the settling tank, receiving the raw sewage from the house and discharging it into a small tank holding about one hour's flow and containing the automatic syphon apparatus for intermittent discharge. This dosing tank must provide for one hour's flow at the maximum rate of flow, and should hold about one fourth of the total daily flow. Then the ground area, either natural or artificial, which receives the intermittent discharge from the dosing tank, completes the installation (see Fig. 73). [Pg 231]

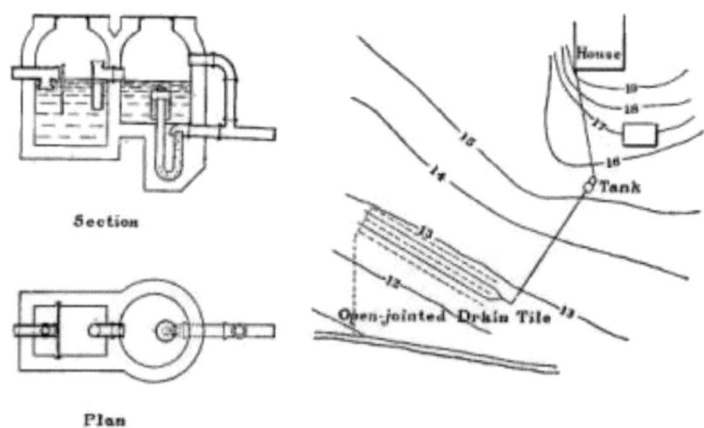

Section

Plan

DETAILS of TANK

Fig. 73.—Plan of sewage disposal for single house with details of receiving tank.

*Underdrains.*

The question of installing underdrains will arise only in cases where the ground water, always to be found below the surface somewhere, comes up so high as to affect the disposal of sewage. Usually no underdrains will be needed unless the ground water gets up to within three feet of the surface, and, in a number of cases, underdrains have been laid under a sewage filter at considerable expense, only to find when the filter was in operation that they were never in use. In clay soils the underdrain is not necessary. In fact, it may be noticed that the underdrain is not for the purpose of taking care of the sewage, but rather of draining off the soil-water and preventing its interference [Pg 232] with the action of soil on sewage. This principle will indicate where underdrains are necessary and where not.

When used, underdrains should be laid from three to four feet below the surface in parallel lines about fifteen feet apart and on grades of not less than one foot in one hundred. It is always better to have the underdrains too large than too small, and drains less than three inches in diameter should not be used, and they should increase in size to four inches and then to six inches as the separate drains are brought together. The writer has seen a six-inch underdrain running full of ground water collected within a distance of a hundred feet, but this was in gravel soil through which the water passed very freely. No exact rules can be given for the size of the underdrains, but it will be noticed that, since water passes through clay soil slowly and through gravel soil rapidly, larger pipes must be used where the soil is coarse.

[Pg 233]

## CHAPTER XI

# PREPARATION AND CARE OF MILK AND MEAT

Milk has long been considered to be one of the most important human foods, particularly for the young, combining within itself all the essential elements necessary for the production of cell tissue and for animal vitality. In composition, it is about 87 per cent water, the remaining 13 per cent being divided between fat, casein, and sugar in equal parts, with a small addition of salt.

As is well known, milk is the sole food upon which it is possible to sustain life for long periods, and while this applies directly to infants, it is by no means confined to them. Many examples can be given of men and women of mature life who, either on account of some digestive disorder or some mental bias, have confined themselves absolutely to a diet of about two quarts of milk a day and have lived thereon for months and years without suffering from lack of nutrition.

In recent years, due to the advocacy of the eminent scientist, Metchnikoff, who asserts that researches in the Pasteur Institute have shown that certain diseases of advanced age are due to auto-intoxication from the larger [Pg 234] intestine and that the consumption of fermented milk acts as an antiseptic, neutralizing this bacterial intoxication, the consumption of fermented milk, or buttermilk, or koumiss, has very largely increased. It is, in fact, rather remarkable to find that in large cities, business men whose digestions have been ruined are devoting themselves to unlimited quantities of buttermilk in the hope that their former excesses and absurdities in the way of food may be counteracted and health restored.

Between these two extremes — the use of milk for the very young and for the aged and infirm — milk plays an important part as food. The consumption of milk in New York State, according to statistics, amounts to about a pint a day for each person for that part of the country. As an article of food, milk has the advantage already referred to, namely, that besides its nutritive power it has a curative effect greatly augmented by fermentation, the modification so vigorously advocated by Metchnikoff. Another advantage which milk possesses as an article of food is that, by sterilization and storage in closed vessels, it may be kept for days and even months in good condition. At the time of the Paris Exposition, milk was sent from America and exhibited alongside of French milk with no preservatives except heat used for removing the bacteria in the milk and then cold storage for keeping others out, and two weeks after the original bottling the milk was in good condition. To meet the need of ailing babies, advantage was taken of this valuable property of milk, by which it could be shipped from dairies near New York to the Isthmus of Panama, and used continually with good results although more than a week old. [Pg 235]

*Bacteria in milk.*

The great disadvantage which milk sustains as an article of food is that the same composition that makes it so useful as a diet for man, also renders it a most admirable culture medium for the rapid development of all kinds of bacteria. Some of these bacteria are, without doubt, benign in their effect upon man; as, for example, the particular species used to produce koumiss and other varieties of fermented milk now recommended by physicians. But there are many other kinds of bacteria that find life in milk congenial, whose effect upon the human system is not salutary, and, if milk infected with those varieties is used for feeding infants, the result is quite likely to be a disturbance of their digestive system, producing diarrhea and cholera infantum and possibly death.

It was at one time common to add to milk certain antiseptics for the purpose of preventing the growth of bacteria, and, except that the preservatives acted quite as injuriously upon man as upon the bacteria, the results, so far as merely keeping the milk went, were all that could be desired. The chemicals added were borax, boracic acid, salicilic acid, sodium carbonate, and other similar disinfectants. Gradually, however, it has come to be known that, inasmuch as the milk when first drawn from the cow's udder is sterile, that is, contains no bacteria, and since it is quite possible to prevent the introduction of bacteria into milk during the processes of milking, straining, and bottling, there is no need of the addition of preservatives, provided particular care is exercised in handling the milk.

*Effects of bacteria.*

Since this care involves the expenditure of both additional [Pg 236] time and money, questions at once arise whether such expenditure is necessary, whether the introduction of a few bacteria into the milk is objectionable, and what the results are upon the persons drinking milk containing bacteria. For our present purpose, the kinds of bacteria which find their way into milk may be divided into two classes, namely, those that are normally in milk and which tend to produce souring, and those which accidentally enter and are able to produce disease in persons drinking the milk. The first kind probably enter the milk from the air or from the surface of the milk-pail, and in the milk increase in numbers very rapidly and have the same effect in the milk and on persons drinking the milk as any large amount of organic matter.

The second kind of bacteria are known as pathogenic; that is, are the direct cause of disease when taken into the human system. Under ordinary circumstances, this latter class will not be found in milk, since these kinds of bacteria must come from some infected person, and if no such person is in contact with the milk at any stage, then it is impossible for the milk to become so polluted. However, those interested in preventing the spread of disease through polluted milk argue that if the conditions in a stable and dairy are so unclean that large numbers of the normal milk bacteria can enter the milk and increase in numbers there, then conditions would be favorable for the introduction of pathogenic bacteria whenever the milker or bottle-washer or the strainer or any of the helpers became sick.

To show the difference in the effect of a clean stable and dairy as compared with an ordinary one, it is only necessary to say that in investigating the quality of the [Pg 237] milk supply of a certain city recently, the writer found one stable where the milk analyses showed from half a million to a million bacteria per c.c., [2] — that is, per half-teaspoonful, — and this was occurring in the dairy regularly from month to month as the analyses were made. Another stable in the same city showed just as regularly a bacterial count in the milk of from 1000 to 5000 per c.c., the difference being due solely to the way in which the stables and dairies were kept, — in the one case with no regard to cleanliness and in the other with the very best attention paid thereto. Certainly, if dirt is so much in evidence that a million bacteria can enter the milk in every c.c., no particular pains can be taken in such a stable to keep out disease germs; while in the clean stable, where so few germs enter, disease germs could hardly find any opportunity for lodgment.

The following example may be given to indicate the effect of impure milk upon a community. The vital statistics of the city of Rochester, including the deaths of children under five years, show that from 1889 to 1896, during the summer, infants died at the rate of 109 per 100,000 population. The health officer of the city undertook to improve the quality of the milk, and from 1896 to 1905, statistics show that the number of children dying, under five years, was only at the rate of 54 per 100,000,—a manifest saving due, without doubt, to the improvement in the quality of the milk. By repeated examinations of the dairies, by rigid enforcement of certain rules governing the distribution of milk, and by detailed lessons to [Pg 238] mothers in the tenement-house districts on the care of milk, the quality of the milk was so improved as to make the reduction in the death-rate already pointed out.

The Honorable Nathan Strauss, of New York City, has taken up the same idea, and, by supplying the poor with milk properly heated so as to destroy the bacteria which may have been introduced by careless handling, has also saved hundreds of thousands of children from premature death.

*Diseases caused by milk.*

Many infectious diseases are propagated by milk, not only among children, whose chief food is found in this supply, but also among those of more mature age who, though drinking only a small quantity, are apparently more easily affected. Four diseases are particularly to be noted in connection with the consumption of milk, namely, typhoid fever, scarlet fever, diphtheria, and tuberculosis.

*Typhoid fever from milk.*

One of the most striking illustrations of the spread of typhoid fever through milk occurred this last year in the city of Ithaca, New York. The city proper lies in a valley between two hills, the milkmen having their farms on both sides of the valley to the east and west, on the hill slopes. One milkman on the west, with a large route, delivered his own milk only in part and bought an additional supply from a farmer on the east. In the family of the latter occurred a case of typhoid fever in September, pronounced by the local physician to be sunstroke, but evidently typhoid fever, since other cases of secondary infection developed in the same family and were then pronounced typhoid. The milk from this east-side farm [Pg 239] was taken down the hillside and turned over to the west-side farmer, who distributed his own milk in his trip from his farm across the valley, his route being so timed as to allow him thus to dispose of all his own milk. Having then loaded up with the east-side supply, he started back across the valley, distributing the milk which was evidently polluted, since on his return route house after house developed typhoid fever, with no cases on the first part of the route and with no other cases in town except those on this milk route. Forty-four cases developed in all, with two deaths.

The Reports of the Massachusetts State Board of Health give a number of cases of the same sort, all showing that milk is easily infected by persons suffering from even mild attacks of typhoid fever, attacks so slight as perhaps not to be recognized or to be worth submitting to a physician, but which are responsible for bacteria passing from the hands or mouth to a can cover or ladle, and so to the milk.

*Diphtheria.*

Diphtheria seems to be well established as a disease transmissible by milk, although its occurrence is not so frequent as that of typhoid fever. Not long since, the writer was much interested in an epidemic of this sort described by a physician who was convinced that the bacteria responsible for the mild form of the disease occurred largely in the nose and throat passages. He noted that as the result of these growths a constant exudation from both passages was present, and that a man with this disease, working over the milk, might easily allow the milk to be polluted by this exudate dropping from his nose. [Pg 240]

The result was a general distribution of a mild form of diphtheria among those using the milk.

*Scarlet fever.*

Many examples have also been given of the distribution of scarlet fever through the agency of milk, the specific contagion probably being discharged by the patient from his nostrils, mouth, or from the dry particles of skin so characteristic of this disease. Unfortunately, mild cases of scarlatina are very apt to occur, so mild that a physician is not called in, and the only positive proof of the disease consists in the subsequent "peeling," although the nasal passages may have been alive with germs.

*Tuberculosis.*

So far as tuberculosis is concerned, nothing seems to be definitely proved. There is little fear of milk becoming infected from tuberculous patients or of the disease being transmitted through milk from one person to another, as with the three other diseases mentioned. The possibility of infection here lies in the fact that a cow, like man, is susceptible to tuberculosis as a disease, and undergoes the same course of prolonged suffering and death. The interesting question is whether the disease may be transmitted from a cow to a man through the cow's milk. With all the refinements suggested by science as to the virulence of the disease thus transmitted, with a study of the comparative symptoms of the two diseases, of the progress of the disease in the cow when the germs are found in the milk, and of the possibility of eliminating these germs by heating or otherwise, the danger from diseased cows is still unsettled.

So far as present knowledge goes, it is probably conservative [Pg 241] to say that although tests made on cows by inoculation with tuberculin show that a large proportion of the animals in the various dairy herds are more or less affected by tuberculosis, yet only a small proportion of the milk from such cows shows the presence of the tuberculosis bacillus. So far as statistics can be given on this subject, it seems probable that not more than ten per cent of the cows reacting under the tuberculin test would show tubercular bacilli in the milk, or would develop tubercular reactions if the milk were used in inoculations. The reason for this is probably that the tubercular growth in the cow does not naturally attack the milk glands until the disease is well advanced, and when the general appearance of the cow indicates severe illness, so that any careful milkman would not use the particular milk, even if the milk flow did not cease. It is not reasonable to assume that all milk from tubercular cows is itself infected, nor yet that all children drinking milk so infected will contract the disease. But the mere possibility of demonstrating that a small percentage of tubercular cows will cause human tuberculosis is sufficient to justify all possible precautions against tubercular animals and against the distribution of tubercular milk. In this connection it is worth while noting that the cows most affected by tuberculosis are those confined in small crowded stables, with no fresh air, with no exercise, and with insufficient or improper food. Unfortunately it is not possible to trace the connection between the particular animal responsible for the disease in a human being, since the period required for the development of the disease is so great that the possible time of onset is forgotten and the cause of the disease entirely out of mind. [Pg 242]

It can only be said, therefore, that laboratory experiments have demonstrated the presence of the tuberculosis bacillus in milk from tubercular cows, and that this bacillus is known to produce tubercular lesions in man. It is wise, therefore, to eliminate the milk of tubercular cows if healthy milk is to be provided.

*Methods of obtaining clean milk.*

Aside from the infection of milk by specific disease-producing bacteria, the milkman of to-day must be very careful to avoid a milk which shall contain large numbers of bacteria of any type which, while not producing any specific disease, nevertheless causes changes in the chemical composition of the milk, which make it at the same time unfit as an article of food for individuals and shows the possibility of other kinds of infection.

There are two axioms to be followed if good clean milk is to be produced, and those are that the milking and straining shall be done in clean stables, from clean cows, by clean persons; and the other that the milk shall be cooled to a temperature of fifty degrees or less as soon as received from the cow. Neither of these requirements is difficult to attain, but they constitute the sole reason why some milk contains a million or more bacteria and other milk less than a thousand; and it is quite possible by enforcing these two requirements to change the number of bacteria in milk from the large figure to the small one.

Probably it is in the stable where the cows are milked that the most important factor in producing large numbers of bacteria is to be found. Not long ago the writer saw a number of stables, the ceilings of which were poles on which the winter supply of hay was stored and the atmosphere [Pg 243] was noticeably dust-laden. A good milk could not be furnished from such a stable, and therefore it may be set down as the first requirement that the ceiling of the stable should be entirely dust-tight. Some of the best stables in the country for this reason have no loft of any sort above the cattle, but if the ceiling is tight, — that is, made with tongue-and-groove boards and then painted, — there can be no objection to the storage of hay in the loft. Hay should not be taken from the loft or fed to the cows just before milking, because the very moving of a forkful of hay through the air of the stable stirs up so large a number of bacteria in the air that quantities of them will later fall into the milk-pail.

*Light and air* in a stable are both important, not so much for the quality of the milk as for the health of the cows that furnish the milk. Ventilation and sunlight are both excellent antiseptics. The ordinary rule for the amount of window area per cow as given by the United States Department of Agriculture is four square feet of window surface. But it is not easy to definitely state any fixed amount of window area, since the value of the window is in its disinfecting power on the bacterial life of the stable, and this is greater or less as the windows receive the direct sunlight or are hidden under eaves where no sunlight reaches them.

The next factor in the production of good milk is the condition of the *walls of the stable*. Like the ceiling, they should be absolutely free from dust, and should be smooth, so that they may be brushed or even washed clean. For this reason, walls with ledges are objectionable, and all horizontal surfaces in a stable are undesirable. Tongue-and-groove [Pg 244] sheeting should never be laid horizontally, but rather vertically, and a smooth brick or concrete wall is better than wood in any case. The same care must be taken to have the floor clean and dry. A floor of saturated wood, containing millions of bacteria which are stirred up by the milker moving around, causes many of those millions to be deposited in the milk-pail. A concrete floor for the stalls and drains is the ideal construction, and both should be thoroughly cleaned morning and night, so that no dried refuse may remain as the living place for bacteria. Nor should the manure thrown from the stalls be left in the vicinity of the barn, but carried away at least 200 feet, in order that the barnyard may be kept dry and clean, that no smell from the manure may reach the milk, and that the flies which come from manure piles may be kept at least that distance from the cows.

The next factor in the production of clean milk is the *condition of the cow herself*, not in the matter of her actual health, but in the matter of the cleanliness of her skin at the time the milking is done. If the udder and sides of the cow have been coated with manure, it is certain that more or less will fall into the milk-pail at the time of milking, and the "cowy taste" of the milk is easily accounted for in this way. In a modern stable, the milkman is careful to clean the cow ten or fifteen minutes before the milking is done by sponging or washing her belly, sides, and udder with a damp cloth or with a cloth moistened with a disinfecting solution. In one set of experiments, for instance, 20,000 bacteria per c.c. were found in the milk when the cow was rubbed off before the milking and 170,000 when the preliminary cleaning was omitted. In another case, [Pg 245] milk from four dirty cows gave an average of 90,000 bacteria, while other cows of the same herd, milked by the same man, but carefully cleaned before milking, gave only 2000 per c.c. The care involved brings its own reward, and it is in most cases a lack of knowledge or an indifference to results which causes the malign effects above noted.

Only a few weeks ago, the writer watched the hired man start the milking and was disgusted to see the old-fashioned practice followed of squeezing a little milk onto the man's filthy hands and then the handful of milk rubbed around on the cow's teats to drip filthy and bacteria-laden into the milk-pail along with the milk itself.

One other factor is involved which, while scoffed at by some of the old-time farmers, has nevertheless proved its value, and that is the use of the *narrow-topped milk-pail*. It is startling when tested by bacterial growths under the two conditions to see how many more bacteria will be found in the wide open pail than in the narrow-topped one, and while, of course, some milkers may not be able to use a pail the top of which is only six inches in diameter, it is quite worth while for milkers who do not know how to use a narrow-topped pail to learn.

The size of the opening is not the whole consideration in the matter of the milk-pail. The way it is washed is even more important. If it is merely rinsed out in cold water and then washed in warm water, it is far from clean, and milk poured into such a pail and then poured out will by that process have gathered to itself thousands of bacteria. For example, some experiments have shown that milk in well-washed pails had, on the average, 28,600 [Pg 246] bacteria per c.c., while that collected in pails of the same sort under identical conditions, except that the pails had been steamed, contained only 1300 bacteria per c.c.

Perhaps the most important factor in the care of these utensils is the necessity of killing the bacteria left in them by the milk itself. Ordinary washing will not do this. Either the washing must be done with some sterilizing agent, like strong salsoda, which must then, of course, be thoroughly rinsed out, or else the inside of the pail must be filled with absolutely boiling water or with steam. The advantage of the latter is that no contamination is possible by the water itself, whereas in washing out the disinfectant the water, unless pure, contaminates the surface again. To show the effects of clean pails, an experiment was made in which milk was drawn from a cow and found to have 6000 bacteria per c.c. It was then poured rapidly from one to another of six other apparently clean pails. At the end of the sixth pouring, the milk was found to be so changed that the number of bacteria had increased to 98,000 per c.c.

The strainer for a milk-pail is preferably made of cheesecloth, since this can always be easily boiled between milkings, and so sterilized. A wire strainer through which the milk has to pass, and where the milk is often stirred by the finger of the milker to make it pass through more rapidly, is in no sense as satisfactory as cheese-cloth.

The straining should be performed as soon as each pail is filled with milk, and pails of milk should never be allowed to stand around in the barn back of the cows, but rather should be taken at once to the milk-room, where it can be strained before any further contamination takes place. [Pg 247]

Then the milk should be cooled, and this, to be effective, must be done in such a way that the temperature of the milk shall at once fall to fifty degrees or less. It is well known that a forty-quart can of milk lowered into spring water cools slowly on the outside, but that hours will pass before the inside of the can has its temperature lowered appreciably. Meanwhile, bacterial growth has started, and that milk can never be as good as when cooled quickly throughout. Special apparatus is made in which the milk is spread out in very thin sheets over a surface cooled by ice or cold water to a low temperature. In this way all the milk is at once lowered in temperature and may then be kept in spring water until time for shipment. Many examples can be given of the value of this kind of cooling. A few years ago, the Cornell University Agricultural Experiment Station determined that a certain milk when fresh contained, about 4000 bacteria per c.c., and fifteen hours later at room temperature had 270,000, and twenty-seven hours later had soured with an innumerable number of bacteria. Another part of the same milk, however, kept at fifty degrees Fahrenheit, showed absolutely no increase in bacteria for twenty-seven hours, and was still sweet with only 12,000 bacteria at the end of three days.

*City milk.*

The value of pure milk is not a matter of individual opinion on the part of the farmer, but it is a vital point with thousands and millions who are dependent upon the farmer for this life-giving food. Unfortunately, to-day the relation between the consumer and the milkman is so remote that it is almost lost sight of, and in place of the personal relationship which formerly existed, which made [Pg 248] the milkman proud of his milk and the consumer proud of her milkman, there is to-day an absolute disregard of the interests of the other side in almost all cases. Even in the smaller cities, consolidated milk companies are being established by which the former independent milkmen are bringing milk to the central station in large cans, where it is dumped into vats along with the milk from a dozen other milkmen. Some may be good and some bad, but what is the use, each one says, of my taking particular pains when my neighbor produces milk of such poor quality? The result is that it is all far from good and likely to deteriorate rather than to improve. To be sure, at the central station it is bottled and distributed to the consumer in apparently clean glass jars, but this is not the same cleanliness that one gets when the bottling is done five minutes after the milk comes from the cow.

When the milk supplied to the larger cities is furnished as in New York, the impossibility of controlling the quality of the supply becomes apparent. The farmer brings to the shipping station his two or three large cans of milk, representing the night's and morning's milkings. These are loaded on a train along with hundreds of others, a few chunks of ice are thrown on top, and the train is started for New York, from points as far as two hundred and fifty miles away, reaching the city in the early evening. There it is received and hauled to milk stations, where it is distributed in different-sized cans and bottles, and the next morning, thirty-six hours old, distributed to the babies of the city as fresh milk. Thanks to the energetic inspection practiced by the officers of the Department of Health of New York City, who have emptied hundreds of quarts of milk [Pg 249] into the city gutters merely because the temperature of the milk was higher than that prescribed, the quality of the milk is not so bad as it might be. In fact, the writer has bought apparently good milk on Long Island, shipped down from New York City, because the local supply was deficient in quantity and inferior in quality, although the latter would naturally be supposed to be fresh and the other was certainly forty-eight hours old on its receipt.

Cleanliness and care are the two watchwords for good milk, and both practices ought to be observed faithfully by the milk producer, whether he has in mind the health of his own family or the health of the dwellers in the city hundreds of miles away.

*Dangers of diseased meat.*

Next to milk, the product of the farm which has most to do with the health of those to whom farm products are sent is the meat which comes from the cows, sheep, and pigs, and makes a large part of the farmer's produce. To be sure, the amount of meat thus sent to market from the farm is by no means as great as in former years, since even the smallest village to-day has representatives of Swift and Co., Schwartzman and Sulzenberger, Jacob Dold, and others of the great western packing houses. There is still, however, a great deal of local butchering, and it is important that the farmer himself should know the characteristics of meat and should be so impressed with the dangers of diseased meat that the temptation to unload a bad carcass on the unsuspecting public may be overcome. There is nothing more certain in sanitary science than that the application of heat destroys animal parasites and micro-organisms, so that, except for diminishing the nutritive [Pg 250] value, there is comparatively little real danger in eating diseased meat when cooked, and the fearful ravages of bad ham have been largely due to occasions where the ham has been eaten raw or semi-raw.

There are two points to be noted in an animal about to be killed, namely, whether the animal is healthy, that is, free from disease, — and whether it is in proper condition, neither too young nor too old, is well-grown and well-nourished. Among the diseases to which animals are subject, some are objectionable because of the possibility of the direct transmission of their disease to those eating the flesh, while others are objectionable because the flesh is spoiled and so causes irritation in the stomach and intestines of those eating it. Among the former diseases may be mentioned trichinosis, tuberculosis, and measles of pigs. In the latter category are animals suffering from such diseases as epidemic pneumonia, foot-and-mouth disease, Texas fever, anthrax, hog cholera, and others in which a general toxic condition of the animal's system results from the disease. Toxins are thus formed in the body which may pass to the human being eating the flesh, and in this way poisons called ptomaines are produced, resulting in so-called toxic poisoning. It is not the function of this book to describe the symptoms peculiar to each of these diseases, and it is here sufficient to say that the flesh of no animal apparently suffering from any disease should be used for food.

The unhealthy animal can usually be recognized by a casual examination, without undertaking to define the specific disease from which the animal is suffering, characterized by such an examination. When sick, according [Pg 251] to Parkes, the coat of the animal is rough or standing, the nostrils are dry or covered with foam, the eyes are heavy, the tongue protrudes, the respiration is difficult, the movements are slow and uncertain, and the various organs of the body perform their functions abnormally. On the other hand, the healthy animal moves freely, has a bright eye and moist nostril and a clear skin, the respiration is not hurried and the breath has no unpleasant odor, the circulation is tranquil, and the appetite good, thirst not excessive, and, if ruminant, when in repose, chews the cud.

There is, however, one exception to this general rule, and that is in the case of tuberculosis, since the most scientific observations have failed to trace any connection between the inception of tuberculosis in man and the eating of meat from tuberculous animals, or to show any evil effects to man from eating the flesh of cows affected in the first stages of tuberculosis. The regulations of the United States Department of Agriculture on this point are as follows:——

"All carcasses affected with tuberculosis and showing emaciation shall be condemned. All other carcasses affected with tuberculosis shall be condemned, except those in which the lesions are slight, calcified, or encapsulated, and are confined to certain tissues ... and excepting also those which may ... be rendered into lard or tallow."

The regulations referred to say in substance that when the lesions occur in a single part of the body, as in the neck, liver, lungs, or in certain specified combinations, the meat may be used; but that where the lesions affect more than one or two parts of the body, the carcass must be rendered [Pg 252] at a temperature of not less than 220 degrees Fahrenheit for four hours into lard or tallow.

This really means that an animal only slightly affected with tuberculosis, where the lesions are slight and are confined to the tissues of certain organs only, may be used for food. This has been decided only after very careful reading of all known facts, and is particularly important in view of the opposition to the use of milk of tuberculous cows. The tuberculin test, on which depends the determination of tuberculosis in cows, is so delicate that a very slight lesion is sufficient to cause a reaction. The lesions are so slight as in many cases to be entirely overlooked by the ordinary butcher. The United States regulations allow such a carcass to be butchered and used for food after the cow has been condemned by the tuberculin test as a milk-producing animal. This does not mean, of course, that those parts of the body affected by the tuberculosis lesions shall be used, but, since these lesions are usually segregated, they can readily be cut out without reference to the rest of the body.

The other point to be noted in selecting or rejecting animals for slaughter is their general condition. This means that they should be of the proper weight,—that is, not emaciated, but with a proper amount of fat,—that the flesh should be firm and elastic and the skin supple. Nor should they be either too young or too old. A prominent example of the first error is in the sale of calves under three weeks old, known as "bob-veal," and while some sanitarians will not object to eating calves under three weeks old, the consensus of opinion is that to be fit for food a calf should be at least that age.

Fortunately, it is for [Pg 253] the interest of the butcher to hold the calf until it has arrived at a certain weight, and the stringent laws of most states prohibiting the sale of bob-veal make it dangerous and expensive for the farmer to slaughter young calves unless they are of the right age.

The most common example of the direct transmission of disease from animals to men is through the development of the parasite in a pig, known as "trichinosis." This disease is due to a minute worm scarcely visible to the naked eye which lives in the muscles of men, dogs, swine, and other animals, and also under other conditions in their intestines. Millions of the young trichinæ may live in the flesh of a pig without producing any particular difference in the appearance of the flesh. After four or five weeks, they become incased in small white spherical capsules which later, after a year or so, become entirely calcified. In this form they live for years in the flesh of the pig and do no harm in that condition. If, however, this flesh be eaten by man without being cooked so thoroughly as to destroy the little worm (about one twenty-fifth of an inch long) which has been living in these capsules, then they become distributed around the stomach of the person eating that flesh, enter the intestines, and attach themselves to the membranes there. They grow very rapidly, and broods of from 500 to 1000 young worms are produced from each one of the entering worms, and, since there may be a quarter of a million or more in an ounce of pork, it is not surprising that the total number deposited in the intestines from a single meal of raw pork is enough to produce great distress, characterized by vomiting and diarrhea. Fortunately, the disease is not [Pg 254] necessarily serious, since after the development of the young worms (and it is at this period when the suffering of the human patient is at its height), the worms begin to form capsules again, as in the pig, and when inclosed, are again inocuous. Professor Sedgwick says that persons in robust health may be able to survive the attack of half a million or more of these flesh worms and recover, but there is a limit to human endurance, and the numbers often contained in the muscles of man from this source are almost incredible. In some severe cases, the numbers contained in human bodies have been estimated by reliable authorities to be as high as forty to sixty millions. Not long ago, the writer was impressed with the severity of this disease by having brought to his attention an epidemic in a herd of swine caused, presumably, by feeding waste which contained rinds of Western pork, infected with trichinæ and many examples may be found of regular epidemics caused by persons eating raw ham infected with this disease. Fortunately the means of prevention is very simple and implies merely the thorough cooking of the meat. If persons will avoid eating raw or underdone swine flesh in any of its varieties, no danger need be apprehended.

In general, it should be remembered that any animals dying of diseases are not fit for food, and this applies to all animals, from the largest to the smallest. Animals dying by accident, of course, are exceptions, but if diseased animals, animals dying a natural death, and animals out of condition are eliminated, the quality of food supplied from any individual farm may be approved so far as the animal itself is concerned. [Pg 255]

*The slaughter-house.*

There is, however, the further question of the sanitary condition of the slaughter-house and the care of the meat after being dressed. It may be that one gets accustomed to the sight of the filthy barns or out-houses so often used for slaughtering. Places infected with flies and other insects, overrun with rats, and the effluvia of which is easily noticeable at a distance of half a mile, are not uncommon and suggest their own condemnation. While it is not possible to directly associate any particular disease with such a condition of the slaughter-house, yet such conditions must result in a rapid development of putrefactive bacteria, in the deposit by flies of different microorganisms brought from the festering heaps of offal and manure in the vicinity, and must prevent the maintenance of the flesh in the clean and wholesome condition in which it may have been up to the time of hanging in such a place. A well-kept slaughter-house will have the ceilings, side walls, and partitions frequently painted, or else scrubbed and washed. The floor of the building, particularly, should be made water-tight, with proper drains so that the blood shall not remain on the floor to saturate the wood and develop decay. An abundance of clean water should be provided, so that the area may be thoroughly washed as often as used, with proper drains provided for carrying away the dirty water. The ventilation of the building should be complete, and provision should be made for lifting and moving carcasses without handling.

In most small slaughter-houses, the obnoxious practice prevails of maintaining a herd of swine to consume the entrails of the slaughtered animals, and a more fearsome [Pg 256] and disgusting spectacle than a dozen lean, active hogs fighting over recently deposited entrails and wallowing up to their bellies in filth can hardly be imagined. Nor is this any fanciful picture. The writer has seen it over and over again, the income from the hogs thus fed being one of the principal assets of the establishment. Such hog meat is not fit for food. The refuse from the slaughter-house ought to be carried away and buried; its fertilizing value will not be lost if it be put in the garden, and the effect of the prompt removal of this refuse will be to improve the character of the entire slaughter-house.

## FOOTNOTES:

[2] c.c. = cubic centimeter, or centister. A centimeter is about 2/5 of an inch (.3937). 1 cubic inch is about 16-1/2 c.c.

[Pg 257]

## CHAPTER XII

# *FOODS AND BEVERAGES*

Before discussing the question of suitable foods for individual needs or the ill-health which is so likely to follow an unrestrained or unwise diet, it will be well to trace briefly the passage of food through the human body, with the various changes which take place in its mass from the time it enters the mouth *until* it is absorbed by the stomach.

*The human mechanism.*

In a little book by Hough and Sedgwick entitled "The Human Mechanism," the authors point out that in many respects the human body is like any machine developing energy by the conversion of certain kinds of raw material. Thus, as the steam engine will use up coal in the development of mechanical energy, so the human body will absorb food and convert it into vital energy, and it is quite as important that the human body shall have its source of energy properly adjusted to its needs as that the steam engine shall be fired with coal possessing a reasonable amount of heat-producing particles.

The human body requires this supply of raw material for several different purposes. In the first place, the very fact of living uses up each minute a number of cells of various kinds in various organs. Each breath taken, [Pg 258] each heart beat, each muscular motion, all tend to the destruction of tissue and involve its reconstruction. Violent exercise uses up cell tissue very rapidly, so much so that a football player will commonly lose from five to ten pounds in weight during a well-contested game. It is a fundamental principle of training for any athletic event involving hard exercise, that suitable food in large quantities must be provided, and a young man training for football or rowing will eat beefsteak, eggs, and other hearty food to an astonishing amount, all of it going chiefly to repairing worn-out and used-up tissue.

In the second place, food is needed to supply material for growth, and so it is that a growing boy eats out of all proportion to his size, and the fact that he seems to be, as it is said, hollow clear to his feet, is only his rational endeavor to supply the material needed for his growing body.

In the third place, food must be supplied for the work to be done by the body, as distinguished from the loss of tissue due to the performance of the work, and finally, food must be provided in order to maintain the bodily temperature, a larger amount being naturally required where the difference between the temperature of the body and the outside air is very great, as in the Arctic regions.

The human body being a special kind of machine, the raw material supplied must be adapted to the needs of the machine, and while a lump of coal admirably supplies energy for a steam boiler, no one would think of feeding a lump of coal to a human being, simply because, by experience, we know that suitable energy is not thereby developed. In the matter of suitability of foods, much depends [Pg 259] upon the local supply. It is not to be supposed, for example, that the Eskimos eat meat and fat altogether because it is the best article of food for them, but rather because it is the only food available. It would be foolish to prescribe fresh fruit or even white bread for the Eskimos because it is out of the question for them to get such food. But, in general, it is possible for the average individual to choose his supply of raw material in accordance with the needs which his experience has pointed out and with the teachings of scientific investigators on this subject. Raw material, however, is not converted into energy by any simple operation. The human body is made capable of taking raw material of most varied kinds and transforming it into nutriment capable of being absorbed by the system and made over into cell tissue. It will be worth while to indicate the steps of this complex process.

*Digestive processes.*

The mouth plays the first part in the scheme of transformation, and here two operations are performed. First the food is crushed and ground by the teeth, exactly as when, in some chemical processes, a fine grinding is essential for the subsequent transformation. In this country, this preliminary process is often sadly neglected, so much so that a distinguished investigator, named Horace Fletcher, has, within the last few years, established a school for the cultivation of the habit of chewing, with the idea that if this practice could be encouraged and at least twenty chews taken with every mouthful, the health of the individual would be vastly improved and sick persons even cured merely through this practice.

The other function of the mouth is to mix with the food [Pg 260] the saliva which drops from small glands in the back of the mouth into the food. The action of the saliva is partly to lubricate the food, so that it will slip down easily, and no better proof of this can be found than trying to eat a cracker rapidly without chewing. But it also acts on starch which is not digested easily unless mixed with this ferment. The action of the saliva on starch is to convert it into sugar, which is easily absorbed later on. Curiously enough, most persons would be more apt to chew a piece of meat thoroughly than to chew a piece of bread, and yet the meat contains practically no starch and therefore does not need the action of the saliva, whereas bread is chiefly made up of starch and therefore needs the saliva as an essential for digestion.

The food then passes down into the stomach, which is a sort of storehouse, preparatory to the really important steps in digestion. Here, the food is acted upon by another element known as gastric juice, which is supplied by small glands found in the membrane of the stomach. The mixture of food and gastric juice is made very thorough by the continual agitation of the food, so that the mass is softened as well as thoroughly mixed. The effect of the gastric juice is to act upon that portion of food known as proteids. Examples of almost pure proteids are found in the fiber of beef and other meat, in the yolk of eggs, and in cheese. Some vegetables, such as peas, also contain large quantities, and coarse flour and oatmeal contain considerable percentages. The effect of the gastric juice on this proteid matter is to break up the complex molecules into small molecules which then pass into solution, making the mass leaving the stomach a uniformly mixed [Pg 261] semiliquid substance of about the consistency of thick pea soup. The food then enters the smaller intestine, at the beginning of which the juices from the pancreas are added. The pancreas is a gland which furnishes a strongly alkaline liquid neutralizing the acid of the gastric juice, so that the gastric agent, pepsin, loses its power. From this gland comes a material which can act on all kinds of food and which is by far the most important of the digestive juices.

When thoroughly mixed with the bile and pancreatic juice, the contents of the intestine are gradually absorbed, in so far as their condition allows, by the surface of that organ and are carried away by the ducts designed for that purpose to the various organs, while that part not suited for absorption is eliminated.

*Teachings of the digestive operations.*

The matter of hygienic eating, therefore, consists in supplying the various organs, the mouth, the stomach, and the smaller intestine with proper food in proper quantity, so that the body itself may be properly nourished from the food supplied. A great deal of scientific investigation in this connection has been made to ascertain any relation which may exist between the different kinds of food and their availability for the body. Scientists have divided all food into four classes, namely, proteids, carbohydrates, fats, and inorganic salts, and they have agreed on the following general statements with reference to these four classes. Examples of almost pure proteids have already been given, and it may here be added that carbohydrates are typically shown by the starchy particles found in potatoes or wheat. Chemically, the difference consists in [Pg 262] the fact that proteids contain nitrogen whereas carbohydrates do not. Fats are self-explanatory, and the group of inorganic salts includes such material as salt, lime, phosphates, and other minerals needed by the body but not requiring digestion.

Just what function each one of these four groups plays in the nutrition of the human body is not definitely understood, but it seems that the proteids are particularly useful in building up cell tissue, that the carbohydrates are particularly useful in providing for muscular energy, that the fats are particularly useful in keeping up the normal warmth rather more by laying on a blanket of fat over the bones than in actually consuming the food in the creation of heat. These statements are not absolute, since experiments have shown that some tissue-building can go on even if proteids are rigorously excluded from the diet, and on the other hand that muscular work, while accompanied by a large consumption of carbohydrates in the body, may come from proteids entirely. This may explain why men can live and even do a reasonable amount of work eating meat and fat altogether, as in the Arctic regions, or dry bread and fruit in other regions, the above facts being complicated by the influence of muscular exercise on the activity of the digestive system.

No principle of hygiene is better established than that men undergoing hard physical exercise need and will take care of a larger amount of coarse food than those occupied in sedentary work. In cold weather what is required is not really more fat as food, but more food. It has been found that there is a limit to the amount of meat food which the body can absorb, and, further, that the excess is not [Pg 263] easily disposed of, as with starchy food, and tends to load up the liver and other organs with the waste products, resulting in general disturbances of the whole body. It is commonly known, for instance, that high-livers, as they are called, are likely to be troubled with diseases like indigestion, rheumatism, or gout, — diseases which are the result of overburdening those organs just mentioned.

*Balanced rations.*

**TABLE XVI**

|  | WEIGHT IN GRAMMES | | |
|---|---|---|---|
| CONDITION | Proteid | Fat | Carbohydrates |
| Child up to 1-1/2 years (average) | 0.71-1.27 | 1.06-1.59 | 2.12-3.18 |
| Child from 6 to 15 years (average) | 2.47-2.82 | 1.30-1.76 | 8.82-14.10 |
| Man (moderate work) | 4.16 | 1.98 | 17.63 |
| Woman (moderate work) | 3.24 | 1.55 | 14.10 |

| Old man | 3.53 | 2.40 | 12.34 |
| Old woman | 2.82 | 1.76 | 9.18 |
| Atwater (man, light exercise) | 3.70 | 3.70 | 13.3 |
| Chittenden (man, light exercise) | 2.16 | 2.83 | 13.0 |

A well-designed food ration, therefore, will be one which will provide the body with the proper amount of food material wisely adjusted to the occupation and the digestive ability of the individual. It has been, in the past, a matter of very exact computation to determine how many ounces of proteid food, how many ounces of starchy food, and how many of fatty foods should be consumed during the day, and experiments have been made in asylums, [Pg 264] prisons, and on companies of soldiers with a view to proving the theoretical figures.

It has always been found that an overdose of proteids results in inability to absorb the excess, and it has been assumed that a ratio of proteids to carbohydrates of one to four is approximately the proper proportion. For instance, Koenig (1888) shows the minimum daily need of food stuffs at different ages and two American authorities, Atwater and Chittenden, have also laid down standards; all three being shown in the preceding table.

The following table taken from Rough and Sedgwick's book, already referred to, gives the percentage composition of some of the more common foods: —

**TABLE XVII**

| | Water | Proteid | Starch | Sugar | Fat | Salts |
|---|---|---|---|---|---|---|
| Bread | 37 | 8 | 47 | 3 | 1 | 2 |
| Wheat flour | 15 | 11 | 66 | 4.2 | 2 | 1.7 |
| Oatmeal | 15 | 12.6 | 58 | 5.4 | 5.6 | 3 |
| Rice | 13 | 6 | 79 | 0.4 | 0.7 | 0.5 |

| | | | | | | |
|---|---|---|---|---|---|---|
| Peas | 15 | 23 | 55 | 2 | 2 | 2 |
| Potatoes | 75 | 2 | 18 | 3 | 0.2 | 0.7 |
| Milk | 86 | 4 | — | 5 | 4 | 0.8 |
| Cheese | 37 | 33 | — | — | 24 | 5 |
| Lean beef | 72 | 19 | — | — | 3 | 1 |
| Fat beef | 51 | 14 | — | — | 29 | 1 |
| Mutton | 72 | 18 | — | — | 5 | 1 |
| Veal | 63 | 16 | — | — | 16 | 1 |
| White Fish | 78 | 18 | — | — | 3 | 1 |
| Salmon | 77 | 16 | — | — | 5.5 | 1.5 |
| Egg | 74 | 14 | — | — | 10.5 | 1.5 |
| Butter | 15 | — | — | — | 83 | 3 |

It will be noted that meats, cheese, and such vegetables as peas are high in proteids, while certain other vegetables, [Pg 265] as rice and white flour, are high in starch or carbohydrates. According to the table given above, a man at moderate work requires 4.1 ounces of proteids and 17.5 ounces of carbohydrates per day. If, then, the carbohydrates were to be made up entirely from potatoes, 18 per cent of which is starch and he should need 17.5 ounces, he must have 100/18 of 17.5 or 97 ounces of potatoes per day, an amount equal to about 6 pounds. If, however, with the potatoes, he should eat half a pound of bread, of which about half is carbohydrates or 8 ounces, the amount of potato necessary would be cut down, and so on with as many combinations as one might choose to make.

It is curious, however, that when different kinds of food are available, one naturally combines different articles of food, so as to make up the well-balanced daily ration, so that the different parts may have the proper proportion. For instance, butter is always used with bread in order to add to the proteid and starch of the bread the necessary fat. With potatoes or rice, either butter or gravy or meat is always used because potatoes and rice are lacking in proteids as well as in fats which the meat supplies. Bread and cheese are well known to make up a good combination, and the table shows why: the bread furnishing the starch and the cheese the proteid and fat. Eggs alone are a very poor article of diet since no starch at all is present, and therefore it is that when eggs are eaten for breakfast, as is so generally the custom to-day, either a generous helping of cereal ought to be given with the egg or else a generous supply of bread or toast ought to be included in the breakfast. Milk is generally considered an ideal article of food, and yet it contains no starch, and it is undoubtedly because [Pg 266] of this fact that milk and bread is more palatable as well as more nutritious than milk alone.

*Human appetite.*

One other factor needs to be considered in this matter of selecting one's daily food, and that is the respect which must be paid to the appetite. The most carefully balanced ration will fail to satisfy the ordinary human being unless it is served attractively and unless sufficient variety is provided. To be sure, soldiers in the army are furnished a carefully computed ration consisting of so much meat, either fresh or salt, so much bread, and so much vegetable food, and the variety being small, the soldier has to put up with his dislike to the same food day after day. The need of fresh vegetables has been proved by the results of a continuous diet of salty food on certain classes of men, such as sailors.

It is well known that a failure to provide fruit or fresh vegetables results in the disease known as scurvy, for which, practically, the only cure is a changed diet. The writer has no doubt but that in many farmhouses a very similar condition, perhaps not so pronounced, exists on account of this very lack of variety in the daily menu. He remembers to this day a week's experience in the house of a well-to-do farmer in the early spring when the winter vegetables were exhausted and before summer vegetables appeared, when the dishes offered three times a day throughout the week were salt pork in milk sauce and boiled potatoes.

Providence intended the different digestive organs of the human body to work, and there is no possibility of condensed or concentrated foods taking the place of ordinary victuals, as has been suggested. The stomach must [Pg 267] have some bulky material on which to work, and similarly the intestine must be comfortably filled in order to exert its forward movements. It is in the same way intended that each organ shall supply the necessary digestive juices to take care of the different kinds of foods taken into the system. It is just as important that the liver should be called upon to act on a certain amount of fat as that the gastric juice should break up the molecules of the proteid, and just as important as both of these is the fact that the saliva should flow freely to decompose the starch before it enters the stomach. It is not intended, however, that the healthy individual should deliberately overload any part of the digestive system.

If a child, in a hurry to get to school, swallows bread and milk without chewing and without allowing the starch to be acted upon in the mouth, then an overburden is placed on the pancreatic gland, making that organ less capable of its regular work. And if, again, the food is drenched in fat, if everything is fried, or if butter is used in large quantities, the liver becomes overworked and cannot keep up with the demands, and digestive troubles follow.

*Effect of individual habits.*

Assuming that the amount and quality of food have been properly adjusted, that each of the several constituents is in proper proportion, and that a suitable variety is maintained, there are still other phases to be considered before the nourishment of the individual may be considered satisfactory. Nature has furnished man with a guide both to the quantity and quality of food that should be taken into the system,—that is, his desire for food, or his appetite,—and, in general, this guide may be safely trusted both as [Pg 268] to the quantity and quality, although, in the latter, the appetite is not so trustworthy as that of the lower animals.

Unfortunately, the appetite is easily distracted by the general conditions of health, and when once the healthy tone of the system has been relaxed, the appetite becomes misleading. For instance, a person not indulging in muscular exercise, but sitting still all day and eating candy or other sweets, has no desire for food, and the lack of appetite in this case indicates, not a failure of the need of food, but abnormal conditions of the system. Also the conditions of housing, lack of ventilation, excessive heat, excess in the use of stimulants or of food, all affect and interfere with the guidance of a normal appetite. Some persons go to the other extreme, and, having been in their earlier years accustomed to heavy exercise and generous feeding, forget that in a more quiet life, less breaking down of the tissue occurs and therefore less food is required. Their appetite is a poor guide since it leads them to immoderate eating, resulting in time in an overloading of the organs and the probable poisoning of the system.

*Cooking.*

Good cooking is as important as any other part of the process of digestion, and, in fact, cooking may be said to be the first step, since there the breaking down of the food tissue occurs, whereby subsequent action by the juices of the body is made easier. For instance, beef may be cooked so long and in such a way as to dry and harden the fibers, making it almost impossible for subsequent digestion; and on the other hand, it is possible to so stew or boil or steam tough meat as to make it quite easily absorbed by the stomach. Cereals, if properly boiled at the right temperature, [Pg 269] and for the right length of time, will have the starch granules so broken up that the saliva will act easily on the broken granules. Raw vegetables containing starch are not acted upon in the mouth and are digested afterwards only with great difficulty, while cooked vegetables are a most desirable article of diet.

A great deal is said nowadays about overeating, and Horace Fletcher affirms that the average man would be much healthier and much stronger if he ate not more than two meals and generally only one meal a day. The relation between the amount of food eaten or the amount of food absorbed or utilized and the need for food cannot be determined for the average but only for the individual. There is no doubt but that men or women doing muscular work require greater amounts of food than those not so engaged. It is a common practice to increase the amount of oats which a horse consumes when the horse has hard work to do and to cut down the amount of grain when the horse stands in the stable. It is curious that this practice, so well known to give good results, is not applied to the human animal as well. But very few men will be found voluntarily to diminish the amount of their breakfast or dinner because on that day or on the following day they are going to stay in the house instead of engaging in vigorous outdoor labor.

No discussion on foods would be complete without a repetition of the frequently given warning, against fried meats and vegetables. Frying coats the outside of the food with a layer of fat not easily penetrated by the digestive juice and not acted on in the stomach. Therefore, all fried food, unless thoroughly chewed and then only when [Pg 270] the frying is done in very hot fat so that it remains on the outside of the whole piece, will pass through the stomach without being acted upon. Frying is a quicker process than roasting, an advantage which appeals to the American notion of haste, but it is better to begin the preparation of the meal earlier and cook the meat by roasting or stewing and the vegetables by boiling or baking rather than to postpone the preparation of the meal until ten minutes before the hour and then fry everything.

*Muscular and psychic reactions.*

Another factor in the power of the body to utilize the food values is the condition of the body at the time of the meal. If the individual is exhausted or even tired, no complete digestion is possible, and particularly is this true if the exercise has involved excessive perspiration. So in hot weather, a heavy meal should not be eaten until after a half hour's rest and after copious water drinking to compensate for that loss of perspiration.

Studies on the digestion of foods and on other matters pertaining thereto have shown that the smell of food, or the mere suggestion of food, stimulates the organs for the production of the digestive juices. It is directly and literally correct, therefore, to say that one's mouth waters for this or that food because the thought or anticipation of the food, if pleasant, will actually cause the saliva to form and flow in the mouth. This is true of the other digestive juices as well, so that an appetizing fritter, for instance, showing the rich, brown crust will stir up the bile, and when the fried cake reaches the opening into the intestine, the bile will be there ready to act. This has been demonstrated by putting into the stomach of sleeping dogs [Pg 271] various kinds of foods and finding that no digestive juices whatever were produced, although with the dog awake and seeing the food before eating, the juices began to flow in the usual fashion.

It follows, then, that the enjoyment of food is quite as important as any other digestive function, and on the contrary, the eating of all sorts of foods with no interest or attention is the best way to induce subsequent indigestion. The fact, then, that a business man eating at a quick-lunch counter does not get the full enjoyment and benefit from his meal as compared with those who sit leisurely over a well-appointed table does not result altogether from the difference in the viands, but rather in the different attitude toward the meal. It would undoubtedly be a great gain in every household if more attention could be given to a cheerful intercourse at meal times — not for the better relationship which would follow, but merely for the effect on the digestion.

After meals, violent exercise is not desirable because thereby vitality is taken away from the muscles of the stomach and intestines and is used up in the other muscles; but it is vigorous exercise after heavy meals only that is condemned, since moderate exercise after ordinary meals is not objectionable. Nor is there any evidence, unless the meal has been excessive, that mental exercise after a meal does any harm. The amount of mental tissue used up in the ordinary processes of mental work is not great enough to call for any large diminution of the supply of blood to other parts of the body.

*Consumption of water.*

A move in the right direction to-day undoubtedly is the [Pg 272] tendency to increase the quantity of water to drink. The body is nine-tenths per cent water, and while a large part of the water in the tissues is made chemically by combinations of hydrogen and oxygen, there must be a constant replenishing of the liquids of the body.

The ordinary person ought to drink, or consume with his food in some way, at least two quarts of water a day, and many difficulties with the liver, kidneys, and other organs would be avoided if this amount of water daily were imbibed. Probably the contention that water should not be taken at meals is not particularly tenable except as the continual swallowing of water increases the tendency to swallow food without chewing, a childish habit sure to lead to distress later. But, to eat one's dinner or part of one's dinner and then drink a glass of water cannot reasonably be assumed to interfere with any digestive process. It is quite likely, in fact, that the greater dilution of the mass in the stomach will tend to easier absorption later on.

*Condiments and drinks.*

There are certain kinds of foods which, though not strictly included in the four elements of food already named, yet are so common as to deserve special mention. Chief among these are the condiments and drinks, particularly coffee and tea. So far as the nutritive value of such materials as salt and pepper, vinegar or spices, goes, they are practically negligible, and yet, undoubtedly, these flavors play an important part in the suggestion of pleasure and therefore in the excitement leading to the excretion of the digestive juices. If one ate salt pork and boiled potatoes always, eating would be a tiresome affair, and it is quite likely that such a sameness of food would fail to [Pg 273] excite subsequent digestion, merely from the monotony of the affair. Salt, however, has a particular rôle in that the human body craves this mineral, and, while its exact value in the body is not clearly known, a certain amount of it must always be provided. The wild tribes of Africa, for instance, away from deposits of salt consider it their most valuable possession and will go to great lengths to procure it. Animals, in the same way, go great distances for a supply of salt.

Coffee and tea are generally consumed merely for the pleasure which the warm drink gives. Both, however, have a certain stimulating effect on the nervous system, and when a tired woman refuses food but drinks cup after cup of strong tea, the exhilarating effect can be produced only at the expense of nerves and muscular tissue which must be later atoned for. Similarly, when a man under stress drinks strong black coffee to keep up, he must pay the penalty for the stimulant. The natural forces of the human body are able to do normally a certain amount of work, their ability to perform this work being directly proportioned to the energy derived from the food-supply taken into the body.

No amount of tea, coffee, or alcohol will add to the living tissue of the system; it merely goads the nerves and muscles to further action, however tired and unwilling they may be. When the stimulant is stopped, or after a time in spite of the stimulant, the exhausted nerves and muscles refuse to continue, and the depleted body stops work and may even die. A certain amount of stimulants at infrequent intervals for particular occasions may do no harm, but the pity of it is that the habit once started, the ultimate [Pg 274] effects are forgotten in the apparent relief of the moment. In the case of tea, besides the stimulating effect, a certain substance known as tannin is developed, particularly when the tea is boiled, and this substance is really harmful on account of its strong astringent property, which acts injuriously on the membrane of the stomach. The bitter taste of the tannin is disguised when milk is used with the tea, and it has been pointed out that tea used without milk or cream is safer than tea with milk, because without the milk the bitter taste would prevent the tea being boiled so long.

Alcohol is stimulating in its nature, because of its setting free from their usual control by the will the unconscious elements of the brain; while the effect of alcohol on the system as a whole is, as has been carefully proved by scientific investigation, unfortunate in every respect. Whether the alcohol be in the form of whisky or brandy or gin or in such milder forms as wines, beers, and hard cider, the continued use of even a small quantity acts adversely on the memory, on the will, on the intellect, on the inventive power, and on all the mental processes. It has a deteriorating effect on all the muscular tissue throughout the body, and while this is sufficiently deplorable, its effect on the mind is by far the more serious. No idea is more false than that a small amount of alcohol aids in the performance of work of any sort, and experience in the army, navy, and in exploring expeditions all go to show that the use of alcohol in any form reduces the capacity, both for activity and endurance. As a protection against cold, it is worse than useless, and the feeling of warmth which drinking alcohol in any form produces, does not [Pg 275] manufacture heat in the body, but is rather a source of danger on account of the reaction of the whole system.

*Tobacco.*

The use of tobacco may or may not be injurious to the human system, and it is said by those accustomed to its use that it is for them a source of great enjoyment and comfort. The essential poison of tobacco is known as nicotine, and experiments are very readily made with this substance, extracted from the plant, to show its deadly character on the heart and nerve cells of animals. It is easy to demonstrate that the use of tobacco affects the heart, since the common "out-of-breath feeling" which comes to users of tobacco when climbing hills or running is well known. No young man training for an athletic event would think of smoking, on account of the danger to his wind.

No boy should smoke, because nothing should be allowed to interfere with the fullest development of the heart and nervous system, and without question tobacco is a potent factor in influencing both. In many individual cases it has been shown that the use of tobacco in excess has a bad effect on digestion, while in other cases the trembling hand and inattentive mind indicate the result on the nervous system. No general law or rule can be laid down, and each man must act as his own individual constitution seems to require.

*The drug habit.*

The use of drugs is, in some cases, so persistent and leads to such dire results that it is well worth while to enter a protest against such practices. The poor creatures who have become fast victims of the morphine habit or the [Pg 276] opium habit or the cocaine habit, or of any one of a dozen which might be named, will not be affected by anything that may be said here. But a word of warning may serve to restrain those who are only at the beginning of this downward path of which the end is positive and certain. The use of drugs once begun is sure to increase until, stupefied by their action, the victim becomes a sot, unfitted for work and a burden to himself, his relatives, and his friends.

Not less dangerous is the use of so-called patent medicines. In most cases, patent medicines are swindles, pure and simple, containing no remedial ingredients and acting only as stimulants. An advertisement some time since, which claimed to cure not only tuberculosis but also cancer, falling of the womb, hair, or eyelids, insanity, epilepsy, drunkenness, disorderly conduct, and pimples was printed in many newspapers. This remarkable remedy was found by analysis to contain ninety-nine parts of water to one part of harmless salts. Many of the vaunted remedies contain morphine or alcohol in such large quantities as to be dangerous, the more so because their presence is not suspected. Such remedies as Dr. Bull's Cough Syrup, Boschees German Sirup, Dr. King's New Discovery for Consumption, Shiloh's Consumptive Cure, Piso's Consumptive Cure, Peruna, Duffy's Malt Whisky, Warner's Safe Cure, and Paine's Celery Compound are all by analysis said to contain large amounts of morphine, chloroform, or alcohol.

Consumptives cannot be cured by any drug now known, and any person who believes it is mistaken. Cancer still baffles the skill of the most clever and the best-trained [Pg 277] scientists. It is perfect folly to believe that any drug or man can cure either disease by a few pills or by a few bottles of medicine. The wise man or woman will avoid patent medicines unless they carry their formula on their label *and unless they are prescribed by some reputable physician.*

[Pg 278]

## CHAPTER XIII

# *PERSONAL HYGIENE*

Whatever the conditions under which one lives, or whatever his abstract knowledge of foods and sanitation, the health of the individual resolves itself at last into a question of his personal habits; and some of these personal questions must be considered in a book of this character.

*Exercise.*

One of the commonly accepted facts of hygiene is that, for the best development and for the perfect health of the human body, a certain amount of exercise should be taken by each part of the body. This is true not only for the larger muscles, such as those of the arms and legs, but also for the muscles of those internal organs less frequently considered. Experiments have been made by tying up some part of the body, such as the forearm, with the result that, in the course of a few weeks, its functions have been so lessened that its usefulness is temporarily at an end. But the general effect of exercise on the body, aside from the beneficial results on the particular muscles engaged, is to promote the building up of new lung tissue. Oxygen is received from the lungs through the blood and is carried to the different parts of the body, where it serves [Pg 279] the useful purpose of carrying off the waste products of the different organs. If the lung action is inadequate, if deep breathing in fresh air is not practiced, or if, through laziness, no exercise is taken, then the amount of oxygen supplied will be deficient and the body will be loaded up with the toxic products resulting from decomposition. The exact effect of exercise upon the lung action may be seen from the fact that under ordinary circumstances a man breathes about 480 cubic inches of air per minute. If he is walking at the rate of 4 miles an hour, he inhales air at 5 times this rate, and if he is walking at the rate of 6 miles an hour, inspiration increases to seven times this rate, or 3360 cubic inches of air passes through his lungs per minute instead of 480, as when at rest.

Of course, it is assumed that in the country a person has no lack of exercise, and that of all men the farmer is in least need of exercise. But, as a matter of fact, the exercise which he gets is irregular and confined to certain sets of muscles, rather than to the development of the whole body. Agility, for instance, quickness of action and immediate control of the muscles, is far less common in the country than is supposed, although there is probably no lack in the actual power of the muscles. It is common observation that among farmers an erect carriage is less frequently seen than an awkward, shuffling gait. The fact is, that exercise, to be beneficial, should affect not one set of muscles, but all the muscles of the body, because the continuous exercise of one set, while leading first to growth, results later in demolition and waste. When, however all the muscles of the body are exercised, there is no demolition or waste, but a healthy growth throughout. [Pg 280] Regular exercise is beneficial, not merely to the muscles involved, but also to the other organs of the body. Exercise sharpens the appetite, makes digestion more perfect, and increases the absorptive power of the intestinal membranes; conversely, lack of exercise, which is found in the country in the winter, lessens both the digestive power and the appetite.

*Clothing.*

Little need be said on this subject, since the amount of clothing needed varies so greatly with the vitality of the individual. It has already been pointed out that in rural communities the death-rate from pneumonia, bronchitis, and similar respiratory troubles is much higher than in urban communities, and it is quite possible that deficient or unsuitable clothing is practically responsible for this.

The object of clothing is twofold: to protect the body against the weather, particularly against changes in the weather, and secondly, to protect the body against injury. Included in the former are the defenses against the elements of cold, wet, and heat; while the protection against injury is chiefly a matter of shoes. As has been pointed out, a large part of the food consumed by the body is utilized in the production of heat, whereby the body temperature is maintained at about 98 degrees Fahrenheit. A large part of this heat is continually being lost from and through the skin by radiation and evaporation, and evidently some regulating influence must be provided so that the amount of heat given off may be adjusted to variations of the external temperature. To be sure, the skin itself acts as a regulator, since a rise in temperature causes the blood vessels on the surface to distend so that a larger quantity [Pg 281] of blood is distributed over the surface and thereby more freely evaporated. Fall of temperature, on the contrary, causes a contraction of the blood vessels and therefore a reduction in the evaporation. But this is not sufficient where external temperature undergoes wide variations, as in the northern and central parts of the United States, and a modification of the clothing is a necessary supplement. The main object of clothing, then, is not to keep out cold or heat, but to preserve and make uniform the evaporation from the body. It is an agent of the same sort as food in so far as the body temperature is concerned, and without doubt light clothing requires a greater amount of food; while, on the other hand, warm clothing will make possible a lighter diet.

The best non-conductor of heat is still air, and if one could always remain in quiet air, no clothing of any sort would be necessary, even in the most severe weather, because the air itself would serve as a garment and would prevent radiation from the body. Therefore, loose, porous garments containing air in their folds and pores are much warmer than a single, tightly woven garment, and the same material made up in three or four thicknesses will give the body far more warmth than an equal weight of texture made up in a single thickness. Similarly, a tight garment is much less warm than a loose one. A practical demonstration of this fact is found in the comparative lack of warmth in an old, much-washed, quilted, bed blanket which is very heavy but quite lacking in warmth compared with a light fluffy woolen blanket, newly purchased.

Much has been written on the advantages of woolen underwear, on the ground that since clothing is intended [Pg 282] to retain the body heat and since wool acts as a more effective non-conductor of heat than either cotton or linen, therefore the woolen undergarment is of the greatest value. Another argument urged in favor of woolen undergarments is that they check the chill resulting from excessive perspiration, since the non-conducting power of wool prevents any rapid evaporation of perspiration responsible for the lower temperatures. For this reason, woolen undergarments are always recommended for those climbing mountains or in occupations where violent exercise is likely to be followed by rest or quiet in cold air. The objection to woolen undergarments at all times is that with sensitive skins irritation may take place, and the odd saying of Josh Billings becomes pertinent, namely, that "the only thing that a wool shirt is good for is to make a man scratch and forget his other troubles." Underwear woolen only in part may take the place of all-wool garments and have the further advantage of being less expensive. The amount of clothing worn in winter depends, or should depend, on the character of the occupation of the wearer.

Formerly, heavy woolen underclothes were almost universally worn throughout the winter without regard to the employment of the individual. When an out-of-door occupation was pursued a large part of the time or when the temperature indoors was hardly above freezing, then heavy clothing was essential; but now that much time is spent in a well-heated house or office, heavy clothing is as objectionable as overheated rooms, and the comfort and health of the body will be much better preserved by not increasing the weight of clothing except when exposed to the outer air. It must be remembered, however, that old persons, [Pg 283] whose circulation is impaired and who are forced to lead sedentary lives, will always have difficulty in maintaining the body heat unless the outer temperature is high, and for such, woolen undergarments are very useful. The outer garments in winter, to be efficient, must have two qualities, namely, an impervious surface so that winds may not penetrate and a loose open weave in which air may be held so that warmth may be secured.

Rubber boots, although very common in the country, are not desirable as a foot covering, because they do not allow the perspiration to evaporate, but rather hold the foot in a moist condition very detrimental to it. Rubber-cloth overshoes or arctics are much better than rubber boots, and felt overshoes are equally satisfactory. Chilblains are fostered by the use of rubber boots, and cloth shoes are a great relief when the feet are thus affected.

*Ventilation of bedroom.*

Since the agitation for fresh air has become so extensive and the knowledge of the dangers of tuberculosis so widespread, much more attention has been given to the ventilation of bedrooms, and whereas formerly the night air was religiously excluded from a sleeping room, it is not at all uncommon now for a window to be kept wide open, even through the coldest nights of winter. From what has already been said on the subject of ventilation, it is plain that to breathe over and over one's expired air is not healthy, and while it is possible that a bedroom may be so large that the concentration of the organic matter in the air may not affect an individual sleeping in the room, yet in most cases it must be admitted that the bedroom is so small or the number of people in the bedroom so large that [Pg 284] this possibility does not exist. It is, again, possible that the structure of the house may be so poor that it is not necessary to open a window to get plenty of fresh air; the writer remembers sleeping in rooms where, with the windows shut, paths of snow across the floor in the morning showed the intimate connection between the inside and the outside of the room.

But the tendency nowadays is to build better houses, to cover the walls with paper, to put on double windows, and even to paste up the cracks to make the room as air-tight as possible. To sleep in such a room without a window open may not be committing suicide, but it is a deliberate method of reducing the vitality, of insuring a headache or a numbed and stupid mental condition, and of loading up the system with poisons which ought to be eliminated by the oxygen which fresh air supplies. It would add many years to the lives of the people of this country if, from childhood up, the habit was formed of sleeping with the window open. Nor need one fear that a cold would result from such exposure. A cheesecloth screen in the window prevents any draft and yet allows perfect ventilation. The face is trained to all kinds of exposure without any danger of catching cold, and there is no reason why, if the bed clothing be sufficient, the night air should not be thoroughly enjoyed without danger. Of course, the bed clothing must be sufficient; two lightly woven blankets are always better than one heavy one. Wool is better than cotton; if a cotton quilt is used, it should be loose and not tied tightly.

*Bathing.*

An important function of the skin is to expel objectionable [Pg 285] elements coming from the breaking down of the cells and from digestive processes; the skin is quite as important a factor in getting rid of this waste matter as those other processes more commonly considered in this connection. This action goes on most energetically when the secretion of perspiration is abundant and when the temperature of the surrounding air is so high that perspiration does not evaporate as rapidly as discharged. All these secretions contain more or less solid material which, unless removed, accumulates on the surface of the skin to clog up the glands and, in some cases, to putrefy and decay. It is this decay of organic matter on the surface of the skin which causes the odors plainly noticeable in a crowd, particularly in the winter time. This accumulation can be prevented only by frequent bathing and by wearing clean clothes, and there is no surer indication of a proper self-respect than the habit of cleanliness, both as to one's person and one's clothes. There is also the very practical feature that cleanliness is an effective method of discouraging infection and disease, partly by the removal of scurf and partly by the greater healthfulness of the skin thereby induced.

Baths have always served as therapeutic agents, and evidences of their use may be found in Roman paintings and in Egyptian sculpture to-day. But from our standpoint it is their hygienic importance that is insisted upon. Ordinarily, the temperature of the bath should be between 90 and 100 degrees, and enough soap should be used to counteract the oily nature of the deposits on the skin.

Unfortunately, facilities for bathing, except in summer, [Pg 286] have not been generally supplied to detached houses in the country. Plumbing in most houses has been lacking, but in these days bath-rooms are being installed with surprising rapidity, and the conveniences resulting are enjoyed as soon as they are understood. Only a few days ago, the writer was told of a small village of perhaps two or three hundred persons where this last summer one house, the first in the village, was provided with a bath-room, to the great interest of all the villagers. The convenience and comfort involved were immediately appreciated, and the plumber, who came in from a neighboring city twenty miles away, secured contracts for and installed twelve bath-rooms in twelve houses before he was allowed to leave the village. This same interest is everywhere noticeable, and the lack of bathing throughout the winter, formerly, alas, so common, is now giving way to a greater cleanliness, thereby improving the health and character of the inhabitants.

A great deal has been written about the value of a cold bath, particularly in the morning, and many people, from a sense of duty, suffer what is almost torture taking a shower bath or a cold plunge bath on rising. When a cold bath (which should not last more than a few seconds) is followed by a good reaction, that is, when after drying, a distinct glow is felt, there is no objection to its use, and undoubtedly it has a tonic effect for those whose vitality is able to endure the shock. But cold baths for their tonic effect are desirable only when the individual is assured of their lasting benefits. Nor must one judge of the effects by the immediate results, inasmuch as the splendid feeling which follows may be succeeded by a [Pg 287] period of depression lasting the rest of the day; in which case, the total effect of the cold bath is bad rather than good. Baths for cleanliness are everywhere desirable, and their frequency should depend upon the individual, his constitution, habits, and work; upon the season and temperature; and on the conveniences for bathing in the house. Baths for tonic effect are not necessary, and if not a pleasure, may very properly be omitted.

One other point to be noted is that no practice is of more value in reducing the ravages of contagious diseases than a frequent and conscientious washing of one's hands. For germs are most certainly transmitted from one person to another, and it is accomplished more frequently by the hands than by any other part of the body.

The invitation, therefore, to a guest to wash his hands before dinner is really an invitation for him to disinfect himself or to get rid of the germs which he is carrying, in order that the host and his family may not be infected during the meal. The guest owes it to his host always to accept the invitation, whether he thinks he needs it or not. Doctors recognize the necessity, and it is surprising to observe how many times during the day a doctor washes his hands, even though he may not come in contact with any particularly infectious disease. An ordinary man, on the other hand, washes his hands only when he thinks they are dirty, although his daily occupation may expose the skin of his hands to infection many times worse than that which the doctor experiences.

*Mouth breathing.*

Children have sometimes wondered why they were made with both mouths and noses, since they could breathe [Pg 288] equally with either, and many years have gone by before they realized that breathing through the mouth was not intended, but that the exclusive province of the nose was to furnish air to the lungs. The reason for nose breathing rather than mouth breathing is twofold. In the first place, no provision for removing or filtering out germs from the air is made in the mouth, whereas in the nose the crooked passages, the moist surfaces, and the hairlike growths all tend to strain out any germs normally in the inspired air.

Further, breathing through the mouth has a tendency to induce inflammation in the tonsils and in the air passage connecting with the ear. This inflammation develops into those growths known as adenoids, which, when enlarged sufficiently, close the nostril entirely and prevent its normal use. A recent examination made by the New York Board of Health of 150 school children, all in some way abnormal, showed that 137 had either adenoids or enlarged tonsils. Example after example could be given of school boys and girls whose mental and moral development has been markedly retarded because of mouth breathing. One need only look at a child or adult who constantly keeps his or her mouth open to be impressed by the listless, vacant, inert appearance of the face thus disfigured. Figure 74 shows a photograph of a schoolgirl just before an operation and the characteristic expression due to adenoids is plainly marked. Earache is largely due to adenoids or to inflammation that rapidly leads to adenoids, and Mr. William H. Allen, Secretary of the Bureau of the New York Municipal Research, reports that in 415 villages of New York State, 12 per cent of the children living there [Pg 289] were found to be mouth breathers. Whenever a child is unable to breathe through his nose, is slow in talking, and then speaks with a stuffy accent, calls "nose" "dose," has a narrow upper jaw, and is either deaf or has inflamed eyes, it is practically certain that enlarged tonsils and a well-developed growth of adenoids are present and should be removed. Not merely do these growths interfere with the mental and physical development of the child, but they also make him more susceptible to contagious diseases, particularly those of the lungs and bronchial tubes.

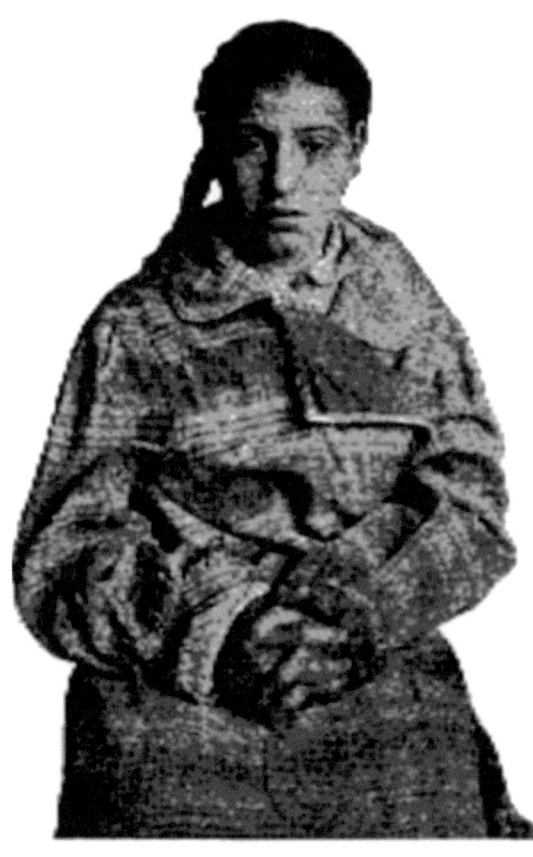

Fig. 74. —
Schoolgirl with adenoids.

The removal of adenoids is a simple operation, lasting not over a minute, and the result of the operation is in some cases almost miraculous. The medical inspectors of the New York City schools consider the removal of adenoids as a most important part of [Pg 290] their work, and groups of children are regularly taken from the schools by the principal to the clinic at the hospital, where one after another tonsils are cut off or adenoids are removed, all fright and commotion being avoided by the gift of five cents as a reward.

*Eyes.*

Another evidence of advancing knowledge in matters pertaining to sanitary hygiene is shown in the greater attention given to the eyes, particularly of children. Such incidental troubles as headache, sleeplessness, or biliousness are frequently due to weak or strained eyes, and in the case of school children a great deal of the alleged insubordination, backwardness, and truancy of the children is caused by their being unable to see written instructions or explanations.

It is not likely that this increased difficulty with the eyes is a new thing, but rather that both physicians and laymen are more careful as well as more expert in diagnosing the trouble. The New York State Board of Health in the fall of 1907 sent out cards for testing the eyes of school children to 446 incorporated towns. The results of using these cards in 415 schools were returned and showed clearly that nearly half the children of school age in the state had optical defects. A similar test in Massachusetts recently discovered 22 per cent of the school children with defective vision, and this knowledge in itself is an advance inasmuch as it suggests to each individual or to all parents that deficient vision is common and that good eyesight is not a thing to be assumed.

In the country it is more difficult, perhaps, to realize these deficiencies, because the constant outdoor life acts [Pg 291] as an offset to the strain during the time when close work is required, and perhaps the distance from a competent oculist serves to postpone the time of consultation, but no greater folly can be indulged in than to suffer inflamed eyes, persistent headache, and imperfect vision, if it is possible in any way to secure the services of an oculist.

Never is it worth while to buy from a jeweler, a grocer, or a hardware store a pair of spectacles, much less to buy them from an itinerant peddler, since an oculist, with his particular apparatus, can measure the seeing ability of each eye and fit each eye with the necessary lens to restore normal vision. It is better to have no glasses than to have glasses that are wrong.

*Teeth.*

A curious result of the recent studies among school children with defective eyes and ears has been the discovery that bad teeth were quite as important in their relation to general health as either bad eyes or ears. One eye specialist went so far as to say that the teeth of school children should be attended to first, because thus many of the eye troubles would disappear.

As has already been pointed out, the first, step in digestion is taken in the mouth, and careful chewing is not less important than the other parts of the digestive process. If one's teeth are not adapted to chewing, if they are bunched, crowded, loose, or isolated, the appearance of the teeth is the least objectionable feature. The real importance comes from the fact that with such teeth perfect mastication is impossible. The teeth themselves harbor germs which actually infect the food and favor its putrefaction. With decayed teeth, infectious diseases find a ready [Pg 292] entrance to the lungs, nostrils, stomach, glands, ears, nose, and membranes. At every act of swallowing, germs are carried into the stomach. Mouth breathers cannot get one breath of uncontaminated air, and dental clinics, organized and conducted in the interests of the health of school children, have been altogether too little inaugurated. The use of a toothbrush should be encouraged in children as soon as they are four years old, and its habitual use twice a day is most desirable for every one.

Only regular examination by the dentist can keep the teeth in good condition, and periodic visits at least once a year to a dentist's office, not to the kind advertised by Indians where they are willing to extract teeth without pain, free, but where a regularly qualified dentist practices, should be the habit. Armenian children, who prize and covet beautiful teeth, are taught to clean their teeth always after eating, if only an apple or a piece of bread between meals, and while probably our American customs would hardly make this possible, there is no question but that a persistent and frequent use of the toothbrush will help much in reducing dentist bills.

*Sleep.*

From many standpoints sleep is the most wonderful attribute of the human body. Our familiarity, from our earliest years, with sleep, closes our eyes to its strange, its awful power. We know that every human being, once in twenty-four hours, will normally close his eyes and for a certain length of time be as oblivious to things present as if already in the sleep of death. It is a common belief that sleep is nature's provision for restoring tired muscles and jaded nerves, and for building up new tissue in cell [Pg 293] and corpuscle. Excessive exertion produces a numbness and exhaustion so that the body becomes "dead tired," and sleep brings back life and elasticity. And yet some parts of the body, some muscles and some organs, do not stop work during sleep, and apparently feel no bad results for their continuous lifelong exertion. Thus, the lungs, whose muscular action is estimated at the rate of one thirtieth of a horse power, have no rest day or night, seemingly without weariness. Similarly, the heart is continually forcing blood under a pressure of about three pounds through the arteries without cessation from birth to death.

Why do the muscles of the arm and leg tire and need sleep as a restorer, while those of the heart and lungs are independent of sleep? Dr. W. H. Thomson, in his book on "Brain and Personality," finds an answer to this question in the fact that the latter do their work independently of the human consciousness, while the former are stimulated and directed by the will. He points out that fatigue comes in proportion to the intensity of the mental effort expended. A baby, to whom everything is strange, whose consciousness is absolutely zero at birth, however well developed his body, sleeps five sixths of the time because of the mental efforts needed in his simplest bodily acts. Brain work, the most absorbing task of consciousness, is always the most compelling in the matter of sleep. Not the muscles themselves but the attention, the skill, the mental effort required to direct those muscles, Dr. Thomson says, constitute the reason for sleep, a reason which, to those who labor only with their hands, must seem unutterably sad. He says that while muscle work is the commonest and the simplest, so it is also [Pg 294] the most poorly paid and the most degrading, and that while brain work is ennobling and the highest type of labor, it is so difficult of attainment and produced only by such grievous toil that most of us shirk it, even while reproaching ourselves at our lack of capacity and purpose. The pathetic burden of unfulfilled possibilities, he says, is the curse of labor, and only in sleep does man have temporary oblivion through which, for a time, he forgets his work and, as it were, uses sleep as an anæsthetic for the pain of labor, to rise therefrom each morning ready to carry his burdens for another day.

Lack of sleep, to those whose brains are active, speedily brings nervous disaster, and the consciousness, from being the active superintendent of the body, becomes inert, and the body drifts like a boat without a pilot. Lack of sleep to those whose work is muscular means a numbness in the nerve cells which guide those muscles, so that they disobey the will or act unreasonably and without direction. But too much sleep, like over-indulgence in any anæsthetic, is only shirking that duty and avoiding that effort to which the higher life calls us, and the sluggard who sleeps more than the tired nerves need is allowing himself to sink deeper and deeper into a slough of despond. He forgets his toil in sleep, but it is only by active, conscious effort when awake that his work may be lifted to the higher plane where the brain is active, where work ceases to be mechanical and a burden, and where that greatest reward of personal satisfaction can be obtained.

[Pg 295]

## CHAPTER XIV

## *THEORIES OF DISEASE*

Disease may be defined as an abnormal condition of the human body, and since there is no one condition of the human body which can be satisfactorily described as normal, there is, therefore, no exact definition of disease.

What is disease for one person because of a departure from his normal health might not be recognized as disease in another person of different normal vitality. Nor is it possible to assign any particular and special cause for disease since the condition recognized as disease is the result, usually, not of one but of a series of causes or circumstances more or less connected and linked together, and in many cases not obviously associated with the resulting disease. Thus, in records of death, it is very common to see reported pneumonia as the cause underlying and fundamental, when the cause was really typhoid fever, the patient yielding to the former disease because of the enfeebled condition due to the latter. Again, many children contract diseases like measles or whooping cough because of reduced vitality due to insufficient nourishment, lack of clothing, and neglect, and their illness is said to be due to measles or whooping cough when under [Pg 296] proper conditions of care and attention they would not have the disease at all. The causes of disease therefore may be divided into two classes, direct and indirect. In the latter class are to be included such causes as environment, heredity, age, and occupation. In the former class are to be found such causes as the introduction of disease germs into the system; the action of poisons, whether introduced into the alimentary canal or into the lungs, and such external conditions as excessive heat and cold and accident.

*Effects of dirt.*

At one time it was thought that diseases could spring up in the midst of dirt, and one of the strong arguments for keeping houses clean, for removing manure piles, and cleaning up back yards, was the fear that without such care diseases might be induced in those living near by. This is possible in a certain sense, but unless the seed or germ of the disease is present in a pile of dirt there need be no fear of the disease being developed. There is, however, a probability that by the organic decay and the consequent pollution of the atmosphere the vitality, energy, and resistance of the individual in the vicinity may be weakened.

It is well known, for instance, that prisoners confined in damp dark cells lose vitality, and when released, have but little of their former physical strength. In the chapter on Ventilation, it has been shown that persons confined in a small room and breathing their own exhaled air may in time become unconscious and die, and therefore it is reasonable to believe that persons living in the immediate vicinity of decaying animal or vegetable matter will suffer a loss of vitality and will have less resistance to disease. [Pg 297]

*Blood resistance.*

It is well known that there are present in the body certain agencies which act as guardians of the body against disease; that there are certain corpuscles of the blood and certain liquids circulating through the system which immediately attack and if in sufficient numbers or strength drive out the advancing enemy, so that "taking a disease" in most cases means that the activity of these resisting organisms is not forceful enough to successfully combat the germs of the disease. These agencies, whether circulating liquids or cells or corpuscles, are most active in the healthy body, and anything that tends to reduce the general health, such as exposure, overexertion, imperfect nourishment, overeating or overdrinking, or lack of sleep, tends to diminish their activity and so makes the individual more susceptible to disease.

*Cell disintegration.*

Although disease is caused by the attacks of germs, another and far more important cause of disease is the breaking down or over-stimulation of some particular organ. This is very plainly seen in diseases involving the stomach or intestines, where habitual excesses in eating lead, sooner or later, to consequent inflammation, disease, and death. This is also true of the lungs; merely living in an atmosphere full of dust will irritate the lungs to such a degree as to cause inflammation. Cancer is presumably the result of local inflammation, although the cause of the original suppuration is unknown. Similarly, appendicitis starts from some irritating cause, resulting in inflammation and the formation of pus. In very many cases the cell-disintegration seems to be a matter of heredity. [Pg 298]

*Heredity.*

Heredity, the second of the indirect causes of disease seems to be assuming less importance as it is more studied. Probably in but few cases is heredity more than a chance factor in the causation of disease. Heredity, formerly considered to be the most important cause of consumption, is now understood to have little to do with this widespread epidemic, although it is agreed that children brought up in the family with a consumptive mother and father are more likely to contract the disease than if they were segregated.

It is a providential arrangement that children inherit the tendencies of both father and mother, and that the good qualities of one parent are known to offset the bad qualities of the other; probably for this very important physiological reason marriage between near relatives, where both parents would be inclined to the same weaknesses, has always been proscribed. However, even with the characteristics of the father offsetting peculiarities of the mother, it is possible for the traits of a parent to be reproduced in children, and this applies to mental traits as well as to physical. In some families there exist tendencies toward nervous diseases, such as epilepsy and insanity, although it is not accurate to say that either disease is naturally inherited. It has been observed that a tendency to cancer, to scrofula, and to rheumatism runs in certain families, but this is hardly more than saying that in certain families, where the predisposition in this direction by one parent is not offset by the tendencies of the other parent, the physical condition of the child is such as to encourage the development of diseases. [Pg 299]

*Age and sex.*

As indirect causes of disease, age and sex cannot be overlooked. It is well known, for instance, that certain diseases belong essentially to childhood, measles and scarlet fever being markedly prevalent among children under ten years of age. In fact, it has been said by experts that if measles could be kept from children under five years old, the disease would be practically stamped out, since beyond that age they are less susceptible and the course of the disease is much milder. No greater mistake can be made than in exposing children to so-called "children's diseases" because of a desire "to have it over with." Not only is such exposure foolish, since it is quite possible to escape the disease altogether if in the first few years of life it is avoided, but also inviting death, since the mortality of the disease becomes markedly less and less as the age of the patient advances.

Many of the diseases of children are due to imperfect and incomplete development; either the lungs or the stomach or some other organ is not equal to its work, and the child remains an invalid or dies. Many children die from imperfect nutrition, especially in the second summer, when teething is at its height, on account of the ignorance of the mother and on account of unsanitary surroundings. No movement is more promising in the way of prolonging the lives of children than that recently inaugurated in New York which undertakes to teach mothers, of foreign nationality in particular, how to dress, bathe, feed, and bring up their children.

Another reason why disease occurs more frequently among children is, as will be seen later, that one attack of [Pg 300] a disease frequently confers immunity upon the patient, so that, for example, a child having scarlet fever is not likely to have the disease later on in life; but this is no argument for exposing one's self to contagion, since it is quite possible that even the first attack may be avoided. Tuberculosis or consumption is preëminently a disease of youth, as is also typhoid fever. It is very rare for the latter disease to appear in children or in adults over forty-five, and for the former to develop until maturity.

In old age, diseases occur due to the gradual failure of the different organs to perform their normal functions. Some of these diseases are connected with the heart and the circulation, others with the liver or with the mucous membranes, so that among those advanced in life, rheumatism, gout, cancer, and diseases of the kidneys are very apt to occur.

One of the objects of sanitation is to eliminate disease due to bacteria and to prolong the normal life, so far as is possible, past the early period when diseases are easily contracted. It is not hoped that death can in any case be prevented, but hygiene will have done its utmost when death occurs only among the aged and when the diseases then causing death are only those which are consequent upon the wearing out of the body.

So far as sex is concerned, the ordinary rules of hygiene or the violation of those rules seem to have but little concern. It is generally understood that males are on the average shorter-lived, by a few months, than females, and all statistics support this position. Some diseases, like typhoid fever, attack males more than females in the ratio of three to two, while cancer attacks females to a greater extent [Pg 301] than males at about the same ratio reversed. Generally speaking, however, excepting in so far as their occupations and manners of living make different their vital resistance, the principles of hygiene are not affected by the incident of sex.

*Occupation.*

Inasmuch as this discussion is a part of rural hygiene and is assumed to apply to only one occupation, namely, that of cultivating the soil, or of raising stock, it may not be considered pertinent to discuss the effect of occupation on disease. It is worth while pointing out, however, that occupation is a very important factor as an indirect cause of disease, and that one's chances of life are vastly greater in the open country surrounded by hygienic conditions than in a city in crowded quarters, confined for long hours each day at some unhealthy occupation.

As a general warning, it may be stated that a factory containing a dust-laden atmosphere is most undesirable, and this is particularly so when the dust is mineral dust. In the country, the only comparison of conditions possible is between that of the outdoor worker and that of the indoor worker; enough has already been said upon the value of fresh air and its improving effect on the vital resistance to make further repetition unnecessary. Unfortunately, in the past the occupation known under the general term of farming has not made itself conspicuous in statistics for healthfulness; but this has been undoubtedly due not to the lack of the value of the outdoor part of the farmer's life, but to the monotony of the work and to the very bad conditions found indoors, particularly in the winter. When this indoor life has been modified so that [Pg 302] plenty of fresh air is supplied day and night, and when reasonable attention is paid to the demands of the body in the matter of food and drink, then the duration of life of farmers will rank high in comparison with other occupations.

*Direct causes of disease.*

The direct causes of disease may be due to the introduction into the human body of a specific microörganism which, if not met by the antagonistic agencies, finally pervades the whole system with its progeny or its virus. The microörganisms thus responsible for disease are commonly divided into two classes, namely, parasites and bacteria. In the first group are included those parasites that cause tapeworm, malaria, trichinosis, and hookworm; in the second group those bacteria that cause typhoid fever, cholera, erysipelas, diphtheria, and probably smallpox, measles, scarlet fever, chicken pox, and a number of others presumably similar.

*Parasites as causes of disease.*

The introduction of worms into the body must come either from impure drinking water, from impure food, or from the bites or stings of insects. When introduced into the body, those parasites that are inimical to man and produce abnormal conditions interfering with usual physiological functions may or may not develop further. In some cases, as in malaria, the very act of hatching the malarial brood is sufficient to throw the host on whom the brood will feed into a violent chill.

In other cases, as with the hookworm, while eggs are produced in the human body, they have no directly detrimental effect, the objectionable feature of their residence [Pg 303] being due to the fact that the continual draught which they make upon the blood vessels of the intestine reduces the vitality, causing anæmia.

In other cases, as with the guinea worm, found in Africa and South America, the worm wanders from the stomach, which it enters toward the surface of the body, and finally breaks through, causing ulcers or abscesses.

In still other cases, as with that form of filaria which causes elephantiasis, the adult worm or the embryos are present in the lymphatics in such numbers as to interfere with circulation, causing the fearful swellings characteristic of the disease named.

Finally, in such cases as trichinosis and tapeworm, there is usually but little inconvenience to the human being harboring them, except when their number becomes very large. Then there may be diarrhœa, loss of appetite, and other digestive disturbances. The different tapeworms are generally responsible for nothing more than indigestion and nervousness. These latter parasites are, however, formidable in so far as their size is concerned. The mature pork tapeworm is about ten feet long, although the eggs, seen in the pork flesh, giving it its name of "measly," are only about a thousandth of an inch in diameter. The fish tapeworm, when mature, measures about twenty-five feet in length, while the beef tapeworm is about the same length. These worms can develop only in the bodies of the animals named, and find their way into the human body only through the medium of imperfectly cooked meat.

If proper precautions be taken in these directions, if only water is used for drinking which is known to be free from such parasites and their eggs, and if insects like [Pg 304] mosquitoes and fleas are kept away by screening windows and doors, and if meat be always thoroughly cooked, the dangers of diseases from parasites will be reduced to a minimum.

By far the most important of the living agencies concerned with the direct production of disease are those small vegetable organisms known as bacteria. Not all bacteria, by any means, produce disease; in fact, it is not too much to say that the majority of bacteria are benefactors to the human race. Their chief agency is not to cause disease, but to prevent it, and they do this because they are able to transform the waste products of animal life, which would normally be dangerous to health, into harmless mineral residue. They are really the scavengers of the earth's surface, not actually carrying off garbage, but rather transforming it, and, in the process, not merely destroying it, but changing it so as to make it available for plant-food. It is through the agency of bacteria that the air, which is being continually overloaded with carbonic acid from the lungs of animals, is reduced and taken up by plants so that an equilibrium is maintained. Otherwise, the atmosphere would be more and more vitiated with carbonic acid and organic vapors, and every one would die as if shut up in an air-tight room. But, because of bacteria, neither is the surface of the earth overloaded with waste organic matter nor do streams, however much polluted, continue to flow without some improvement being traced in their quality.

In some of the ordinary manufacturing processes, bacteria are all-important, as in making vinegar, wines, [Pg 305] cheese; in fact, in any of the fermented food products. In agriculture, they are entirely responsible for supplying an adequate amount of food material to growing plants. Fresh manure is not suitable for plant-food and would be of no value on the fields or in the garden except as improved and modified by bacterial action. One of the greatest discoveries of their importance recently made has to do with the way in which peas and beans are able to absorb nitrogen from the air through the agency of bacteria. One knows that plowing under a crop of peas or clover enriches the soil, and that peas or clover make the best growth for this purpose. The reason is that these plants, through the activity of bacteria, are able to absorb nitrogen from the air and afterwards to convert it into food material.

But with all these good qualities a few bacteria, gone bad, perhaps, are associated with diseases, and by a series of experiments, chiefly those of a Frenchman named Pasteur and of a German named Koch, and of their followers, it has been ascertained that certain bacteria, and those only, will cause certain diseases. These diseases, that is, these caused by bacteria, are generally spoken of as epidemic or contagious, of which typhoid fever and cholera are examples.

All contagious diseases cannot at present be definitely associated with bacteria, probably for the reason that the methods employed to find the bacteria have not been adequate. For instance, the bacteria of smallpox has never been found, although the disease is so characteristically one of bacterial origin that no one can doubt the cause. Similarly, the bacteria responsible for measles, scarletina, and whooping cough have never been discovered, although the [Pg 306] cause of each is also presumably bacterial. More definite information on the subject of the individual and responsible bacteria will be given in the subsequent chapters dealing with specific diseases. Inquiries into the method of growth and into the life history of specific bacteria serve our present purpose only as they teach methods for the prevention of the disease. For example; when it was found that the parasite of yellow fever, in the course of its life, spent fourteen days in the mosquito's body in such a condition that the mosquito during that time was harmless, it made possible exposure to mosquitoes laden with yellow fever for a period of thirteen days from the time of the preceding case.

*Antitoxins.*

But the methods of combating the different diseases when once contracted in the human body, based on the knowledge obtained of the life history of these germs, have been the most important result of their biological study. A large part of this knowledge has been acquired by the study of animals which have been found susceptible and so available for experimental investigation, and it may be that the impossibility of studying measles, for instance, in animals, may be one reason why the germ has never been discovered.

There is no evidence that animals suffer spontaneously from such diseases as typhoid fever, Asiatic cholera, leprosy, yellow fever, smallpox, measles, and so on; but it seems that in animals, as in man, the disease is the direct result of the life and growth in the animal of the characteristic disease-producing germ. The fact that diphtheria or tuberculosis can be experimentally given to rabbits or [Pg 307] guinea pigs is without doubt the chief source of our knowledge of those diseases, although, in general, it is impossible to produce diseases in any animal which will be, clinically, precisely like the disease as it appears in man. The converse of this is also true, namely, that when it has been found impossible to experimentally inoculate an animal with a disease supposed to be bacterial in nature, then but very little of that disease is known.

The most important result of bacterial studies has been the production of what are known as antitoxins, and no more wonderful discovery has ever been made. To understand as best we may the principle involved, it is necessary to explain the process of bacterial attack. When bacteria capable of producing disease are introduced into the system, either through the mouth or into the lungs or into the blood through some skin abrasion, the bacteria, finding there a congenial habitat, thrive, grow, and multiply. In some cases, this bacterial growth results only in breaking down the cell tissues at the point or in the vicinity of the place where growth occurs; for instance, if a cut is made with a dirty knife, that is, one carrying bacteria on the blade, and is not immediately washed out with an antiseptic solution, bacteria will grow and pus will form in the cut. Similarly, a splinter, if not removed and cleansed, will produce a pus-forming wound. But unless a very extensive suppuration starts, the difficulty is all local. So it is with consumption, when the bacteria are localized in the lungs and by their growth destroy the lung tissue without, at least for many weeks, affecting the general health.

There are germs, however, like typhoid fever and diphtheria, which do not produce any particular local disturbance [Pg 308] with the growth of bacteria, but the whole body becomes sick, the circulation of the blood is affected, and a general disturbance ensues. This is due to the action of a poison, called a toxin, which is set free as a result of the growth of the bacteria in some one part of the body, which poison is then carried by the blood throughout the entire system, inducing fever and a general debility.

Just how these toxins are formed is not certain. They are not the bacteria themselves. This we know because the disease-producing bacteria can be grown in broth and the mixture can be strained through fine porcelain, fine enough to strain out the bacteria. Yet it has been found that the clear liquid passing the porcelain filter is capable of producing disease and is a deadly poison without the presence of any bacteria at all. During the incubation period of a disease, as, for example, in the three-week period when typhoid fever is developing, these poisons are being formed and are being scattered through the body, and it is during this time that the fight takes place between these poisonous forces and the defending forces always present in the human system. As already pointed out, these defensive forces are powerful or not, according as the general health of the individual is good or bad, and we see the familiar sight of persons said to be run down taking a disease, while those not so depleted of vitality are able to resist or remain immune.

So certain are scientific men of this power and of the fact that the power resides generally in the white corpuscles of the blood that, in the presence of a dangerous infection, a person's blood may be examined, and, if the white corpuscles are not present in sufficient quantity, [Pg 309] proper means must be taken for developing this element in the blood, or else the person must take himself away from the infection, if the infection is to be avoided.

As a result of the conflict between the toxins and the defensive forces of the body, certain vital processes are set free in the blood and in the cells which seem to possess a highly specialized power of defense against any subsequent attack. Pasteur, in his researches on the subject of rabies, developed this power of resistance by inoculating into rabbits the rabies infection of a monkey. Monkey rabies is not a severe form and is scarcely felt by the ordinary rabbit, but if the infective material (usually part of the spinal cord) of the monkey-infected rabbit is transferred to a second rabbit, the disease becomes more severe; and if the disease is passed from animal to animal, it may be built up into as severe a form as desired, up to the maximum. Pasteur found that by inoculating an individual with a one-day rabbit, that is, with the weakest brand of infection killing a rabbit in one day, and the next day with a two-day rabbit, that the person could receive this two-day inoculation without discomfort or danger because of the greater antagonism acquired by the preceding inoculation. Continuing the inoculations for fourteen days and making the strength of the infection stronger each day, at the end of the period it was found that the fourteenth inoculation, strong enough to produce the disease and kill a fresh subject, had, on account of the preceding inoculations, produced ability to withstand or counteract the actual disease developing perhaps at the same time. Fortunately, in the case of this disease, the shortest period for its development is fifteen days, and often it is a month or more after [Pg 310] the bite of the dog before the disease develops. By successive inoculation of increasing strength for fourteen days, the system will have acquired a habitude to the disease which prevents the normal effects.

Diphtheria is prevented in much the same way, except that in this case horses are used, their blood being strengthened to resist the disease by successive inoculations of the diphtheria poison. It is probable that all the bacterial diseases which exert their influence through the transmission of toxins in the blood may be counteracted by the production of an antitoxin when once the method of building up this antitoxin has been learned. At present, rabies, tetanus, diphtheria, and cerebrospinal meningitis are the four diseases for which antitoxin is made commercially and generally used. For a great many years, scientists have labored without success to find an antitoxin for consumption, and within the last year extensive experiments have been made in the American army on the use of antitoxin for typhoid fever.

*Natural immunity.*

It may be worth noting that not all resistance to specific diseases needs to be acquired in the roundabout way just described. The state of being free from disease is known as immunity, and the way of securing immunity just described is known as artificial immunity. This artificial immunity may also be obtained in the course of events by having the disease as a child, thereby generating the antitoxin in one's own body instead of in the body of some cow or horse or rabbit.

There is, however, a natural immunity which is due to long-continued environment or to protracted heredity. [Pg 311] The negroes in the South have, by a lifelong proximity and struggle with the disease, acquired a practical freedom from typhoid fever, although it remains with the negro sufficiently to form a focus for the spread of the disease among others not equally immune. Creoles in yellow-fever districts have a natural immunity from the hookworm disease, although probably the class are responsible for its generous transmission to the poor whites with whom they associate. Racial immunity from certain diseases may be shown by statistical studies.

*Chemical poisons.*

Instead of the introduction of toxins into the body by the agency of bacteria, it is quite possible for chemical poisons, not formed originally by bacteria, to be set free in the body. Sulphate of copper, for instance, is essentially a mineral poison which acts on the human system in such a way as to produce death, and certain other mineral substances may be mentioned, such as phosphorus, arsenic, and mercury, which are well-known poisons. There are also many vegetable products, not bacterial, which are poisonous in their nature, that is, distributing to the blood and lymphatics certain substances in solution which act on the cells of the various organs of the body in such a way that the activity of those organs is stopped. Opium, cocaine, alcohol, and some of the coal-tar products used for headaches, as phenacetin, are deadly poisons when a limited dose is exceeded.

There are also certain poisons engendered in the body itself whose action is similar to that of chemical bodies and which can hardly be called bacterial. These poisons represent generally stages in the process of nutrition where for [Pg 312] some reason the normal process is arrested and chemical bi-products are set free. Also, tissue which has been thrown off, in or by any organ, begins to decompose, thereby sending throughout the system the poisons of decomposition. Inflammation too generally results in the breaking down of the cells and the distribution of the resulting poisons. Of late years, much has been said of the poisonous property of the body waste not disposed of by excretion, and the theory of auto-intoxication, so-called, has received many adherents. The great scientist, Metchnikoff, has even gravely contended that it would be well for children to have their larger intestine removed entirely, because in that organ putrefaction occurs, the cause of the auto-intoxication he would try to prevent.

*External causes.*

The external causes responsible for disease are due to conditions of weather so severe as to be outside the possibility of self-protection. Excessive heat is responsible each year for deaths from sunstroke, and other conditions of weather are often the direct causes of disease, if not of death.

Accidents are the indirect cause of death, and there will always be a small proportion of the deaths occurring each year due to violence or accident. But, inasmuch as these deaths are clearly preventable, it is the duty of those interested in rural hygiene to study the reasons for accidental death, and, if the number of such accidents can be reduced, to strive for that reduction. As an example, it may be mentioned that each year a number of deaths in New York State, and probably in other states, occur from accidents at culverts and bridges, due to insufficient [Pg 313] protection in the way of railings and fences. A method of reducing the deaths from accidents, therefore, would include a proper survey of all the roads of a vicinity to make sure that no danger exists in this regard. Other precautions against preventable accidents will readily suggest themselves.

[Pg 314]

## CHAPTER XV

# *DISINFECTION*

Inasmuch as more than 10 per cent of all deaths are due to bacterial or to various infectious diseases, it is of considerable interest to study the various means by which these germ diseases may be prevented. In this chapter it is proposed to discuss the different ways in which the active agents concerned in the spread of disease may be captured and put to death. It has already been pointed out that infectious diseases can be acquired only by the introduction of the specific germs into the human body, either through the mouth or lungs or through some skin abrasion. Further than this, it is quite as definitely known that the vitality of the germ after leaving a diseased person depends primarily upon its condition at the time of leaving the body and afterwards upon the environment which that germ finds outside of the affected person, while waiting for a chance to make its next human resting place.

It is evident, therefore, that if during the interval which elapses between the time when the germs leave a sick person and the time when they enter another person some method could be found by which these germs could be killed, the progress of the disease would be effectually stopped.

This, in the most general sense, is what is meant by [Pg 315] disinfection. It is a determined effort to destroy the carriers of disease while temporarily absent from the human body which is their natural home. This process of killing bacteria, however, is not so simple a matter as it might at first seem. They are, unfortunately, such minute beings that they cannot be seen, so that the warfare is waged against an invisible enemy, not, however, to be despised on that account. The methods of warfare must be uncertain, since the exact location of the enemy cannot be known, and it is manifestly impossible to disinfect the universe. What is done is to fix upon the location or surroundings where the original patient was confined, and, assuming that the germs, if any, which have escaped ready for further infection are somewhere near, to poison the air and the wall and floor of the room in question so that happily the germs may be killed.

*Disinfecting agents.*

The various agents used to destroy those germs which are carriers of disease may be divided into two groups, namely, heat in its various forms, and chemicals. Literally, the word "disinfection" means "doing away with infection," so that to disinfect a room is to do away with the infection present in the room. It has, however, come to have a more general meaning than this and is commonly used instead of the word "destroy," so that a disinfecting solution is the same thing as a destroying solution, applied, of course, to bacteria.

It has already been explained that by far the majority of bacteria are useful if not essential to human life, and one of the difficulties in employing disinfecting or destroying solutions is that they put an end at the same time to both [Pg 316] useless and useful bacteria. As an example, the fermentation processes in the human intestines are accompanied if not produced by certain kinds of bacteria, although on occasion these harmless or useful bacteria may develop into most obnoxious germs, producing unpleasant fermentation. It might be easy enough for a doctor to make a patient swallow some antiseptic solution, like carbolic acid or corrosive sublimate or nitrate of silver, for the purpose of getting rid of certain undesirable bacteria in the intestines, but it does not need a doctor to know that for a patient to swallow such active poisons as these would not merely kill the harmful bacteria and the good ones as well, but probably the patient himself.

*Antiseptics.*

There is another word often used in connection with bacteria, namely, "antiseptic," and the common significance of this word applies to a substance which interferes with or retards the growth of bacteria without actually destroying them. Doctors, for instance, use antiseptic instead of disinfecting solutions on wounds, not because they do not wish to kill the pus-forming bacteria, but because the antiseptic solution will prevent their growth and not be, as a disinfecting solution, harmful to the cells which he is trying to repair. It would be folly, for example, to inject a strong 50 per cent solution of carbolic acid into a wound on the arm produced by a saw, because all the energy of the vital forces at the seat of the wound are needed for repairs, and there is none to spare for so active a detergent as carbolic acid. An antiseptic, on the other hand, is mild enough so that it does not act on the tissue at all, but merely prevents any undesirable growth of bacteria. [Pg 317]

*Deodorizers.*

There are substances used, perhaps not so much around country houses as around city houses and in water-closets, which are neither disinfectants nor antiseptic, but act as deodorizers only. Such a substance, for example, may be thrown into the kitchen sink, not at all for the purpose of killing bacteria, but for disguising the smell from the cesspool into which the sink-wastes discharge. It has no disinfecting properties and is good for nothing unless the material is so scented as to be agreeable on that score. One of the frauds perpetrated on the public is the preparation and sale of the various appliances designed and regulated to produce a perpetual smell and claimed on that account to be either disinfecting or antiseptic agents. The smell is worth nothing.

*Patented disinfectants.*

The poison of the disinfectant or antiseptic, whether it be in liquid or in gas form, is the essence of the material, and since the value of disinfectants is based on the crude raw materials which any one can buy, it is clearly unnecessary to buy expensive patented solutions for disinfectants when ordinary lime or carbolic acid are equally as good and can be had at much lower prices.

A disinfecting solution, to be successful in its action, must be reasonably proportioned in volume to the amount of material to be disinfected, whether this be a liquid or clothing or the air of a room. It is the height of absurdity, for instance, to pretend to disinfect the air of a large room by burning a tablespoonful of sulfur on a shovel in the center of a room without even taking the trouble to close the door. It is absurd to attempt to disinfect the bed [Pg 318] linen in a single pailful of hot water, since even if the water was hot at the beginning, it would be so reduced in temperature by the first piece that went in that its efficacy would be lost for everything else. It is equally absurd that a liquid from a bottle, no matter how much advertised, can effectually disinfect a room, either by a gentle sprinkling of the liquid on the walls and floor or by a more thorough spraying of the air with an atomizer containing the liquid.

*Disinfecting gases.*

Two gases are available for use in disinfection, and these are valuable particularly in killing germs left in a room after a patient suffering from an infectious disease has been removed. The diseases referred to in the following chapters are all of this nature, and one of these two gases ought to be used in every case; otherwise the room may continue to harbor germs of the disease for months or years with the possibility of infecting a future tenant at a time when his vitality was such as to make him an easy prey. Nor must the contents of the room be overlooked.

The writer was recently told of a large family where one child had scarlet fever, recovering in September. The sick room was thoroughly disinfected, but the careful housewife, fearing damage to her blankets, had taken them to the attic before disinfection began. In the cold weather of February these blankets were brought down, and in six days the two children sleeping under them had contracted the disease.

*Sulfur as a disinfectant.*

When sulfur is burned, a gas is formed known as sulfurous acid, and until the last few years, it was the most common of all disinfecting agencies. The writer well remembers that when about to visit a city in South America infested [Pg 319] with yellow fever, he was seriously advised to fill the inside of his shoes with sulfur as a precaution against the disease. He might as well have worn a red ribbon on his hat so far as any protection went, but it illustrates the confidence formerly shown in sulfur as a disinfectant.

It is now known that in the dry, powdered state, sulfur is of no value unless, perhaps, the germs be smothered with the sulfur flour. When burned, however, the gas given off has a certain disinfecting property, although this is limited. It has almost no power of penetrating into curtains, blankets, and upholstered furniture, although the penetration is decidedly increased if these objects are moistened either by steam or by water vapor. The proper amount of sulfur to be burned for any room is at the rate of 3 pounds per 1000 cubic feet of air space in the room. Thus, if a room be 12 feet by 15 feet and 8 feet high, containing 1440 cubic feet, it would be necessary to burn 144/100 of 3 pounds, or 4-1/3 pounds.

Before undertaking to disinfect a room with sulfur, it should be made thoroughly air-tight, and this must be done carefully, not merely by closing the larger and obvious openings, like doors and windows, but by pasting strips of paper over every crack which might allow air to escape. Thus the four edges of the window sash must be pasted up, and a strip must close the crack between the two sashes. All the doors but the one reserved for exit should be pasted up from the inside, and finally this last door pasted up on the outside. If the floor has settled away from the base-board, the cracks thus made must be pasted up. In short, the room must be made absolutely air-tight. The room should be left thus closed for at least twenty-four hours, [Pg 320] and since there is some danger from fire, a proper provision should be made for the burning sulfur. This can be done by placing an old milk pan (a most convenient object in which to burn the sulfur) on a couple of bricks, which may be set inside a wash tub with perhaps three or four inches of water in the tub. The most convenient way of ignition is to moisten the sulfur with a little alcohol which can be readily set on fire.

Since clothes of every sort are more effectually acted upon when moist, they should be sprinkled with a hand atomizer just as the sulfur is lighted, and this should always be done in the case of any stuffed furniture or hangings. Anything that can be removed should be taken out and sterilized by steam, since live steam is the only disinfecting agent which will penetrate such things as mattresses, pillows, and rolled-up bundles of every sort, and with these last even steam is not certain. It is far safer to send a mattress to the cleaner to be steamed than to try to sterilize such bulky objects at home. It requires about twenty-four hours with the room tightly closed to generate enough gas so that the bacteria which may have found their way onto the walls or floor or ceiling or into the air of a room will be surely killed. After that time the room can be opened and then the usual household cleansing processes carried out as an additional safeguard. It is a wise measure in the case of infectious diseases, even after a room has been fumigated with sulfurous gas, to wipe off the woodwork and the walls, if their construction allows it, with a solution of carbolic acid, since in this way the germs which have accumulated on the woodwork will certainly be killed. [Pg 321]

*Formaldehyde disinfectant.*

Formaldehyde is the other gas which is commonly used for disinfecting the air of a room. It is most readily produced by buying solidified formaldehyde and then decomposing it by the action of heat. Formaldehyde candles, as they are called, may be purchased at almost any drug store, and while special forms of generating stoves may be found in the open market, an ordinary heating apparatus of almost any sort will answer the purpose of decomposing the solid formaldehyde. About 20 ounces of the formalin should be used for each 1000 cubic feet of space. With this agent, however, as with sulfur, the penetrating power of the gas is not very great, and such things as mattresses and clothing should be sent to a steam sterilizer rather than be trusted solely to the power of the formalde-hyde.

In using this gas, the same care about pasting up cracks and crev-ices in the room should be followed as already prescribed for the use of sulfur, and, as with sulfur, a reasonable precaution against fire should be taken by placing the apparatus in a tub of water or in a large pan of sand where accidents cannot happen. The room should be kept closed for at least twelve hours, and then should be thoroughly aired, and if the room is to be used again soon, the disa-greeable odor may be removed by the free use of ammonia, either sprinkling it around in the room or by placing about saucers of ammonia.

*Liquid disinfectants.*

More common than gases and most readily suggested as disin-fectants are certain liquids which have been proved both by labora-tory experimentation and by actual experience to have the power of killing bacteria when brought [Pg 322] into contact with them. Those liquids which have commended themselves particularly have additional advantages in not destroying fabrics, metals, or tissue with which they are brought in contact and in being purchasable at moderate prices.

There is little choice between a number of such liquids, and the number of modifications or combinations which are made and bot-tled and sold under some fancy name is legion. But the label, the name, and the additional price add nothing to the value of the basic chemical from which they are all compounded, and except for their convenience, they have little to recommend them.

*Carbolic acid as disinfectant.*

Carbolic acid is one of the most useful of these liquids, and in its various forms appears in almost all disinfectants. It may be obtained from the drug store in two forms, either as a crystal or as a concen-trated solution.

A 2 per cent solution, that is, one pint of carbolic acid to six gal-lons of water, is the proper strength for all such uses as wiping off wooden surfaces, furniture, floors, etc. A stronger (5 per cent) solu-tion is used when it is intended to destroy organic matter containing large quantities of germs. This is practically a saturated solution, so that if a bottle be partly filled with the crystals of carbolic acid and then completely filled with water, the water will absorb enough of the carbolic acid to make a 5 per cent solution, and the water may be poured on and off as long as the crystals remain. This 5 per cent solution is the proper strength to receive sputum from tuberculous patients, material ejected from the stomach in diphtheria, and fecal matter from typhoid and cholera patients. [Pg 323] This strong solution should not be used on the living human body, since it is powerful enough to eat directly into the flesh, and being a violent poison, it should be kept out of the way of the household and carefully labeled to avoid accidents.

Carbolic acid has no value at all in the way of disinfecting the air, although fifty years ago surgeons were accustomed to use a spray of carbolic acid around the operating table before an operation in order to destroy any germs of the air lingering in the vicinity. It is equally futile to pour carbolic acid into sewers or to stand it around on the mantelpiece for the purpose of disinfecting a room. Nor are sheets wet in carbolic acid and hung over doorways and at the end of passages anything more than a remnant of medievalism.

*Coal-tar products.*

There are certain preparations made from coal-tar which, either alone or combined with carbolic acid, have very strong disinfecting properties and which are the bases of most of the patented disinfecting solutions now sold. They are commonly called cresols or creosols and a 4 per cent solution of any of the three ordinary forms will destroy bacteria in a few hours. They are commonly used for receiving organic excretions of sick persons in the same way as carbolic acid is used, and have about three times the power of carbolic acid to destroy bacteria.

They have one great advantage besides the strength mentioned, in that they are not materially affected or interfered with by the presence of albuminous material. Carbolic acid in the presence of albuminous material, like sputum, for instance, has the strength of the disinfectant [Pg 324] partly used up in combining with this albuminous material so that the strength remaining for disinfection is weakened, and the result is not as satisfactory as it would otherwise be. The coal-tar products, on the other hand, are not so interfered with, and the solution acts in full strength upon the bacteria.

*Mercury for disinfectant.*

Corrosive sublimate, or bichloride of mercury, is one of the most active poisons known and is as effective in dealing with the microscopic organisms known as bacteria as it is in dealing with the larger animals for which it has been used for years past,—the destruction of bed-bugs.

For general cleaning purposes, such as scrubbing woodwork, floors, and walls, it should be used in strength of about 1 part to 3000 parts of water. This means that for 1 ounce of corrosive sublimate 3000 ounces of water or 25 gallons must be taken. This solution is very active in its effect on all metal, so that it must be kept in brassware or earthenware, and when mixed with the material which it is intended to disinfect, it must be kept from tin or iron. This solution is also affected by albuminous material, although this may be counteracted by the addition of salt. It is a good plan, therefore, to add to the solution salt at the rate of about 4 teaspoonfuls to each gallon of solution. On account of the very poisonous action of this solution great care must be taken to keep it away from children, and it has been suggested that it is desirable to add some coloring matter to the liquid, since without this it may be mistaken for clear water.

*Lime for disinfecting.*

Chloride of lime is one of the most useful as well as one [Pg 325] of the cheapest disinfectants available. It costs about $25 a ton, although by the pound this wholesale price would not be obtained. It is effective in a 1 per cent solution, that is, 1 pound of chloride of lime to 100 pounds or 12 gallons of water. To be effective, the solution must be well stirred into the organic matter to be disinfected, since it is the chloride rather than the lime which is the disinfecting agent. Saucers or soup plates of chloride of lime standing around the room have no effect upon the germs in the air and on the floor and are of no more value than sulfur, or roses for that matter. Chloride of lime is commonly known as bleaching powder, and its effects on clothes or on any substance which can be eroded is well known. It is, therefore, not a suitable material for disinfecting towels, because the action is on the towel as well as on the bacteria, differing in this respect from mercury, which does not hurt the fiber of clothes.

Milk of lime is produced by slaking ordinary building lime until a fine white powder is obtained, about an equal quantity of water to the amount of lime to be slaked being necessary. When the powder has formed and steam has ceased to be given off, then about four gallons of water should be added to each gallon of the powder and the mixture well stirred. This will probably always leave some lime in the bottom of the vessel, since limewater is a saturated solution, and these proportions furnish more lime than is necessary. If not too thin, it is a good whitewash and is a most important agent when used as a whitewash in disinfecting walls and ceilings of such rooms as hospitals and cellars and other places where have been contagious diseases. Milk of lime is an admirable disinfectant in the [Pg 326] sick room and generally in houses where infectious diseases have been. It may be poured down drains, into water-closets and privies, and used liberally in all places where bacteria may be supposed to thrive. It must come into intimate contact, however, with the bacteria, and merely sprinkling a little lime dry around the borders of a gutter or drain is of no value. The writer saw, not long ago, a chicken yard where the inspector of a health department had undertaken to secure disinfection by a generous sprinkling of white lime powder around the yard. Such a procedure, however, is not effective, but in a drain the dry powder might be of value because it would later become effective when washed in solution into the drain. Ordinarily, the dry powder is to be avoided.

*Soap as an antiseptic.*

No better antiseptic exists than ordinary soap, not altogether because of the properties of the soap, but because of the action of the soap combined with hot water. Washing soda, dissolved in water and used for boiling clothes which have become polluted, adds to the disinfecting power of the hot water the disinfecting properties of the soap, and the result is most effective. Ammonia has not the same value as the soda or potash soap, although it has the power of destroying bacteria in the course of a few hours.

It may not be out of place to emphasize the value of soap, not particularly in times of epidemic or contagious disease, but as a continual safeguard against infection. A large proportion of the contagious diseases are probably the result of infected fingers or hands coming in contact with the mouth and leaving there the germs of infection. One [Pg 327] of the first things a surgeon learns, in order to avoid any possible infection of wounds or of openings which he makes for an operation, is to thoroughly wash his hands in order to remove therefrom all possible germs. He scrubs his hands, particularly his finger nails, with soap and water and then bathes them in a solution of bichloride of mercury before touching the patient in any place where infection might occur. The difficulty, even with this great care, of freeing their hands from bacteria has been found to be so great that, in late years, surgeons have preferred to use, during operations, thin rubber gloves which can be boiled before using and can be soaked in a stronger antiseptic than the hands could bear.

It is extraordinary, from the standpoint of self-infection, to see how men can be so careless as to sit down to dinner, after having worked in places where their hands have come in contact with all sorts of organic filth, without stopping to wash those hands even in cold water. It is certainly providential that disease germs are as uncommon as they are, for with the careless habits of most people in putting their hands to their mouths, the death-rate from infectious diseases would be much higher than it is except for the fact that most of the germs thus introduced into the mouth are not disease-producing.

*Disinfecting by heat.*

Better than any chemical agent known to be a destroyer of bacteria is heat in one form or another. This may be steam or hot water or dry heat. If a high enough temperature is maintained for a sufficient length of time, the action is absolutely destructive to all germs. Fire does, of course, destroy bacteria along with whatever material the bacteria [Pg 328] are concealed in, but such a disinfectant is of little value for ordinary purposes, since the object of disinfection is to destroy bacteria without destroying the surface on which they are lodged. In some old buildings, where consumption or smallpox, for example, has become permanent, it may be that the surest way of killing all the bacteria is to burn up the house.

*Dry heat.*

Unfortunately, even a moderate heat cannot always be applied. One's hands, for example, can neither be heated in an oven to the necessary temperature for destroying bacteria in their pores, nor can they be immersed in boiling water or steam for a sufficient time to secure thorough disinfection. Therefore, with the body, chemical means for disinfection must be employed. Also when it is desired to disinfect a liquid, such as beef broth, in which the experimenter desires to grow some particular species to the exclusion of all others, dry heat is inapplicable because it would evaporate the liquid, nor is chemical disinfection possible because of its antiseptic effect on the bacteria to be cultivated. Moist heat, therefore, must be used. When dry heat is used, it is usually for the disinfection of glassware or earthenware or metallic objects, the quality of which will not be affected by the necessary temperature, namely, 150 degrees Centigrade, or about 300 degrees Fahrenheit. This temperature must be maintained for at least an hour, and it is not certain even then to penetrate in full power to the middle of blankets or comfortables. Except for glassware to be used in a laboratory, dry heat, such as would be obtained by a kitchen oven, is not to be recommended. [Pg 329]

*Boiling water.*

Boiling water, on the other hand, is the most effective and penetrating disinfecting agent available. One has only to expose an object to boiling water for five minutes to absolutely kill all disease-bearing bacteria contained, and since bed linen, clothes, blankets, and such articles as are naturally used in a sick room have to be washed after a patient's recovery, it requires but very little additional trouble to subject the soiled articles to that temperature of the water which will secure disinfection at the same time. But the water must be boiling. The mere fact that it was once boiling water gives it, half an hour later, no disinfecting properties, and complete disinfection can be secured only by actually boiling the garments or articles for at least five minutes. The apparatus necessary therefore — and no better piece of disinfecting apparatus can be secured anywhere—is a good old-fashioned wash boiler. The action is more certain, that is, more penetrating, if a little washing soda is added to the water at the rate of a tablespoonful of soda to a gallon of water. This solution is admirable for washing dishes, spoons, knives, forks, and other eating utensils used by sick persons. It is always a mistake to wash dishes from the sick room in the same vessel with other dishes. They should not only be washed separately, but they should be washed in boiling water, and preferably in a soap solution as just described.

*Steam.*

For some purposes, steam is better even than hot water; its effect on cotton and woolen garments is not so disastrous. A comfortable or blanket, for instance, may be subjected to steam without losing its elastic quality, and [Pg 330] for small garments, an ordinary steamer, such as is used for puddings, answers admirably. Cities use steam sterilizers because of the greater convenience in furnishing steam to a large tank as compared with filling and emptying a tank with water and then providing sufficient heat to boil that water. The exposure to steam should last from half an hour to an hour, depending on whether the objects to be disinfected are small, open, and loose, or large, compact, and dense. Some articles, like bales of rugs, rolls of wool, and large bundles of cloth, cannot be sterilized at the center by ordinary steam, and while it is not likely that infection at the centers of such tightly rolled bundles has occurred if exposure took place while rolled up, yet it is certain that the disinfection does not reach these centers. In the case of such bundles as rugs from infected countries, where any single rug may become the medium of infection, it is requisite to thoroughly sterilize all parts of the bundle. For this purpose, it is necessary not merely to expose the articles to live steam, but to have the live steam under pressure so that it is forced into the inside of the packages by an excess of external pressure. This is probably not available in an ordinary house, where boiling must continue to be the method of disinfection.

*Drying, light, and soil.*

Before leaving this chapter, three agencies for disinfection may be pointed out, not perhaps to be depended on, but in order that the kindly provisions of nature may be appreciated. All germs removed from the body, which is their natural home, and exposed to the air are subject to drying and thus are killed. Unfortunately, this does not become true except after long periods of time, nor is it [Pg 331] equally true with all germs, but it is certainly one of the methods by which the evil effects of disease germs may be lessened. The germ of consumption lasts as long as any germ, and yet this, when dried in the street, loses its vitality after about a week. Similarly, the typhoid fever germs, unless kept in a moist condition, dry up and die in a few days. With the drying, however, comes the danger that in the process they may be lifted by the wind and carried in the air to the mouths or nostrils of well persons, so that it is not wise to depend solely on this method of disinfection.

Sunlight is more positive than the wind, and the exposure to direct sunlight of a bottle filled with disease germs will kill them all in two or three hours. The surface layers of a pond never have as many bacteria in them as the lower layers, partly on account of the sedimentation, but largely because they are killed by the direct action of sunlight. The bacillus of consumption and bacillus of diphtheria are both killed in an hour or so by direct sunlight. This is one reason why living rooms should have sunny exposure and why, on the other hand, disease thrives in dark tenements.

The soil is the third natural method of disinfection, not because the soil itself destroys bacteria, but because in the soil are to be found millions of non-harmful germs and these germs are hostile to the disease-producing germs, so that they destroy their virulence. It is on this principle that the wastes from typhoid fever patients are buried in the garden, the presumption being that the bacteria there present will destroy the typhoid fever germs before they can escape and do any harm. While this action undoubtedly exists, it is not positive enough to depend upon, and disinfection by the use of chemicals should always be practiced.

[Pg 332]

## CHAPTER XVI

## *TUBERCULOSIS AND PNEUMONIA*

These two common widespread diseases affecting the lungs may be discussed together, although they are not closely related in origin or effects.

*Tuberculosis.*

That form of tuberculosis known as consumption is at present the most prevalent and the most dreaded of all infectious diseases. In 1908, in the Registration Area of the United States (about one half of the whole country), it caused 67,376 deaths. Deaths from other infectious diseases are shown in the following table, together with the population: —

## Table XVIII. Showing Deaths From Various Infectious Diseases In The United States, 1908

| | |
|---|---:|
| Population of Registration Area | 45,028,767 |
| Deaths in Registration Area | 691,574 |
| Deaths from tuberculosis | 67,376 |
| Deaths from pneumonia | 61,259 |
| Deaths from diarrhœa (chiefly of babies) | 52,213 |
| Deaths from cancer | 33,465 |
| Deaths from typhoid fever | 11,375 |
| Deaths from diphtheria and croup | 10,052 |
| [Pg 333] | |
| Deaths from scarlet fever | 5,577 |
| Deaths from whooping cough | 4,969 |
| Deaths from measles | 4,611 |
| Deaths from smallpox | 92 |
| Deaths from hydrophobia | 82 |
| Deaths from leprosy | 11 |
| Deaths from bubonic plague | 5 |

Pneumonia is second in fatality, the two diseases of pneumonia and tuberculosis carrying off 128,635 persons, or about one fifth of all persons dying in the year. While these have both been great plagues to humanity from the very earliest days, it is only within the last ten years that their ravages have been appreciated and, especially with tuberculosis, their causes actively combated. There are two phases to be considered in discussing tuberculosis or consumption, namely, first, the method of prevention and second, the method of cure. It follows also that, since the cure of advanced cases is impossible and since every case which exists is a menace to the health of the community on account of the danger of the spread of the disease, the prevention is far more important than the cure.

Until the discovery by Robert Koch, in 1882, of the germ causing consumption, little could be done in the way of prevention, but since that time, only one quarter of a century ago, we have learned and applied the knowledge that, in the vast majority of cases, the disease is spread by the sputum of consumptive patients, which becomes dry, forms dust, and so is carried into the air to be breathed by persons not otherwise affected. It seems so simple a method, then, to prevent the spread of consumption. All that need be done is to take care of the expectorations of [Pg 334] persons suffering with the disease. It is thoroughly believed by experts that if this were done carefully and faithfully, the disease would be stamped out within a few years, and the slogan of a certain sanitary organization is "Complete Control of Tuberculosis in 1915." Too much emphasis cannot be placed on the direct and simple method of infection, and while other factors enter, as will be shown later, a thorough recognition and control of tuberculosis sputum would practically stamp out the disease.

The following circular, issued by the Committee on the Prevention of Tuberculosis of the Charity Organization Society of New York City, indicates the procedures advised by them to prevent the spread of the disease and, as will be seen, the essence of the axioms there expressed are summed in the words "Don't spit!": —

DON'T GIVE CONSUMPTION TO OTHERS.

DON'T LET OTHERS GIVE IT TO YOU.

*How to prevent Consumption.*

The spit and the small particles coughed up and sneezed out by consumptives, and by many who do not know that they have consumption, are full of living germs too small to be seen. These germs are the cause of consumption.

Don't spit on the sidewalks; it spreads disease, and it is against the law.

Don't spit on the floors of your rooms or hallways.

Don't spit on the floors of your shop.

When you spit, spit in the gutters or into a spittoon.

Have your own spittoons half full of water, and clean them out at least once a day with hot water.

Don't cough without holding your handkerchief or your hand over your mouth.

Don't live in rooms where there is no fresh air. [Pg 335]

Don't work in rooms where there is no fresh air.

Don't sleep in rooms where there is no fresh air.

Keep at least one window open in your bedroom day and night.

Fresh air helps to kill the consumption germ.

Fresh air helps to keep you strong and healthy.

Don't eat with soiled hands; wash them first.

Don't neglect a cold or a cough.

To be sure, the precept of "Don't spit," as applied in cities, has other reasons for enactment than to prevent tuberculosis. Spitting is a filthy habit, and its practice should be decried on the score of cleanliness whether on the streets or in any public place, so that the signs now seen in street cars and railroad trains, in halls and office buildings, are intended not altogether for consumptive patients, but also for those who need laws to force them to observe ordinary rules of cleanliness and decency. It is, however, the main step towards doing away with consumption, and the faithful observance of the injunction ought to be insisted upon quite as much in the individual home as in a city street or public building. Case after case has been cited of instances where one consumptive patient in a family has spread the disease through the household, and, at intervals of a year or so, one after another of the family has succumbed to the attacks of the consumptive germ, when by proper precautions and suitable care of the sputum of the first sick person, the other deaths might have been prevented.

*Individual resistance to tuberculosis.*

There is a remarkable difference in the ability of individuals to withstand the attacks of this disease, and it will [Pg 336] be found always that the first to succumb are those whose vitality has been in some way depleted. The women of the family, who are generally confined to the house, who do not have their lungs reënforced by a continual influx of fresh air, who are tired and worn out with their household duties, give themselves an easy prey to the attacks of the bacteria, while the men and boys, who are more outdoors, who are vigorous and strong, throw off the attack and are not affected.

It is a significant fact that by examination, dead bodies, so far as was known, not afflicted with tuberculosis in life, have, to the extent of 60 per cent, been found to have evidences of consumption in their lungs; that is, the edges of the lungs have been found affected, although the vitality of the individual was such that the action of the germ had been stayed before any serious injury was done. Most of us, at one time or another, have had, unknowingly, mild cases of consumption. It would be strange, indeed, if we did not, in view of all the tuberculous infection flying around in the air. But most of us are able to successfully combat the disease, so that the germs are destroyed before they are able to affect the entire body.

The other part of prevention consists in building up and holding up the vitality of the individual to a point where the vital forces can successfully oppose the attacks of the germs. Probably the decrease in the number of cases of consumption in the last quarter of a century has been due quite as much to the improved sanitary conditions of living, whereby the germs have been unable to secure a foothold in the individual, as to any precautionary measures taken against the germ itself. [Pg 337]

*Precautions by the consumptive.*

But the chief factor in the future restriction of the disease, as in the past, must be the disinfection of the germs immediately after they are thrown off from the consumptive patient, and it is well worth while to emphasize just what the consumptive should do or have done for him in order that he may not be responsible for the further spread of the disease. In the first place, when he spits, he must appreciate and act on the fact that the sputum is alive with consumptive germs, each one of which may possibly transmit the disease to whoever may come in contact with it. The patient must keep in mind continually that this sputum is poison, a deadly poison, and that it is his duty to see that every particle of it is disinfected or destroyed by one of the methods already indicated. He may expectorate into a vessel filled with a carbolic acid solution or he may expectorate into a vessel filled with water which may afterwards be boiled. He may use a cloth or paper, like a Japanese napkin, which may later be burned in the fire. But, above all things, he must not expectorate anywhere and everywhere, regardless of the consequences.

The consumptive patient must not cough without holding a handkerchief over his mouth, since small particles of sputum may become dislodged and distributed in this way.

The eating utensils used by a consumptive patient must not in any way be allowed to infect other people. The consumptive must have his own dishes reserved exclusively for him, and they must be, after each meal, carefully disinfected. With these precautions and with avoidance of such practices as kissing or otherwise directly infecting others, there is no reason why a consumptive [Pg 338] patient should be in any way an object of dread or why he should not live with his family in as much comfort as he can obtain, in perfect safety to himself and to them.

*Cure of consumption.*

The chief factor in the cure of consumption is the time at which the attempt at cure is started. Consumption is not an incurable disease, as was once thought, and there is no reason for so considering it. There is no such thing as galloping or quick consumption as distinguished from slow or lingering consumption, since the consumptive germ is the same in all people. The same germ may act differently in different people, and if one's power of resistance, as happens with those accustomed to drinking liquor, is low, the action of the germ is rapid, although the disease is identical with the form in which death comes only after years and years. If taken in time, that is, before the germ has so infected the body as to be beyond all possible restraint, as large a proportion of consumptive patients may recover as of patients from typhoid fever or diphtheria or any other infectious disease, but the cure must be started early. For instance, at one of the sanitariums in the Adirondacks, out of 267 patients admitted, who had the disease in an incipient stage, complete recovery was had in 219 cases, the disease was arrested in the case of 42 others, and in only 6 was the treatment not effective. Where the disease had become advanced, however, it was found that out of 192 cases, only 32 apparently recovered and 140 were improved to some extent. These are the significant facts in an institution for incipient cases only, where advanced cases, such as are met with by the practicing physician, are not received. [Pg 339]

Unfortunately, the ordinary physician does not always recognize the disease in its first stages, and a person may suffer for months with consumption, and even pass the time when the cure of the disease would be possible, without its being recognized. Such sick persons are treated for catarrh, for an obstinate cold and bronchitis, for grippe or malaria, whereas a proper diagnosis of the disease would be a recognition of the early stages of consumption and thus would prompt the patient to start at once on the necessary methods for cure. Nor is it possible to recognize the disease by any one definite indication. The cough which was once thought to be the deciding symptom is very often absent until the last stages of the disease. Expectoration of blood is similarly one of the last symptoms, exhibited only when too late for remedial measures. The presence of the tuberculosis bacillus or "T. B." in the sputum is also not generally found until the tissue of the lungs has become well advanced towards destruction, too late for remedy.

Experts in diagnosis attach great importance to family history, and have learned to expect the disease in persons when exposure to contagion is inevitable. They will recognize the disease from evidence not discernible to regular practitioners. For instance, if one member of a family is known to be affected, any chronic indisposition in another member, involving, perhaps, a daily rise in the temperature of the body, not sufficient to arouse alarm, but apparent in the listless behavior of the person, may be enough to suggest the beginning of the disease. An expert may detect the clogging up of the lung tissue by an examination of the lungs themselves, and probably this direct [Pg 340] examination, with a record of the daily rise and fall of temperature, particularly if the suspected patient has a listless feeling and a gradual loss of weight, would be sufficient to suggest the ordinary remedies.

The three remedies, which are nature's own methods, are good food, fresh air, and rest. It is difficult to say which of these three items is the most important. Certainly no hope of building up the resistance of the patient against the inroads of the disease can be expected unless the patient is thoroughly nourished. One of the sad facts in connection with those unfortunates whose fight against tuberculosis is nearly over and who in desperation have fled to Arizona, hoping that the dry air might afford relief, is that the lack of nourishing food, inevitable in those deserts, hastens on the disease, so that the expected benefits from the dry air are entirely offset. Likewise, in tenement-house districts in cities, the fight against consumption is practically useless because of the impossibility of securing for those starved or underfed helpless ones the nourishing food necessary. In the country, this part of the treatment ought to be the simplest, and yet one fears that the habit of eating through nine months of the year only salted and dried foods has not furnished patients in the country with the kind of nourishment necessary. Experience indicates that eggs and milk should be the bulwark on which the patient must depend for food, and in the sanitariums of New York State it is not uncommon for patients to be stuffed with two dozen raw eggs every day in addition to other food.

The next important factor is rest, since the effect of tuberculosis is to break down lung tissue, and for the prevention [Pg 341] of this it is necessary to give the forces of the body every aid in preventing this destruction. All exercise taken by a tuberculous patient means the withdrawing of that much blood from the lungs, where is the strategic point of the disease, to the part of the body being exercised, and one of the most striking features of sanitarium treatment is the absolute rest enjoined on the patients. Flat on their backs, day and night for months, without so much exercise as walking across the room, is the ordinary treatment, and the effect of disobedience is plainly seen in the rise in temperature or increase in fever which follows a violation of these rules. Even when the patients are allowed to sit up, they do not sit straight, but rest on couches or reclining chairs, so that their heads are down and their feet up, making the passage of the blood to the lungs easier. Even where the patient, determined to recover, is not able to place himself in the hands of a hospital physician, he can adopt this important method of arresting the disease by strictly avoiding exercise and exertion of every sort. The Massachusetts General Hospital in Boston has tuberculosis clinics, where patients who are not far enough advanced in the disease to require absolute rest are inspected daily, their condition noted, and advice given for the following twenty-four hours. One of the most common violations of the prescriptions given is overexertion, and yet the rest condition is essential for building up the diseased lung.

The third method of treatment involves fresh air, in order to improve the oxygenating character of the blood. If one remembers that the oxygen in the blood is the chief scavenger of the body and that the vitality of the red corpuscles [Pg 342] and their abundance is an essential factor in curing the disease, it will be seen why fresh air is so important. The tendency to-day is to insist on fresh air and to lay less stress on the climate than was formerly done.

It was not uncommon a few years ago for a physician, recognizing consumption, to send his patient away, partly because he honestly believed the climate of Arizona or Colorado or the Sandwich Islands was better than that where the patient lived, and partly, without doubt, because he was glad to get rid of a disease which he knew it was not in his power to cure. To-day, unless the patient can go to a properly equipped and maintained sanitarium, physicians recognize that conditions may be as beneficial at home as elsewhere and, provided the three factors mentioned — good food, rest, and fresh air — can be obtained, the chances for recovery are better because of better care at home than elsewhere.

But fresh air is essential, and this means that the patient must spend twenty-four hours a day in the open. He must eat and sleep out of doors. He must not go into the house when it rains, nor when it snows, and even with the thermometer at zero he must still stay out, wrapping himself up, to be sure, so that his body is not cold, but breathing into his lungs the life-giving, vitalizing, oxygen-bearing air. The side porch of a house may be very easily transformed into a room with a cot bed and an easy chair, where the consumptive may stay continually, and while it is convenient to have a window or a door opening from the porch into a room where the patient may be dressed and bathed, this is not essential, although customary in sanitariums. If no side porch exists, it is possible to build [Pg 343] such a porch, and the picture shows how such a construction may be added to even a small house in the city (Fig. 75). If this is out of the question, the windows of a room may be left open all the time, or the patient may lie on a bed, the head of which either extends through the window or is arranged to admit fresh air by a specially devised window tent.

Educational campaigns have been vigorously prosecuted for the past ten years, and gradually through the world is spreading a growing appreciation of the dangers of this disease. The effect of this increasing knowledge is reflected by a continually decreasing number of deaths in proportion to the population. The following diagram (Fig. 76) shows how this law is obeyed in New York State, the downward tendency of the line since 1890 being very plainly marked.

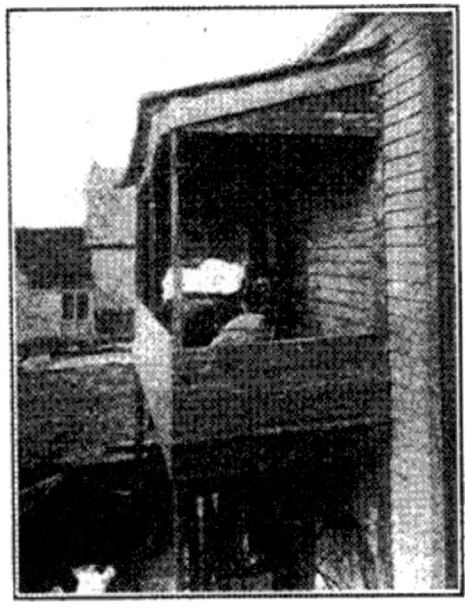Fig. 75. — Outdoor sleeping porch for tuberculosis patients.

The results being so manifest, the prophecy of Dr. Biggs of New York, written in 1907, is certainly justified: —

"In no other direction can such large results be achieved so certainly and at such relatively small cost. The time is not far distant when those states and municipalities [Pg 344] which have not adopted a comprehensive plan for dealing with tuberculosis will be regarded as almost criminally negligent in their administration of sanitary affairs and inexcusably blind to their own best economic interests."

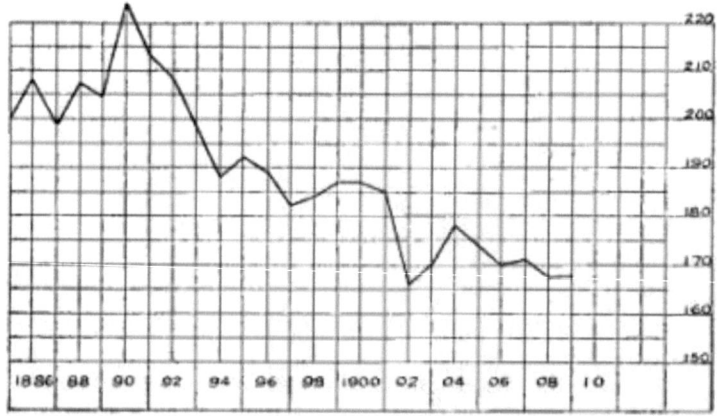

Fig. 76. — Mortality from pulmonary tuberculosis. Deaths per 100,000 population.

*Pneumonia. – The germ.*

In New York State in the year 1908, the largest number of deaths from any specific disease was due to consumption, the number of deaths in the rural population alone being 2906. The next largest number of deaths in the rural communities, and always a close second to consumption, was from pneumonia, the number being 2191; so that pneumonia justly ranks as highly important in the list of diseases which are at present most deadly in their effect on the human race and against which a vigorous fight should be made.

While pneumonia, like tuberculosis, is due to the action of a specific organism, the germ itself is not so generally [Pg 345] infectious; that is, the germ has not the power of remaining vigorous when out of the human body in the same way as has the germ of consumption. Like tuberculosis, the germ is expectorated and remains virulent when dried into dust, but the germ is much more sensitive to temperature changes and does not live longer than two or three hours when dried and exposed to the sun. It is, very curiously, a normal resident in the mouths of at least one third of all healthy persons, and it is only necessary for the body of these persons to become weakened for the germ to be able to secure a foothold and produce the disease. Unlike tuberculosis, which attacks chiefly those in the vigor of life, from fifteen to forty-five years of age, pneumonia attacks generally the very young and the very old; those under five and those over forty-five, the time of life when the vital resistance is the least.

*Weather not the cause of pneumonia.*

One of the sources formerly believed to be largely responsible for pneumonia, that is, exposure to severe weather, is curiously negatived by the fact that children and old people are not those generally exposed to weather. Perhaps no fallacy in any disease has been more prevalent than that pneumonia is usually contracted by exposure to wet or to cold. It has, indeed, been noticed that the disease has been practically non-existent under conditions where it would be prevalent if exposure alone were the cause. For instance, in the Arctic zone, where the temperatures are very low and where no adequate provision against the rigors of a severe climate are possible, pneumonia is practically unknown. During Napoleon's retreat from Moscow, when thousands of soldiers died from [Pg 346] physical exposure, from frost bite and starvation, where if exposure were the predisposing cause of pneumonia, it would have raged as an epidemic, it seldom appeared, proving this opinion.

Perhaps one reason why the disease has been supposed to result from exposure is the undoubted fact that it is chiefly prevalent in the winter and spring rather than in the summer. This argument is, however, modified by the fact that the majority of cases do not occur in January or February when the temperature is lowest, but in March, when the opening of spring is in sight. The reason for this is evident when we remember that the cause of the disease is a germ, generally present in the body and needing only a reduced vitality for its successful inroad on the human system. When, therefore, a person shuts himself up in an overheated house, without ventilation, takes insufficient exercise, and lives with an apparently determined effort to do everything possible to reduce his bodily vigor, then it is no wonder that the germ, almost in exultation, finds an opportunity for successful development.

*Preventives in pneumonia.*

Much as in tuberculosis, then, the best remedy and the best prevention for pneumonia is a careful attention to the needs of the body in order that it may preserve its normal vigor. Regular hours, sufficient sleep, and good food will, in most cases, keep the body in such a condition that pneumonia need not be dreaded, no matter what the exposure or what the temperature. Further than this, if the disease does once start and gain a foothold in the lungs, the best cure is, as with tuberculosis, a plentiful supply of oxygen or fresh air in order to remove the toxins formed [Pg 347] by the disease and give the lung tissue an opportunity to recover.

Formerly medical men treated pneumonia by confining the patient in an overheated room in which steam was generated, with the idea that the lungs would be most helped by an atmosphere of moist heat. Now, a pneumonia patient is supplied with all the fresh air possible, the windows of the sick room, even in winter, being kept continually open, and every effort being made to give the patient fresh air even when every breath means a shooting pain, and apparently untold suffering. In some of the New York City hospitals, the ward for pneumonia patients is on the roof, and children and babies suffering with pneumonia are at once taken there, even with snow piled all around the tent in which they are kept. The nurses and physicians are obliged to don fur coats, and heavy blankets must be provided to keep the patients from freezing to death; but the pneumonia germ, under these conditions, is worsted almost as if by magic, and within a few hours after leaving the warm wards of the hospital the patients start on the road to recovery.

The remedy, then, for the 2000 cases of pneumonia which occur in New York State each year, is an improved regulation of the health conditions of the separate families throughout the state—a better hygienic regulation of the everyday life. Care must be taken to provide better ventilation in the houses, more fresh air in the sitting room and in the sleeping rooms, more outdoor life in the winter time, and more exercise by which the blood circulation will be kept active. Then more varied and more suitable food must be consumed, food which will be capable of absorption [Pg 348] by the tissues and not clog the intestines and poison the system. More bathing, by which the pores of the skin can be relieved of the organic matter which otherwise clogs them and prevents their effective action in the removal of waste products, must be indulged in. With these three factors properly evaluated, with more fresh air, with better food, with ample bathing, pneumonia need not be dreaded, since then it would attack only those few whose constitutional vigor was impaired, and in the course of a generation or two the number of these would be so decidedly diminished that pneumonia would find no one susceptible.

*Infection of pneumonia.*

It must not be forgotten that a pneumonia patient is a source of infection quite as much as is a tuberculous patient, and the same precautions against infection should be followed. The nurse should be particularly careful not to infect herself. She should be careful to exercise enough self-control always to get daily exercise and fresh air and must, as a matter of self-protection, avoid overfatigue. The eating utensils, food refuse, and soiled clothing may all be infectious and must be sterilized by boiling as soon as removed from the sick room. The severe epidemics which have occurred from pneumonia have occurred in camps where sanitary conditions are grossly violated. Under such conditions pneumonia has become a most alarming epidemic, sometimes called the black death. In a single house, however, disinfection of the wastes of the patient and a proper care of the personal hygiene of the rest of the family will avoid the spread of the disease, and if the patient has sufficient vitality, sustained by good food and fresh air, he will recover without serious after affects.

[Pg 349]

## CHAPTER XVII

## *TYPHOID FEVER*

The two diseases already described, tuberculosis and pneumonia, are by far the most serious of all the infectious diseases, being responsible in New York State alone, in 1908, as already stated, for 5727 deaths. No other infectious disease even approximates the virulence and deadliness of these two, and while some of the constitutional disorders, such as Bright's disease, diarrhœa, and irregularity of the circulation, each result in from 2000 to 3000 deaths, the cause and prevention of these are so little understood as to baffle the hygienist. There are a number of contagious diseases which, while comparatively unimportant in the number of deaths, yet are of concern because the cause of the disease is so well known that the means of prevention is quite within our power. Of these, typhoid fever, in New York State in 1908, among the rural population alone resulted in 437 deaths, a rate of 18.7 per 100,000 population. The facts substantiate the assumption that for every person dying with typhoid fever there are ten cases of it, so it is a fair statement that in the rural part of New York State, in 1908, there were not far from 5000 persons afflicted with this disease. [Pg 350]

Perhaps one of the reasons why so determined a fight against this particular disease, involving only 5000 cases of illness during the year, has been made, is on account of the length of the illness in each case and on account of the fact that the disease usually attacks those in the very prime of life, from 15 to 40 years. It is also to be economically considered by reason of the loss of time involved in an illness of nearly two months and the loss of money implied in the nursing, doctors, and medicine. The movement against the disease is most encouraging because the line of attack is well known, and there is, humanly speaking, no reason at all why the disease should not be stamped out.

*Cause of the disease.*

Typhoid fever is a modern disease, and only for the last fifty years has it been recognized in medicine. It is caused by bacteria, and its manifestations are the results of bacterial growth in the body, chiefly in the smaller intestine. Here the toxin produces a violent poison which results in an attack of fever, lasting about six weeks. Owing to the bacterial growth, serious failings, commonly known as perforations, may develop after a severe attack, in the membranes and linings of the intestine, and the resulting inflammation is not infrequently the immediate cause of death. It is a thoroughly established fact that the disease is caused by a special type of bacteria and that if the bacteria could be killed outside the body, no transmission of the disease could occur. It is also true that if the disease germs could be destroyed within the body the patient would recover immediately, provided the toxins had not been already distributed through the system.

There are, therefore, two possible methods of doing [Pg 351] away with typhoid fever, one by eliminating all possibility of transmission outside of the body of the patient and the other by killing the germs while in the body of the patient. The latter plan is not feasible, since no antiseptic has been found which will kill the germs without killing the patient. It has been discovered that a drug called utropin will act on the germs when located in certain parts of the body, as in the kidneys; but this drug, although very effective in destroying germs in those organs, has no effect elsewhere. In general, we must eliminate the disease by preventing its transmission from the sick to the well.

*The bacillus of typhoid.*

Unfortunately, the typhoid fever germ is comparatively hardy and is not so easily killed by unfavorable environment as is the germ of pneumonia, for instance. It lives in water and in the soil, although probably it does not increase in numbers in either place. Nor will it live in the soil or in water indefinitely, and a great deal of study has been expended in trying to determine just how long typhoid fever germs will live under different conditions. It has been found, for example, that drying kills the typhoid bacillus in a few hours, although a few may survive for days. Experiments have also shown that it cannot leave a moist surface. It cannot, for instance, jump out of cesspools and drains and take to flight through the air, conveying the disease.

There is no possibility of contracting typhoid fever because a drain near the house is being cleaned out, since, so far as is known, the typhoid fever germ does not get into the air. The direct rays of the sun will kill typhoid fever germs within a few hours, although the value of this [Pg 352] sort of disinfection is limited, because where typhoid fever germs are apt to accumulate, the turbidity of the water prevents the penetration of the sun's rays for more than a few inches.

It has been found that a high temperature kills typhoid fever germs, and even so moderate a temperature as 160 degrees Fahrenheit is sufficient to destroy them. This is the principle employed in pasteurizing milk, since it is assumed, justly, that by raising the temperature of the milk to 160 degrees Fahrenheit, for ten minutes, it will be possible to kill any typhoid fever germs present. Boiling, of course, since this involves a temperature of 212 degrees, will kill the germs, and it is for this reason that wherever a water is suspected of typhoid pollution, it should be boiled before being used for drinking. It has been found that in distilled water, that is, in water where no available food is to be had, the germs will live about a month, and that in water with organic matter present, but without other bacteria, this period may be extended two or three times. In water rich in organic matter, but where other antagonistic bacteria are also present, the typhoid germs are usually driven out or killed at the end of three or four days.

It is not unreasonable to expect that at least half of the germs discharged into a stream will live a week, and if the stream has a uniform current, so that the germs are continuously carried downstream, they will be found below the point of infection, a distance equal to that which the stream will flow in a week. This is important because it shows how unlikely it is that the germs once placed in water will die out or disappear without infecting those who subsequently drink the water. There is evidence that [Pg 353] the typhoid germs, like all other germs for that matter, are likely to settle to the bottom of a lake or pond, and so a stream passing through a pond will lose a large part of the bacterial pollution with which it entered. This is not positive enough, however, to insure a good water-supply, since in the spring the heavy flow of the stream will wash this deposited material out through the pond, carrying the infectious matter downstream. In addition, the upheaval of the settled material from the bottom of the lake, which occurs twice a year on account of the variation in temperature at different depths, will bring the settled germs to the top.

It has been found also that just as a high temperature destroys the germs, so a low temperature has the same effect. Typhoid fever germs in ice are practically harmless after two weeks, and since in natural ice the impurities of the water are largely eliminated mechanically, so that frozen water is purer than the water itself, there is very little chance, even when ice is cut from a polluted pond, for typhoid germs to be found alive after being in an ice house for three or four months. In the ground, the life of the bacteria is longer, and while experiments do not agree very well as to the exact length of time that the germ may live there, there seems to be evidence that they may live several months, if not a year or more. Cases have come under the observation of the writer which seemed to show that certain well waters were polluted by germs which could only have been deposited in the near-by soil nearly a year before the time of the consequent outbreak.

Entirely to deprive the germs of life, therefore, it is necessary, inasmuch as they are so widely distributed, to [Pg 354] act promptly and at once disinfect the fecal discharges from the patient rather than to wait until those discharges have been thrown into a stream or onto the ground and then attempt disinfection. There is probably no more important thing in stopping the spread of typhoid fever than to practice carefully disinfection in the sick room, using bichloride of mercury and chloride of lime, as already described in Chapter XV. Since, however, such disinfection is not always practiced and since care must be taken to avoid the introduction of the germs into the system, it is well to know how, assuming that they have not been killed in the sick room, they make their way from that place to a healthy individual.

*Methods of transmission of typhoid.*

There are three main avenues used by the germ, namely, water, milk, and flies, and of these three, the first is by far the most important and includes probably 80 per cent of all the cases. The reason for this is twofold. First, that water is so universally used, and second, that it is so easily and generally polluted. There are many historic examples which show definitely that water once polluted by typhoid germs is able to spread the disease far and wide.

The epidemic in Ithaca, New York, is a good example and ranks as one of the most serious that this country has ever known. The water-supply of the city is taken from a small stream, Six Mile Creek, which is a surface water with a drainage area of about 46 square miles. The stream is polluted to a large extent. About 2000 persons live on the watershed, and there are many houses practically on the bank of the stream which runs for a large part of its course at the bottom of a valley with steep side slopes. At [Pg 355] the time of the epidemic, 1903, a dam was being built on the stream about half a mile above the waterworks intake, and while no proof of the fact could be found, it was generally supposed that some of the Italians working on the dam were affected with typhoid fever and had polluted the water. However, there were on the banks of the stream, farther up, no less than seventeen privies, and it was known that there were at least six cases of typhoid fever during the season just previous to the epidemic. During the month of December, 1902, a heavy rain occurred, so that any pollution on the banks would naturally have been washed down into the stream. On the 11th of January, the epidemic broke out through the town and by the middle of February there were some 600 cases reported in a population of 15,000. The number of deaths from this epidemic was 114, and there is reason to suppose that the number of cases was double the number reported by the physicians. After the water from the creek was shut off and after the citizens had been persuaded to boil all water used, the epidemic stopped and the installation of a filtration plant has prevented any recurrence of the epidemic.

In 1880, a severe epidemic occurred in Lowell, Massachusetts, and was traced to an infection of the river from which the city's water-supply was taken. This was definitely shown to have come from a small tributary of the Merrimac River, and the particular infection responsible for the epidemic was traced to a small suburb named North Chelmsford, where one case of typhoid fever occurred in a factory, the privy of which was located directly on the bank of the small tributary.

In 1900, an epidemic of typhoid occurred at Newport, [Pg 356] Rhode Island, through the pollution of a well, and about 80 persons were affected, most of whom lived within a radius of 300 feet of the well and all of whom used the well water. The well was a shallow one with dry stone sides and a plank cover, and surrounding the well were about 20 privies, the nearest one only 25 feet away. The water in the well was 2 feet below the surface of the ground. It was found that a month before the epidemic broke out, there had been cases of typhoid fever in houses adjacent to the well, and that discharges from the typhoid patients found access to the privy vault which was only 25 feet from the well. It was practically certain that the well was infected by the leechings of these privies, particularly from the one only 25 feet away.

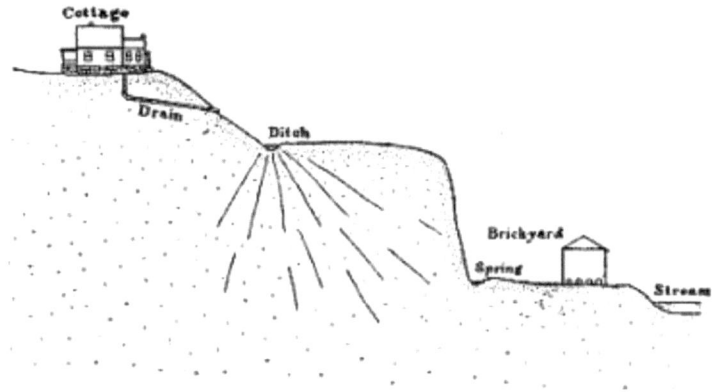

Fig. 77.—Spring infected by polluted ditch.

Another example of the way in which underground waters, such as springs, may become contaminated is described by Whipple as occurring at Mount Savage, [Pg 357] Maryland, in 1904. Through this village ran a small stream known as Jennings Run, which was grossly contaminated with fecal matter. In July, 1904, a woman who had nursed a typhoid patient in another town came home to Mount Savage, ill with the disease. She lived in a cottage on the hillside above the stream, and the drainage of the cottage was conveyed through an iron pipe onto the ground just above the stream. Figure 77 (after Whipple) shows the relative positions of the cottage and stream. Heavy rains occurred during the first week in July which probably washed the infectious matter from the ground into the ditch and then through the ground into a spring just below down the slope. A week afterwards twenty workmen who had been drinking water from the spring came down with the fever and new cases occurred daily for a week or two.

An interesting epidemic occurred in Massachusetts, caused by a farmer's boots carrying infectious matter from recently manured fields onto the well cover, whence it was washed into the well by repeated pumping.

The moral of these incidents is very plain, namely, that where any possibility of the infection of drinking water occurs, that water ought either to be avoided or else to be thoroughly sterilized before using. This applies particularly to the old-fashioned well, — the kind with loose board covers and chain pumps.

*Construction of wells in reference to typhoid.*

Two points already mentioned are essential if well water is to be kept pure. One is to line the well with a water-tight masonry lining, and the other point is to have the cover of the well made with a thoroughly water-tight [Pg 358] coating. This does not always give full protection, since in some cases polluting matter may pass through even ten feet of soil. This would be particularly true if the well was in a fissured or seamed rock, and very recently the writer found a well dug in a laminated granite, where a near-by sewer, leaking at the joints, contaminated the water of the well, although the well was cased with an iron casing twenty-five feet deep. The sewage escaped into a crack in the rock and followed the crack down vertically and horizontally into the well. Limestone is even more dangerous if any pollution exists in the vicinity. In cases where a well goes down to a horizontal layer of limestone and where a privy vault is dug to the same rock, it is found that pollution will follow the surface of the rock horizontally a long distance, and this condition of things always makes a well water suspicious. In sand or fine gravel, on the other hand, the danger of contamination is almost negligible; on Long Island, for example, the cesspools and well are both dug ten or fifteen feet deep and only fifty feet apart without any trace of contamination being detected.

*Milk infection by typhoid.*

Milk is responsible for perhaps 5 per cent of the cases of infection. Although the infection is always foreign to the milk itself, — that is, enters the milk only after the milk is drawn from the cow, — milk frequently becomes infected because infected water has been added to it or because the cans have been washed in infected water, or because some persons in contact with a typhoid patient have had their hands infected and then handled the milk or the milk utensils. There are a number of epidemics [Pg 359] which have been clearly traced to milk polluted in one of these ways. In Somerville, Massachusetts, for example, in 1892, 32 cases occurred, 30 of which were on the route of a single milkman. It was found that the milkman had two sons, one of whom had typhoid fever just before the outbreak. This son washed the milk cans and mixed the milk in a milk house in the city, and the inference was that in some way this man infected the milk, probably in one of the mixing cans.

In Stamford, Connecticut, in 1895, an epidemic occurred which caused 386 cases and 22 deaths. Ninety-five per cent of all the cases occurred among those who took milk from one dealer, and it was probable that in this case the infection came from using a badly polluted water to wash the cans. In Montclair, in 1902, a small epidemic involving 28 cases occurred, where the health officers decided, after having found out that the cases were all among those customers taking milk in pint bottles, that the infection came from a house on the route, where typhoid fever had occurred. It appeared that this family infected the bottles left at their house, and since the milkman failed to sterilize the bottles before re-filling them, the infection was passed on to others also taking milk in pint bottles.

*Infection by flies.*

Flies also transmit typhoid fever chiefly because they are essentially such unclean insects. They are born in filth and they delight in living in filth, and if privies and cesspools and manure piles and garbage piles could be shut out from flies, the fly pestilence would be at an end. The feet of the flies are suction tubes, and when a fly lights on any object, it causes more or less of that material to [Pg 360] stick to his feet, and then when he flies elsewhere, he may leave the particles on the object on which he alights. This has been proved by allowing a fly, caught in the house of a typhoid fever patient, to walk over a gelatine plate, leaving on the plate not merely his tracks, but the germs which his feet had carried. When the plate was exposed in an incubator, it was found that, within two or three days, millions of bacteria had grown from the number deposited by the one fly.

It is believed that the number of cases of typhoid which occurred in our Spanish-American War, at the military camps, and which were so disastrous, were due largely to flies. Among the 107,973 soldiers quartered in military camps at that time, there were 20,738 cases of typhoid fever, and the number of those which were fatal constituted 86 per cent of all the deaths from disease during this campaign. It was shown by the commission appointed to investigate the matter that the spread of the disease was not due to water or to food, but in most cases to the direct transmission of the germs through the agency of flies. In the Japanese and Russian war, where in the Japanese army of over a million men only 299 deaths from typhoid occurred, strict measures were taken to do away with all the breeding places of flies, and Major Seaman, who writes most interestingly on the success of the Japanese in avoiding typhoid, describes the ways in which the Japanese soldiers made flycatchers of themselves and waged war against flies quite as actively as against the Russians.

### Other sources of typhoid fever.

There are other sources of the disease; for instance, there have been a number of small epidemics undoubtedly caused [Pg 361] by infected oysters. One of the unpleasant habits of the oystermen is to bring in oysters from the ocean and leave them for a few days in shallow water where they may plump up or fatten, and they have found by experience that this fattening occurs more rapidly in dirty water. If the oysters are fattened in sewage-polluted water, the typhoid germs get inside the shell in the oyster liquor and are thus transmitted to those persons who eat the oysters raw.

Some kinds of food may transmit the disease: lettuce and celery, for instance, if washed in contaminated water or handled by persons with unclean hands or perhaps fertilized with manure containing typhoid germs. Finally, it is possible to acquire the disease by direct contact—not that the germs of typhoid are in the air in the room where a typhoid fever patient is lying, but rather that the nurse in some way soils her hands and then infects herself by putting her fingers in her mouth, or handles dishes or food afterwards used by other people, and so infects those others. It is not uncommon, for example, to see food partly consumed by a sick person given to children, or it may be that a child in the sick room is fed dainties prepared for the use of the patient. The result of such division of food is very apt to be a division of the sickness to the injury of the child.

### Treatment of typhoid fever.

So far as present knowledge extends, the disease is one best treated by being let alone, with some moderate modification. When germs have been swallowed and when the vitality of the individual is such that the disease is contracted (happily, as has already been said, only about [Pg 362] 10 per cent of those into whom the germ effects an entrance are inoculated), the first stage in the disease is a multiplication of the germs. This constitutes what is known as the incubation period, and lasts about ten days. During this time, the individual feels uneasy, has more or less headache and backache, and loses mental energy. The typhoid bacillus during this time spreads into almost every organ and tissue of the body, and towards the end of the period, when the resisting forces of the body have been proved unable to counteract the attack and the fever is well developed, the condition of the patient is deplorable. The bacteria are everywhere throughout the system, although they are especially active in the small intestines. This inflammation may produce ulceration and the blood vessels may be attacked, so that hemorrhages or even peritonitis may occur. A slight rash appears on the body, and a peculiar appearance of the tongue is to be found in severe cases. In from two to four weeks, the battle has been decided, and if the resisting forces prevail, the fever stops, and the patient begins to get well. This means probably, not that the bacilli are all dead, but that the patient has developed in his blood a sufficient antidote to the poison, so that the effects of the latter are no longer noticeable. The period of recovery, if the patient does recover, is most tedious, since the condition of the alimentary canal is such that great care must be exercised lest serious disorders there occur, and, although the patient is excessively hungry and really in great need of nourishing food, no greater folly can be committed than in allowing his desire for food to lead to indiscretion.

Injudicious exposure or fatigue will also cause a relapse, [Pg 363] and while recovery is usually a simple matter, it is only so when under the eye of a judicious and careful nurse. The only treatment required is plenty of water for drinking, to make up for the enormous loss by perspiration from the skin, which helps to wash out the poisons from the body. Then baths, where such methods of treatment can be used, as in hospitals, are also used both to lower the skin temperature and to add water to the surface. Sponge baths in water or alcohol are valuable and in some cases tub baths with the temperature as low as 40 degrees are used. Then a proper diet to keep up the strength of the patient, liquids always, and usually milk, forms the only other treatment possible. No drug is of any avail, and uninterrupted watchful care is the only way of combating the disease.

In concluding this chapter, it may be mentioned that certain army officers interested in medical work have discovered what they believe to be an antitoxin for typhoid fever, and they have inoculated hundreds of soldiers as a preventative. The results are not yet conclusive, but there seems to be great promise. It is hoped that the time may come soon when people will be so educated that there will be no opportunity of the germs escaping from the sick room, and that food and drink will be so cared for that there will be no possibility of infection. The writer feels that it is in these last two methods of prevention rather than in the use of antitoxin that the hope of the future lies.

[Pg 364]

# CHAPTER XVIII

## *CHILDREN'S DISEASES*

There are four diseases, scarlet fever, measles, whooping cough, and chicken pox, which are recognized as belonging preëminently to the period of childhood and which are supposed to be the result of bacterial contagion, although, curiously, the specific bacteria concerned in any one of these four diseases has not been detected. They may be rationally grouped together for two reasons. First, because of their attacking, in the majority of cases, children under the age of fifteen years, and second, because the first stages of these diseases are very similar, so that the recognition of them is not easy except for the practiced physician. It must not be thought, however, that because these are diseases of childhood and because a majority of children have them at one time or another, without great suffering and without serious after effects, they are on that account to be despised. Scarlet fever, for instance, is to-day probably the most dreaded of children's diseases, not because so many children die of it, — although the death-rate is large, about 20 per cent of the cases finally succumbing, — but because of the large number of complications and consequences which are directly due to this disease. Measles, also, though not to the same extent, is frequently followed by serious after results. In the United States, about 13,000 children die every year of measles and about half as many die of scarlet fever. It is a significant fact that the [Pg 365] death-rate is much higher among younger children, so that if, by carefully keeping children from the possibility of infection, the disease can be postponed until they are well along in years, the danger of fatal termination is much reduced.

The following table, for instance, shows the number of deaths from measles and scarlet fever at different ages, and it is very evident from this table that if the former disease is contracted by a child under five years old, the danger of death is four times as great as if it were postponed until the child were ten years old:—

**Table XIX. Table showing Deaths and Percentages from Measles and Scarlet Fever for Different Ages in United States Registration Area for 1907**

| Measles | | | Scarlet Fever | | |
|---|---|---|---|---|---|
| Age Period | Number of Deaths | Per cent of Total Deaths | Age Period | Number of Deaths | Per cent of Total Deaths |
| All ages | 4302 | 100 | All ages | 4309 | 100 |
| Under 1 yr. | 1058 | 24 | Under 1 yr. | 175 | 4 |
| 1-2 yr. | 1315 | 31 | 1-2 yr. | 474 | 11 |
| 2-3 yr. | 626 | 14 | 2-3 yr. | 639 | 15 |
| 3-4 yr. | 343 | 8 | 3-4 yr. | 640 | 15 |
| 4-5 yr. | 189 | 4 | 4-5 yr. | 511 | 12 |
| 5-9 yr. | 350 | 8 | 5-9 yr. | 1213 | 30 |
| 10-14 yr | 89 | 2 | 10-14 | 315 | 8 |

| | | | yr. | | |
|---|---|---|---|---|---|
| Under 5 yr. | 3531 | 82 | Under 5 yr. | 2439 | 58 |
| Under 15 yr. | 3970 | 92 | Under 15 yr. | 3967 | 92 |
| Over 5 yr. | 771 | 18 | Over 5 yr. | 1870 | 42 |
| Over 15 yr. | 332 | 8 | Over 15 yr. | 342 | 8 |

The table shows also that the dangerous age period for scarlet fever is later than for measles. It indicates that [Pg 366] while 82 per cent of all deaths from measles are of children under five years of age, only 58 per cent of the deaths from scarlet fever are in that period; but that the number of deaths of the latter between five and nine years is so great that the percentage of deaths under fifteen is the same in both cases. The moral is plain, namely, that a child should be carefully protected from infection by measles until he is five years old and from scarlet fever until fifteen, if the danger to the child's life is to be reduced to a minimum.

*After effects of scarlet fever and measles.*

In themselves, these diseases may not be severe, children often having mild attacks of scarlet fever, called scarletina, and apparently suffering only from a cold, but exposure, by which a cold is developed either during or after the disease, may lead to serious troubles. Inflammation of the kidneys often occurs, which may develop into chronic Bright's disease and ultimately cause death. Inflammation of the ear is another incident of scarlet fever, in which abscesses are formed, resulting not infrequently in permanent deafness.

The consequences of measles are not so serious usually, and a more common after effect is trouble with the lungs or bronchial tubes. Pneumonia, croup, and bronchitis very often follow measles, due, as already indicated, to exposure before the body has regained its normal condition. In both scarlet fever and measles the eyes are apt to be affected, and it is very important in both diseases to keep the patient in a darkened room and to forbid use of the eyes in reading or other close work. On account of the complications following scarlet fever and measles, as [Pg 367] well as for their greater death-rate, these diseases are more serious than the other two included in this discussion, — whooping cough and chicken pox.

*Preliminary symptoms.*

The beginning of each of these four diseases is much the same, and the symptoms are likely to be mistaken for those of an ordinary cold. In all of them, the first indication of illness is redness and itching on the inside of the nose and throat with snuffling and discharging from both eyes and nose. Sometimes the throat is affected, and the patient complains of sore throat. Then the cheeks become flushed, headache may follow, and fever begins, so that the patient is in a sort of stupor, unwilling to do anything and glad to lie in bed. In severe cases vomiting may accompany or precede the outbreak of fever.

At the outset, the probable reason for the similarity of these four diseases as well as their likeness to a common cold is that the germs responsible for all of them enter the body through the nose and throat and begin their attack upon the membranes there. The action of the germ is followed by the formation of poisons or toxins which are distributed by the blood through the body, causing the fever and what are known as "general symptoms." At the beginning it is not possible to determine to which particular germ the distress of the patient is due, and probably the continued prevalence of these diseases is chiefly owing to the fact that in the early stages and in mild cases throughout, the sufferer is allowed to be at large with every opportunity for spreading the disease.

*Contagiousness.*

If, whenever a child has a cold accompanied by a fever, [Pg 368] the mother would promptly put him in bed in a room by himself, keeping the other children of the family away from the sick room and the invalid under restraint until all possibility of transmitting the disease is over, the number of cases would be greatly diminished. Unfortunately, there seems to be a general impression that such precautions are useless, and that sooner or later every child must have these children's diseases. This is a mistaken notion, and the table already referred to is sufficient evidence to prove the error of this way of thinking.

All these diseases are affections of the whole body, caused by poisons generated by germs, for which so far scientists have found no antidote. The reason is plain. The germ itself is not known, and no animal has been discovered on which scientists can experiment. If we could only produce measles in a rabbit, for instance, we could very soon detect the germ and would no doubt be able to procure an antidote to the measles poison. But this has not been done, and therefore in measles and in the other diseases mentioned we can only hope that the sick person will be able to generate in his own body sufficient antidote to secure his own recovery. Physicians therefore are almost helpless in treating these diseases. They keep the patient in bed in order that all his strength may be kept for fighting the disease. They insist on ventilation in abundance, so that oxygen may be applied to the lungs in large quantities in order to neutralize the poison. They advise sponge baths in cold water and alcohol to allay the fever, and they prescribe nourishing, easily digested food, such as milk, eggs, fruit, and plenty of water to drink. In the hope of diminishing the chances of infection, [Pg 369] particularly in measles and scarlet fever, they recommend antiseptic sprays for the nose and throat and antiseptic ointments, such as carbolized vaseline for the skin when peeling or desquamation is going on.

*Quarantine for scarlet fever.*

Scarlet fever, while the most violent, is also the shortest lived, in the majority of cases not more than three or four days, although the full period of recovery is much longer. The peculiarity of this disease lies in the abundant peeling which takes place usually from the entire body and particularly from the hands and feet; in fact, in a number of cases where the disease is light, the peeling from the hands and feet is the only positive proof that the malady has been scarlet fever. During this process of peeling contagion seems most active; therefore, although recovery seems entire so far as the fever is concerned, the patient should remain strictly isolated during this time. It is a slow process, lasting from two to five weeks, and is very tiresome for the child who feels perfectly well; yet, in the interests of other children, the child must be kept strictly at home until at least a week after the last sign has disappeared. It is also for the child's own sake very desirable to observe this quarantine, since it is during this period of recovery that most of the complications of scarlet fever occur, and if the patient is kept under observation, either in his sick room or on some porch where atmospheric exposure is not too great and where the child is certain to eat nothing harmful, the chances for avoiding lung troubles and digestive disturbances are minimized.

There is such a striking difference in the severity of cases of scarlet fever that the name "scarletina" was for a [Pg 370] long time applied to mild cases with the feeling that possibly it represented an altogether different disease. At the present time the disease is more intelligently diagnosed, and while there is vast difference in the severity of the sickness, it is all the same thing. Of the ordinary cases, about 5 per cent terminate fatally; that is, in a village or a community where a hundred cases occur, there would be five deaths. If the epidemic, however, is of the severe form, a larger percentage of deaths occur, often reaching 20 per cent of those affected. It has been noted that as an epidemic progresses, the disease becomes more serious, and a death-rate of only 5 per cent may, in the course of an epidemic lasting several months, gradually increase to one of 20 or 25 per cent. For this reason strong efforts ought to be made to stamp out an epidemic while it is in the first stages.

Besides the possibility of contagion from the skin as it comes off, to prevent which the antiseptic ointment is used, contagion also occurs through clothing used in the sick room. In fact, the contagiousness of scarlet fever is probably as malignant as any other infectious disease. It has been observed that a year after a case of scarlet fever in a house, the unpacking of a trunk or the unrolling of a bundle would set free the contagion and would result in new cases of the disease. The writer learned recently of a family in which a child had died of scarlet fever and some of its clothing had been packed away in the attic. A younger sister grew up, married, moved away, and some twenty years after the death of the child, came back to her former home on a visit with her own little girl. The grandmother, visiting the attic, found the clothing packed [Pg 371] away so long before, gave it to her grand-daughter to wear, and in ten days the child was dead with the same disease.

There are a number of cases where scarlet fever seems to have been carried by infected milk, and great care must be taken on dairy farms to avoid any possibility of this kind of infection. To prevent the disease being transmitted after apparent recovery, thorough disinfection should be practiced. The patient's body should be very carefully and completely and continuously covered with antiseptic ointment which prevents the distribution of the contagion in small particles of skin. The sick room, after the patient's recovery, should be thoroughly disinfected, and all bedding steamed or boiled. All the surfaces in the room should be washed with a solution of carbolic acid, 1 in 50, or corrosive sublimate, 1 in 1000.

*Measles.*

If the disease is measles, one may expect a general epidemic, since its power of direct contagion is nearly equal to scarlet fever, although the fatality is much less. It is unfortunate that so little pains are taken to prevent the spread of this disease and fortunate that, except in the case of very young children, the effect of the illness is only a temporary inconvenience. Curiously, however, if measles attacks savage tribes where it has been before unknown, the severity of the disease is very great. Cases are on record where measles have broken out on the frontier and whole villages were wiped out; where the insignificant measles, so innocuous in civilized communities, became a plague similar to a scourge of the Middle Ages. It apparently has been modified by its passage through generations of individuals, just as any bacterial disease germ is modified [Pg 372] by successive transmission through the bodies of different animals. When, however, the disease breaks out in a community which has not suffered from the disease for many years, it is, on that account, likely to appear in a far more virulent form.

*Characteristic eruptions of measles.*

Measles, like scarlet fever and chicken pox, is an eruptive disease; that is, is accompanied with a rash, differing slightly in the three diseases of which the presence of the rash and its progress over the body is one of the distinguishing features. In scarlet fever, for instance, the rash appears first on the neck and chest or back and spreads outward to the extremities. In measles, the rash appears on the extremities, beginning on the face usually, and spreads to the chest and trunk. In scarlet fever, this rash appears as fine scarlet pin points scattered around on the reddened skin, and on the second or third day the entire body may look like a boiled lobster. In measles, the rash appears as blotches, while the skin is not flushed but retains its natural color. In chicken pox, the rash appears generally on the body first and consists of small red pimples which develop into whitish blisters about as large as a pea and well separated. They are much more distinct and separated than the rash of scarlet fever and measles, and are much more likely to be mistaken for smallpox pustules than for an ordinary eruptive rash.

One of the old-time fancies connected with these eruptive diseases is the belief that an abundant eruption is a sort of guarantee against the severity of the disease. The old nurse was careful to keep the child in bed, well covered, steamed in fact, until the eruption appeared, and it was [Pg 373] commonly thought that nothing should be done to check the rash or to prevent its coming out. This is not sustained by later science, and the appearance of the rash, whether it strikes in or strikes out, has nothing to do with either the disease or with its severity. No possible connection can be traced between the dissemination of the poison through the system by the action of the bacteria and the appearance of the skin, which is a minor factor in the disease. It may be worth while to repeat that the greatest danger from measles consists in the possibility of lung complications, and infinite care should be taken to keep the patient shielded from drafts and free from overexertion until recovery is complete. Like scarlet fever, the skin peels off, although not to the same extent, and the small particles are capable of transmitting the disease. Probably, also, the secretion from the nose and throat will transmit the disease, so that it is the height of folly to allow a sick person to use a handkerchief, for example, and then to use the same handkerchief to wipe the baby's nose when he comes into the sick room. All dishes and clothing of every sort should be boiled or steamed, and to be rendered harmless they should be soaked in a disinfecting solution before being taken from the sick room. The room itself, after being vacated, should be disinfected and the walls washed, as already prescribed.

*Whooping cough.*

Whooping cough is unlike the other three diseases in that it is a nervous trouble, and probably the germ or the poison formed by the germ attacks the nervous system, and particularly one great nerve connecting the lungs and stomach. This is why the spasm of coughing is frequently followed by vomiting, and the only remedy which is of [Pg 374] value in whooping cough is a nerve depressant which will diminish the activity of the nervous system without at the same time interfering with the strength or vigor of the patient. On account of this connection between the lungs, whose spasmodic ejection of air seems to threaten the entire collapse of the little patient, and the stomach, so alarming do the repeated fits of vomiting appear that often this feature of the disease is even more serious than the coughing, pathetic as it is with younger children. In some cases the stomach cannot retain nourishment long enough to feed the body, and the child literally wastes away unless the period of the disease runs out before the child starves to death.

It is often weeks instead of days before the disease can be recognized. Then, if it develops in its usual form, begins the coughing so characteristic of the malady and the hard straining whoop so painful to listen to. Occasionally this coughing may be severe enough to cause a rupture of a blood vessel; but ordinarily, unless the stomach is affected by sympathy, no great danger need be feared. Fresh air, moderate exercise, good food, and some mild nerve depressant is all that can be done. The disease is very contagious and is usually transmitted directly from the sick person to the well person. It may, however, be carried in clothing, particularly in handkerchiefs and towels. Like measles, if it gains a foothold in an uncivilized community, it attains the size of an epidemic or plague with very fatal results. It seems to have a great power over girls and children, particularly those whose vitality is below the normal. Like measles, one does not generally have two attacks of this disease. In the winter, [Pg 375] and this is the time when the whooping cough is most common, it is often followed by lung troubles, such as bronchitis and pneumonia. The death-rate from whooping cough is as large as from scarlet fever and measles combined, but chiefly because the disease is common among the smallest children. It is not unusual for babies under a year old to have whooping cough, and when their vitality is low, they scarcely ever recover.

*Precautions against spread of whooping cough.*

Probably the disease does not become contagious until the cough starts, and there is no reason why the disease should not be arrested in the first victim, provided proper isolation is practiced. The idea of a child with whooping cough, even when he whoops only once or twice a day, being allowed to attend school and mingle with the other scholars and to distribute the disease among them seems in these days of sanitary knowledge almost criminal. As soon as the first whoop occurs the child should be put in a room by himself and kept there until the last whoop has been whooped, and no other child should be allowed to go into the room, and the nurse or mother who is in charge should be careful about contact with other children after coming from the sick room until she has changed her outer garment. A big apron with long sleeves, fitted closely around the neck, which may be slipped on and off easily, is an admirable protection. The same precautions about disinfecting dishes, napkins, towels, handkerchiefs, and bedding should be observed here as already referred to.

*Chicken pox.*

Chicken pox is the mildest of eruptive diseases. It has no relation to smallpox, so that the theory sometimes [Pg 376] held, that an attack of chicken pox prevents any attack of smallpox later, is a mistake. Instances are on record where a person has had both diseases almost at the same time. The appearance of the eruption is the characteristic feature of this disease, and it is so well distinguished that there is no danger of failing to recognize it. It is not common in grown people, and while it should not arouse suspicion in children, it is so uncommon in adults that a suspected case is probably a mild case of smallpox, and should always be quarantined as such.

With children, the accompanying cold and fever is often very mild, so that the appearance of the rash is the first and only symptom of the disease. The eruption is a progressive thing, each day's crop coming to full bloom and dying out as the next day's crop develops. This is, by the way, a distinguishing characteristic of this disease, differentiating it from smallpox where the pustules are more persistent and where the breaking out is more general. The pustules are sometimes extremely irritating, and it is very hard to keep children from scratching, the results of which may leave deep scars and so should be avoided. An antiseptic ointment should be used as with scarlet fever and measles, carbolized vaseline being suitable, although sometimes a strong solution of soda is substituted. It is not common to disinfect in chicken pox to the same extent as in the other diseases, the contagion being apparently in the air rather than in clothing and short lived. In New York State, in 1908, no deaths are recorded from chicken pox, and it is because of this lack of fatal results that the disease is regarded so indifferently and no particular pains taken to prevent its spread. [Pg 377]

## CHAPTER XIX

# PARASITICAL DISEASES (MALARIA, YELLOW FEVER, HOOKWORM, BUBONIC PLAGUE, AND PELLAGRA)

*Malaria.*

From time immemorial, malaria (or fever-and-ague) has been one of the great plagues of humanity. No advance outpost of civilization but has suffered, more or less severely, from this disease. Dickens, in one of his novels, describes graphically the disease as it existed in the early American settlements, and vividly portrays its ravages, both mental and physical, among the pioneer settlers. Certain sections of the world have been especially noted for the prevalence of this disease, making extensive regions practically uninhabitable. The vicinity of Rome, with its swampy marshes and low-lying areas, has been one of these plague spots. The jungles and swamps of the equator and the coastline of Africa and South America and the valley lands of the Mississippi River have all been noted as most dangerous districts for human beings to live in. Even in civilized communities the ravages of the disease have, under conditions most conducive to malaria, been fearful, so that only most urgent requirements of mining, manufacturing, or similar material processes have prevented the obliteration of entire communities.

The cause of the heavy death roll resulting from a bold [Pg 378] defiance of the reputation of these localities—a defiance bravely adopted by hardy pioneers, by agents of trading companies, and by representatives of governments—has been, up to the last ten years, assigned to the water-laden condition of low-lying ground. Swamps and stagnant pools, moisture-laden air, and a hot climate have been universally considered to be the cause of the fever, and the transmission of the disease has been supposed to be due to the passage through the moist air of the germs of the disease, although the exact form and behavior of these germs was unknown. Certain specifics have been proved by experience to have some value. For instance, it has been found that planting a row of trees between the house and a pool from which malaria might come has been of aid in warding off the disease. In a number of cases a thick row of eucalyptus trees, so associated in the popular mind with this purpose that they are known as the malaria tree, have been planted as a tight hedge with apparently very useful results. Drainage or filling up the low lands has always been found to reduce the prevalence of the disease.

Many years ago the use of quinine in large doses was found to be a specific, and the writer well remembers, on the occasion of his visit to a malarial region, buying quinine at the grocery store by the ounce in the same way that one would buy spices or tea, the dose being a teaspoonful. Why quinine should prevent the daily or periodical chills characteristic of the disease was not known, or why a row of eucalyptus trees interfered with the development of the disease was not known, and people generally were content to rest with the knowledge of these facts only. [Pg 379]

*Mosquitoes and malaria.*

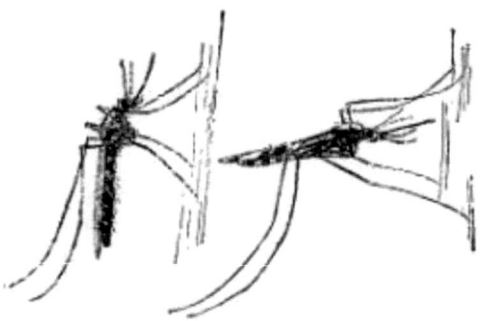

Fig. 78.—Resting positions for ordinary mosquito (left) and malarial mosquito (right).

In the year 1900, however, English scientists, working in the Roman Campagna, demonstrated conclusively that which had been vaguely suggested before, namely, that the cause of malaria is a parasite composed of little more than an unformed mass of protoplasm, not floating in the air at all, but transmitted only by the bite of a mosquito. By a series of most interesting experiments, conducted by them and by other scientists in other parts of the world, it has been definitely proved that when a mosquito bites an individual suffering from malaria, the mosquito draws up into his body, along with the blood of the bitten person, some of the malarial parasites. In the body of the mosquito, the parasite develops, requiring for a full-grown specimen about seven days; then, if the mosquito bites another person, the parasite is injected into the skin of the victim, and in the course of about a week a good case of malaria ensues.

Fortunately, only a small proportion of the number of [Pg 380] mosquitoes in the world are capable of nourishing the malaria parasite. Under ordinary conditions about 5 per cent of all mosquitoes found are malarial, and a particular name has been given to those capable of transmitting the disease. The ordinary mosquito is known as the "culex," while the malarial kind is known as "anopheles." Figure 78 shows the characteristic attitude of the two kinds by which the one can be distinguished from the other when resting on a wall or ceiling. As will be noticed in the drawing, the culex carries his body parallel to the wall with his hind legs crossed over his back. The harmful mosquito, the female anopheles, always hangs on by her front legs and has her body at an angle of about forty-five degrees to the surface to which she clings, her hind legs hanging down. The wings of the harmless mosquito are usually mottled, while the wings of the malarial mosquito are of an even color. The details of the behavior of the parasite on its long journey from the original malarial patient through the body of the mosquito and into the body of the person bitten is full of interest to the scientist, who must, however, be provided with a good microscope to follow such minute bodies; but the methods of avoiding the disease are more pertinent to our present purpose.

While quinine is still recognized as the particular antidote for the malarial poison, efficient as we know now because it is poisonous to the parasite and not because it has any particular effect on the person, of late years more and more stress is being laid on the elimination of the mosquito. Naturally, if the mosquito can be destroyed and the transmission of the disease thus prevented, there will be no further need of quinine. The general impression that [Pg 381] swampy land is favorable to the development of malaria is correct, but not because the damp air is itself pernicious. The significance of the damp ground lies solely in the fact that mosquitoes in one stage of their existence require water for their development. They breed only in water and always deposit their eggs in water, on the surface of which the eggs float in very small layers. The eggs hatch into larvæ or wrigglers, which also must remain in water for development, and it is not until the third stage, that of the full-grown mosquito, that the animal leaves the water which was his birthplace. Obviously, therefore, if there is no water there can be no mosquitoes.

*Elimination of mosquitoes.*

Another pertinent fact discovered by scientific research is that the development of the malarial mosquito is confined to the vicinity of stagnant pools, because in fresh water, where fish are to be found, the eggs and larvæ of the mosquito are a most acceptable fish food. One of the most practical ways, therefore, of getting rid of possible mosquitoes is to make sure that the pond always contains a number of fish. Woods Hutchinson gives the following interesting description of the way this fact was discovered: —

"It was early noted that mosquitoes would not breed freely in open rivers or in large ponds or lakes, but why this should be the case was a puzzle. One day an enthusiastic mosquito student brought home a number of eggs of different species, which he had collected from the neighboring marshes, and put them into his laboratory aquarium for the sake of watching them develop and identifying their species. The next morning, when he went to look at them, they had totally disappeared. Thinking that [Pg 382] perhaps the laboratory cat had taken them, and overlooking a most contented twinkle in the corner of the eyes of the minnows that inhabited the aquarium, he went out and collected another series. This time the minnows were ready for him, and before his astonished eyes promptly pounced on the raft of eggs and swallowed them whole. Here was the answer at once: mosquitoes would not develop freely where fish had free access; and this fact is an important weapon in the crusade for their extermination. If the pond be large enough, all that is necessary is simply to stock it with any of the local fish,— minnows, killies, perch, dace, bass,— and presto! the mosquitoes practically disappear."

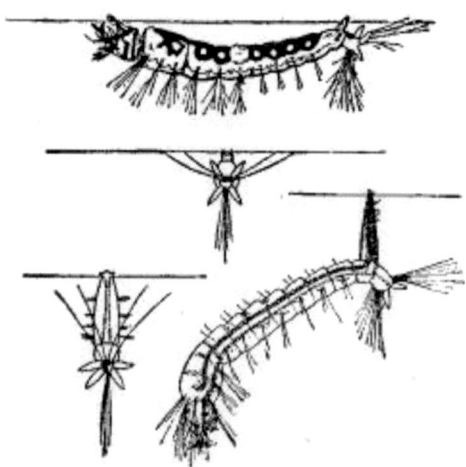

Fig. 79.—Top view is of larva of Anopheles. Bottom view is of larva of Culex.

Another factor in the development of the mosquito from the egg to full-grown mosquitohood is that in the larvæ stage air must be supplied, curiously enough, through the tail which projects slightly above the surface of the water as the larvæ hang head downwards (see Fig. 79). If the surface of the water is covered with some impervious material, the mosquito larvæ will be suffocated, and it has been found that oil lends itself most readily to this desirable purpose, applied at the rate of one ounce per fifteen square feet of water surface. The oil spreads out over the surface [Pg 383] in a very thin film, but persistent enough to keep off the air supply from the mosquito larvæ. This method, about which much has been written and said, is perhaps the one most commonly employed, and its results have been most satisfactory. In the vicinity of the city of Newark, New Jersey, for instance, is an area of about 3500 acres, 8 miles long and about 3 miles wide, practically all marshland. In 1903 ditches were dug throughout this marsh in such a way that the surface water was drained off, drying the ground so that hay can now be cut where formerly rubber boots were necessary to get onto the ground at all. The consequence has been that the mosquitoes have practically disappeared from this region, formerly frightfully infested, and the cost of the 70 miles of small ditches dug has been amply repaid by the freedom from malaria as well as from the nuisance of the ordinary mosquito.

Other campaigns have been waged, using kerosene or crude petroleum for the coating of ponds or pools. Wherever clear water exists the kerosene treatment is probably best. Where marshland is found, through which the kerosene penetrates with difficulty, drainage is a more useful method.

The size of the pools required for the development of the mosquito is very small. Thousands of mosquitoes may be formed in the amount of water contained in an old tomato can, and barrels half full of rain water or pools of water in the vicinity of an old pump or in the barnyard will afford golden opportunities for mosquitoes looking for a place to lay their eggs. While the ordinary culex requires from one to two weeks only for the complete [Pg 384] transition from egg to mosquito, so that a pool filled with rain water and not dried up within that period will be sufficient to develop a brood, the malarial mosquito requires much longer — two or three months — for the full completion of her development. It is, therefore, a simple problem for an individual householder to search out the pools which remain filled with water for a period of two months, and either stock them with fish, drain them entirely, or coat them with kerosene. No hesitation need be felt about the result of this treatment. It will positively eliminate all malaria in the vicinity if the work is thoroughly done.

*Limitation of mosquito infection.*

The distance that the malarial mosquito can fly is of interest as indicating the distance which one must go from a house, hunting for available pools. All mosquitoes are unable to fly against the wind, so that, as already noted, one side of a swamp may be comparatively free from malaria, while the other side may be overrun with it, merely on account of the direction of the prevailing winds. Some mosquitoes that breed in salt marshes may be carried for miles, so that a land breeze will bring millions of the pests to seashore cottages which, with a sea breeze, are quite free from them. The anopheles has a habit of clinging to weeds, shrubs, and bushes when the wind blows, so that it is seldom carried more than about two hundred yards from the place where it is hatched. If all pools of water, therefore, within this radius are disposed of, the elimination of malaria will logically follow.

If one is obliged to be in a region where malaria is common, the disease can be avoided absolutely by protecting [Pg 385] one's self from mosquitoes, and since the anopheles prefer the early morning and evening hours, it is at those times of the day particularly when precautions must be taken. It was once thought that the night air caused malaria, and this had some foundation in fact, because it is in the early evening that the anopheles is on the wing. By staying in the house after sundown and by carefully screening the doors and windows, one may live in a malarial country with perfect immunity. Volunteers have lived for months in the worst malarial regions in the world without a trace of the disease, the only precaution being to keep the doors and windows screened and to prevent mosquitoes from biting.

An interesting experiment was made some years ago by sending a malarial mosquito by mail from Italy to England, where an enthusiast allowed himself to be bitten by the insect. He had had no trace of malaria before, but a week after the mosquito's bite he came down with the disease. It has also been noted that in such parts of the country as Greenland and Alaska, where mosquitoes are as thick as in the far-famed New Jersey marshes, malaria does not result from the mosquito bites unless a malaria patient from other countries starts the infection.

The disease itself may be mild or severe. It takes about a week after the mosquito bites before the symptoms appear, and sometimes the attack is postponed for weeks or months. Chills are the usual accompaniment of the disease; in children under six, convulsions are more common. The chill lasts from a few minutes to an hour, and directly after the chill comes the fever, which lasts three or four hours. The attacks usually occur every other day and sometimes [Pg 386] every two days, generally at the same time of day. When persons have lived for a long time in malarial regions, the intermittency of the chill and fever is less noticeable and the continuous character of the fever often leads the disease to be mistaken for typhoid. The intermittent regularity of the fever, however, although between attacks the temperature never falls to normal, distinguishes this type of malarial fever from true typhoid. The positive determination of the disease is possible by an examination of the patient's blood, in which the malarial parasite can readily be found. Quinine is the remedy and the only remedy, and, fortunately, it does no harm, even before the character of the disease is positively known. The chill seems to be due to the development of a new brood of parasites in the blood of the malarial patient, and in order that the quinine shall have its effect on the blood, it must be swallowed three or four hours before the time of the expected chill, and then it will probably prevent, not the next chill but the one after. If the quinine cannot be taken directly with reference to an expected chill, then it must be taken regularly, sometimes for months before the chills cease.

*Yellow fever.*

Yellow fever, although not common in this country, is interesting as being almost exactly similar in its mode of infection to malaria. It is transmitted through a parasite, as is malaria, and can only be passed along through the agency of another kind of mosquito, known as stegomyia. In 1899 there was a serious outbreak of this pestilence in the cities of our southern coast, and the terrors of the plague of the Middle Ages were revived for a number of months. Trains going out of the infected regions were stopped by [Pg 387] crowds armed with guns and the passengers prevented from proceeding, lest thé disease might spread. No goods or freight were allowed to pass out from the infected area, and the prejudice against intercourse with the outside world went so far that guards even forbade the carrying of disinfectants to the victims.

Like malaria, the disease is one requiring a hot climate, generally because it is favorable to mosquito growth. It is most common in the seacoast cities of the South, and is probably transmitted often by mosquitoes brought on board ship. Since Havana has been cleaned up by Americans, the danger formerly existing from intercourse with that city has ceased, although only three years ago the writer stopped in a hotel at Havana, where two persons had died of yellow fever a week before. The smell of disinfectants in the hotel was so great that not a fly or insect of any sort was visible, and no other hotel in the city could have been safer or more comfortable. It has been proved positively that yellow fever cannot be transmitted by direct contact, since, in the interests of science, volunteers have slept in beds from which the dead from yellow fever had just been removed without contracting the disease. That the infection is due only to mosquitoes is proved by the fact that later, when bitten by mosquitoes, they succumbed to the disease. It requires about two weeks for the disease to pass through its regular stages in the body of the mosquito, so that there is no possibility of its transmission for that time after the mosquito has come in contact with a yellow fever patient.

The symptoms of yellow fever are characteristic and very severe. The eyes first become bloodshot and, in the [Pg 388] course of two days, yellow, whence the name of the disease. Severe vomiting is also characteristic, the discharge being sometimes discolored like coffee or even tar and known as black vomit. The skin appears yellow, a condition which lasts for some time and is particularly noticeable if by the pressure of the finger on the skin the blood is made to recede. Among persons previously in good health, the death-rate is about that of typhoid fever, but among those in unfavorable surroundings and among those given to the use of alcohol, the rate will be much higher. Practically, it may be expected that this disease, like malaria, will disappear from the face of the earth. When the only requirement is the destruction of the mosquitoes and when mosquitoes can be so easily killed as already explained, it is only a question of time before mosquitoes and the diseases they cause will be stamped out. In Havana, before 1901, the number of the deaths yearly was about 750. In the year after the American intervention, when Colonel Gorgas, by military command, insisted on the thorough cleaning of the houses and the general use of kerosene in all drains and cesspools, there was not one single death.

*Hookworm disease.*

The third parasitical disease common in some parts of the United States has received much attention during this last year and is known as the hookworm disease. It is a new discovery in medical science, and whereas the physical condition of the victim is usually a clear indication of the disease, a positive diagnosis is always obtained by the use of the microscope. Several years ago it was announced in the United States that the laziness and shiftlessness of the poor whites living in the sand lands and pine [Pg 389] barrens of the South was due, not to any inherent cussedness but to the presence of a parasite in the intestine, known in Italy and Germany as the hookworm, the disease being called Uncinariasis.

The development of the disease is interesting. The worm, which is about an inch long and looks not unlike a bit of thread, lays eggs by the thousand in the intestinal tract of a human victim. Afterwards they pass out in the excreta and, favored by heat and moisture, develop in the soil in about three days into minute larvæ. These larvæ have a most extraordinary power of attaching themselves to and penetrating into the human skin and body. They may also enter the human body in a drink of water or on unwashed vegetables. In infected regions the soil becomes fairly alive with these larvæ, and it is hardly possible for a child to walk barefoot outdoors without becoming infected. When the larvæ have penetrated the hand or foot, they begin a long and circuitous journey through the body, moving from the extremities through the veins to the heart and thence to the lungs. From here they are carried through air cells into the bronchial tubes, thence along the mucous membrane up the windpipe and down into the stomach and finally, from the stomach, they pass out into the intestines, the goal of their long journey.

This all takes time, and probably from the time they enter the skin to the time they begin their murderous work on the lining of the intestines requires about two months. In the intestine the larvæ develop into adults; but before this final stage an intermediate existence is reached, at which time they attach themselves to the mucous lining and bore into it, presumably for the purpose of making a [Pg 390] nest in which later to lay their eggs. The burrowing parasite causes a great loss of blood, and it is on account of the resulting anæmia that the poor whites show always such incapacity, indifference, and apparent laziness. That this disease is of importance in considering the hygienic condition of the country is apparent when it is pointed out that in the southern part of the United States, chiefly in the rural districts, there are at least two million persons at present infected with the disease, and that should these hookworms be blotted out of existence, two million incapables would be changed into two million active Americans, ready to raise the southern districts to a commercial elevation which their natural resources seem to justify.

The treatment of the hookworm disease is simple, and the donation by Mr. Rockefeller of $2,000,000 is intended to be sufficient to furnish the opportunity at least for a complete cure of all the cases. It has been found that a small dose of a preparation of thyme known as thymol stupefies the parasites with which it comes in contact, so that they unloose their claws and are set free in the intestine after its use. A dose of epsom salts shortly after clears them out, and except for the loss of blood, the disease is finished. Sometimes, however, in long-continued cases the worms have penetrated so far into the membrane that the use of thymol cannot withdraw them. In fact, in autopsies, it has been found necessary to take tweezers and to use considerable force in order to pull them out.

The prevention of the disease is really the cure of the disease, an apparently simple matter, as already described. An improvement of sanitary conditions so as to make impossible further pollution of the soil should be also [Pg 391] undertaken. Wherever the disease has prevailed in this country or in Europe, it has been because of an utter neglect and disregard of what are now known as ordinary sanitary conveniences, and the report of the Country Life Commission, although many charges were made against the conditions of living in different parts of the country, was far from telling the whole story in the matter of the shortcomings in parts of the southern states. There is, therefore, every reason why the farmer and others living in the country should be urged to make themselves comfortable with all known modern sanitary appliances. This is desirable, first, for the sake of others on whom their sins of unhygienic living might be visited, and then for their own sake, because there such sins would also have an effect to a degree tenfold more severe.

*Pellagra.*

Another disease peculiar to country life, and which has only within the last few years been recognized, is known as pellagra. Not yet is it even known through what agency the disease is transmitted, but it has been beyond question established that in some way corn is responsible for its spread. Apparently, spoiled corn is necessary, and while presumably the corn itself is not the agent, the parasite or organism that is responsible lives only on corn which has been spoiled. Scientists have long worked on the disease, and it would be a merely speculative pursuit, one of interest to scientists and medical men only, except for the fact that within the last few years it has broken out in this country and is increasing to a most alarming degree. The disease itself is almost hopeless when once established, physicians being yet utterly unable to grapple with it; and [Pg 392] while in Italy, Spain, and Egypt it has been known for a century, there is still a death-rate of over 60 per cent, and these deaths occur after most horrible suffering and agony.

As in rabies, the parasite, if it is a parasite, acts through a poison which penetrates to the nervous centers, producing mental disturbances culminating in an active insanity. At the same time, the agent attacks the skin, whence its name "pell'agra," which means "rough skin," so that the body appears as if it were affected with a severe attack of eczema, large patches of skin peeling off and leaving the raw surface. In fact, in one of the Illinois hospitals, only a few years ago, some insane persons, infected with this disease, died, and because the effect of the disease on the skin was not known, the nurse in charge was accused of scalding the patients with boiling water, the appearance of the skin being the only proof. The nurse was discharged, although, without doubt, she was innocent, and the appearance of the skin was due solely to the disease. It has been estimated that there are at present in the United States five thousand victims of pellagra, with the number constantly increasing, although physicians of standing make estimates largely in excess of this.

Apparently preventive measures must consist in eliminating the possibility of the use of spoiled corn. Indications are that the disease appears only when such corn has been used, and in parts of Mexico where corn is always roasted before being used, pellagra is never known. It has been described as a disease of the poor, because the disease has flourished chiefly in districts where poverty is so extreme that corn, and spoiled corn at that, is the only [Pg 393] food within reach. Usually, where a mixed diet with meat is possible, pellagra never appears. In other places, as in Italy, where the peasants live on a porridge of corn meal cooked in great potfuls, a week's supply at a time, and during the week exposed to dirt and flies and often spoiled before eating, pellagra is most common. Experiments have shown that in these districts, by excluding corn from the diet and furnishing a substantial fare, the disease has been banished. Unfortunately, the taint of the disease passes from parent to child and even to the third and fourth generation, and the physical deformities commonly seen in pellagrous districts are due to this hereditary taint. Dr. Babcock, Superintendent of the City Hospital at Columbia, South Carolina, after discussing the disease, sums up by saying, "Pellagra is a fact, and the United States is facing one of the great sanitary problems of modern times."

*Bubonic plague.*

The bubonic plague, or "The plague," as the importance of the disease has caused it to be called, is one of the oldest of known epidemics. In the third century it spread through the Roman Empire, destroying in many portions of the country nearly one-half of the people. Its immediate origin is a bacillus causing symptoms similar to blood poisoning, although in some cases, where the lungs are attacked, the disease has some of the characteristics of pneumonia.

A description of this disease is included here because, while bacterial in its nature, it is transmitted largely, if not entirely, by fleas and by a particular species of flea known as the rat flea. These fleas harbor the plague bacilli [Pg 394] in their stomachs and inject them into the bodies of those they bite, in the same way that the anopheles or stegomyia mosquito transmits malaria or yellow fever. Elaborate experiments made in India in 1906 show conclusively that close contact of plague-infected animals with healthy animals does not give rise to any epidemic, so long as the passage of fleas from infected to healthy animals is prevented. When opportunity, however, was given for fleas to pass from one animal to another, the bacillus and the disease was generally carried over. It has also been found that while this species of fleas have their normal residence on the body of rats, they will also desert a rat for man, if the infected rat is dying and no healthy rat is in the vicinity to receive them. It is, then, obvious that to eliminate the disease, the most direct and positive course is to destroy the rats which are the home of the disease.

In India, where the plague appeared in 1896, causing about 300 deaths, it rapidly increased in virulence until in 1907 it caused 1,200,000 deaths. The ports of the Pacific coast became much alarmed, and when cases of the disease were actually found in San Francisco in 1906, the matter was so terrifying that the United States Marine Hospital Service was at once instructed to stamp out the disease if possible. This procedure was directed almost entirely against rats. Deposits of garbage on which rats might feed were removed, rat runs and burrows were destroyed and filled in, and stables, granaries, markets, and cellars where rats might abound were made ratproof by means of concrete. Rats were trapped and poisoned by the thousand, nearly a million being thus disposed of. As a result of such thorough work, the plague was stayed, and in [Pg 395] 1909 not a single case of the disease among human beings was found, and although 93,558 rats captured were examined, only four cases of rat plague were found.

In southern California, however, the fleas deserted the rats for ground squirrels, and one county in particular, Contra Costa County, had an epidemic which caused the squirrels to die by the thousands. The attention of the scientists was thus turned to the squirrel as a host of the flea, and a warfare similar to that against the rat has been for a year past carried on against the infected squirrels. Between September 24, 1908, and April 12, 1909, 4722 ground squirrels were killed and examined for plague infection, and from June 4 to August 13, 1909, the work being continued, 178 squirrels were found to have the plague.

Now that the relation between fleas and their hosts and the transmission of the disease is known, there need be but little fear in the future of this old enemy of man again getting control and spreading without hindrance throughout a whole country.

[Pg 396]

## CHAPTER XX

## *DISEASES CONTROLLED BY ANTITOXINS (SMALLPOX, RABIES, TETANUS)*

*Smallpox.*

A hundred years ago, the most dreaded disease in this country or in Europe was smallpox; and even yet writers of fiction, when they desire to expose their hero to the most harrowing conditions possible, leave him in a deserted hut with a man dying of smallpox. But to the educated person of to-day smallpox is encountered absolutely without dread, since it has been robbed of its terrors by the introduction of vaccination. As far back as 1717, Lady Mary Montague, writing home to England, described the eastern method of taking smallpox deliberately, under comparatively agreeable conditions, in order that severe cases of the disease might be prevented.

Why one attack of the disease should prevent a subsequent case was not known, nor why inoculation with other virus than that of the disease itself should be efficient was not known. But the fact was thoroughly established then that in some way, in the process of the disease and recovery, there was left in the body some substance or agency which was sufficiently powerful to ward off subsequent attacks.

In 1796, Dr. Jenner discovered that a disease very similar to smallpox existed in the cow, and that if the scab from a pustule on the cow was used for inoculation instead [Pg 397] of similar material from a smallpox patient, the resulting disease would be less severe and the protection against subsequent attacks equally efficient. Since that time, therefore, cowpox matter or vaccine has been used to develop a mild form of disease for the express purpose of preventing subsequent attacks.

This is the fundamental principle involved in all antitoxin treatment, and the only difference between vaccination and the injection of diphtheria antitoxin is that with vaccination the disease and the consequent protection is developed in the individual during the course of the disease, while with diphtheria the first attack of the disease and the resulting protective agencies are developed first in the horse and then the essential elements of the blood are introduced into the patient, thereby increasing his resistance to the disease. Smallpox, of all diseases, formerly claimed the largest number of deaths. A hundred years ago, persons marked with smallpox were a common sight. Among the Indians, whole tribes were wiped out with it. It is computed that in Europe, during the eighteenth century, 50,000,000 people died of smallpox. In England, the death-rate was 300 per 100,000. As late as 1800, Boston was visited by severe epidemics of smallpox.

*Value of vaccination.*

Owing to vaccination, the extent and intensity of the disease has continually grown less until to-day attacks of smallpox are not serious and the results are seldom fatal. For this reason and because of the chronic objection of uneducated persons to submit to governmental or outside restrictions, there has been, in recent years, a serious outcry against vaccination, with the result that in New York [Pg 398] State, during the year 1908, there were in certain parts of the state epidemics of smallpox with, however, but two deaths. The disease may, however, at any time become serious, and, because of its virulent contagiousness, no objection ought to be made to reasonable requirements in the matter of vaccination.

Vaccination is usually not the cause of any serious inconvenience or illness, and, while some slight swelling of the arm may result, the protection afforded is so great in comparison with the temporary inconvenience that the latter ought not to be even considered. The protection afforded by a successful vaccination lasts usually from two to seven years, and it is understood that after ten years the protection is certainly lost, and in the presence of a smallpox epidemic one ought to be re-vaccinated after the minimum time named. Whether every person always ought to be vaccinated at intervals of five years or so is open to discussion. If one were on a desert island in a large or small community without intercourse with the outside world, vaccination would be of no value since smallpox would be impossible. There are communities where smallpox has been for years unknown, and consequently where the need for vaccination is not apparent. On the other hand, where smallpox is prevalent in the vicinity, and the disease is continually recurring, it is of the greatest importance, in order that it may be promptly suppressed, that every individual lend himself readily to vaccination.

Whatever harmful results formerly came from vaccination were due to a lack of cleanliness on the part of the person vaccinated or in the vaccination material itself. More care is now used in disinfecting the surface of the [Pg 399] arm and in protecting the exposed skin after the inoculation. If the vaccination "takes," a certain amount of inflammation follows, the spot on the arm suppurates, the suppuration, however, disappearing at the end of about three weeks. If this does not occur, that is, if the vaccination does not take, it may be either because the vaccine was not good or because of the unsusceptibility of the person. In the largest proportion of cases, however, the difficulty is with the vaccine or with the doctor who does the inoculating, and when smallpox is prevalent in the vicinity a person should be re-vaccinated until the vaccination does take. The disease itself, while disagreeable, is not as hopeless as was formerly thought. There is no particular heroism in being physician or nurse to a smallpox patient now, inasmuch as vaccination absolutely prevents contraction of the disease, and the isolation practiced is the most serious objection from the standpoint of the attendants.

*Characteristics of smallpox.*

The disease first shows itself as does measles and scarlet fever, with the appearance of a severe cold accompanied with a high fever. On the second day a rash resembling that of measles and scarlet fever breaks out on the body; this preliminary rash almost immediately disappears and is followed by the real characteristic smallpox eruption, usually about the fourth day. This eruption appears first on the forehead or face and then on the other extremities, the hands and feet.

In mild cases, it is very difficult to distinguish between smallpox and chicken pox, and the only safe measure is to consider all cases of chicken pox in adults to be smallpox, [Pg 400] as they probably are, since the former disease almost never attacks grown-up people. The pustules which form in smallpox are first hard and red, and then two or three days later they are tipped with little blisters which later fill with pus and appear yellow. About the tenth day of the eruption this yellowish matter exudes, forming the scar or scab which later dries up and falls off. Often this eruption is accompanied by excessive swelling of the face, so that the eyes become closed, it is impossible for the patient to eat, high delirium prevails, and the task of the nurse in such cases is an unenviable one. Although usually the pustules are separate and distinct, sometimes in severe cases they run together, so that the hands and face present one distorted mass of suppuration and crust.

The disease is particularly prevalent among negroes, perhaps because they are seldom vaccinated, and in recent epidemics in New York State it has been chiefly through negroes that the disease has been kept alive. The method of prevention for this disease is almost entirely vaccination. Just how the disease spreads is not clearly understood, although it is supposed that it is transmitted chiefly by clothing, dishes, and other articles in contact with the infection. These should, therefore, be thoroughly disinfected. The hope of eliminating the disease, however, comes rather in the use of vaccination. In New York State, in 1908, only two deaths from smallpox occurred, although twenty years before, with the smaller population, the number of deaths ran up into the hundreds.

*Treatment of smallpox.*

The actual treatment of a case of smallpox consists in little more than providing suitable food, in sponging the [Pg 401] body to reduce the fever, and in anointing the skin to allay the irritation of the pustules. As in measles, the eyes are badly affected, and a darkened room is essential for the comfort of the patient as well as for the avoidance of permanent injury to the eyes. Carbolic acid solutions or ointments are to be used continually on the surface of the body, relieving the irritation and to some extent preventing pitting, which is a lasting mark of the disease.

*Diphtheria.*

Diphtheria was also formerly a much-dreaded disease, physicians standing helpless before severe attacks and in all cases unable to do more than suggest ameliorating remedies.

The disease usually begins with a cold, sore throat, and local inflammation, which develops sometimes with alarming rapidity. In the days of our grandmothers, the first thing that the anxious mother did when a child complained of sore throat was to get a spoon and look for white patches in the back of the throat. With severe cases of diphtheria which these white patches foretold, the growths of membrane would be so rapid as to obstruct the breathing, and the child—for the disease is preëminently one of childhood would be in danger of dying of strangulation. The doctor's remedy for this condition was to make an incision in the throat below this accumulation and insert a tube through which the breathing might continue. The writer will never forget having lived through a sickness and death of this sort in his family, seeing as a boy a bottleful of the membrane which the doctor was taking away after the death of the victim, and, while doubtless the size of the bottle and the amount of the membrane has been [Pg 402] magnified by the lapse of years, it still remains to him as a terrible visitation and an inevitable cause of death.

*Cause of the disease.*

The immediate cause of diphtheria has been known only within recent years. Sewer air was for a long time thought to be responsible, and overcrowding or congestion in tenements was believed to be a fruitful source of the disease. Some years ago, when diphtheria had been epidemic in one of the state institutions and when experts had been called in to suppress the disease, the elaborate reports which they made dwelt on the quality of the drinking water and on the method of disposal of the sewage as if those factors would account for the disease. About twenty-five years ago, it was shown definitely that the disease was due to certain bacteria, and that while the membrane in the throat was the result of the rapid development of these bacteria, yet the mortality from the disease was not due to the suppression of the act of breathing, but to the development of a poison by the bacteria which went into the circulation of the body and produced death, just as any poison, as strychnine, for example, would do.

When once this fact was accepted, namely, that the disease was dangerous because of the poisons involved, scientists undertook to find a way to neutralize these poisons, and it was soon discovered that such neutralizing substances could be grown in the blood of guinea pigs. It was found that if a small dose of diphtherial toxin was injected into a guinea pig,—a dose small enough so that the guinea pig would recover,—it could then be given a larger dose from which it would also recover. This process might be repeated, until at the end of several weeks it could be [Pg 403] given a dose the size of which would have been sufficient to have killed it almost instantly at the beginning, and which it could take and enjoy at the end of the series. The point was that evidently, as with smallpox, successive inoculations resulted in the formation in the body of some substance or agent capable of neutralizing the poisons of the disease, subsequently formed. The guinea pig is so small that the amount of restraining substance available made it desirable to find a larger animal, and the horse, equally susceptible to the disease with the guinea pig, was selected as the animal best suited for producing what is now known as diphtheria antitoxin.

*Production of diphtheria antitoxin.*

In laboratories, to-day, sound horses incapable of ordinary labor are devoted to this life-saving task, and, without serious injury or inconvenience to themselves, they develop artificially in their blood this agent which neutralizes the effect of the diphtheria germ. The blood of the horse, when removed, precipitated, and strained, contains this property which is used almost exactly as vaccine in the case of smallpox, except that in the case of diphtheria the development of the disease is so slow that it is not necessary to use this treatment until the disease has appeared. In smallpox, on the other hand, the disease is so rapid that when contracted it is too late for vaccination to be of much value. In New York State, the Department of Health furnishes this horse antitoxin free of expense to health officers to use with persons or families unable to purchase the preventative, so that no longer does any need exist for the continuance of diphtheria as a cause of mortality. [Pg 404]

If the disease is early recognized and a proper amount of antitoxin injected, that is, forced in under the skin so that it may be absorbed by the blood, the probability is that in all cases the patient will recover. It is equally useful with vaccine as a preventative of disease, and in a school, for instance, where diphtheria has broken out, it is only a reasonable precaution to use antitoxin freely to prevent infection of those exposed to the disease.

To make use of the antitoxin at the proper stage of the disease, early recognition is important, and fortunately science here can be of great service. By wiping out the throat with a sterilized swab of cotton, the bacteria present in the throat, if any, will adhere and may be wiped off onto a gelatine substance in which the germs can grow. In twelve hours, they will have developed, if present, so that with a microscope they can be positively recognized. In Massachusetts, and particularly in the city of Boston, the Board of Health maintains a laboratory with a medical expert in charge, to whom physicians may refer these smears for diagnosis. No excuse exists, therefore, in such a city for failure to recognize and prevent the further development of diphtheria, since every wise physician would take a sample of mucus from a throat in case of any irritation there, the Board of Health would furnish accurate diagnosis, and the use of antitoxin will prevent the disease.

*Symptoms of diphtheria.*

The disease itself acts on the human body through the formation of poisons which the bacteria generate by their growth. If the germs have secured a foothold in the upper throat, then the well-known membrane is formed and the toxins produced spread through the blood and cause [Pg 405] headache and fever, even before any experience of sore throat is felt. The temperature rises very high, the child begins to vomit, and the pulse becomes weak, and after about seven days a large percentage of these throat cases begin to improve. The membrane breaks off, the fever declines, and the child begins to recover. If the localized attack is in the larynx, a harsh cough is one of the symptoms, and this is soon followed by a serious difficulty in breathing.

The poisons are formed, as before, in the blood, and, while a surgical operation has been performed often in the past to afford relief from the tendency to strangulation, the bacterial poisons are not affected thereby, and, while the operation might be successful, the child was quite apt to die as the result of the poisons. Now, in either case, antitoxin is administered at the very outset of the attack, with the result that the poisons are counteracted, the temperature drops rapidly, the membrane is apparently at once affected and lessened, and the child recovers at once. No greater boon to the human race in the matter of disease has ever been discovered, and it is certainly most absurd for parents to refuse the use of this wonderful antidote. Not long since, the writer found a family of four children in a home where diphtheria was rampant. The mother and two children were sick with diphtheria in its worst form, and the father refused to allow the doctor to administer the antitoxin even to those sick, much less to those who had been, up to that time, only exposed. Apparently there was no direct law requiring the administration of the antitoxin, and the physician in attendance and the health officer were obliged to stand by and wait for the death of the children, which actually happened, knowing that a [Pg 406] dose of the antitoxin ready at hand could have been administered and the children's lives, in all probability, saved.

The diphtheria poison is so virulent that in many cases it acts on the different organs of the body, particularly on the kidneys and the heart, and the recovery from this poison may take weeks. It is very necessary, therefore, for the patient to be kept quiet, and this can best be done in bed, for at least three weeks after the crisis has passed. The nervous system is often affected, so that the child may squint or stutter or perhaps not be able to see, but these effects are usually temporary and pass away as the effect of the poison disappears.

*Rabies.*

Rabies is the third assumed bacterial disease which is reacted upon by the administration of an antitoxin. When it occurs in man, it is generally known as hydrophobia, although it is the same disease as that known as rabies in dogs, skunks, wolves, and other animals. The virus of the disease is in the saliva of the animal, so that when a dog bites another animal or human beings, the poison is injected into the wound made with the teeth.

The actual germ has not been found, and while there is no doubt that it originates with some specific bacterium, it is probable that the transmitted disease is due rather to the toxin of the germ than to the germ itself. The greatest number of cases, by far, are caused by the bites of dogs, and the most obvious and plainest method of preventing the disease is to prevent dogs from biting. That this is efficient in stamping out the disease has been proved by the records of cases in England and Germany. There, a quarantine on all the dogs in the country, that is, the strict [Pg 407] enforcement of laws requiring muzzling, has eliminated the disease except on the borders of other countries where such quarantine is not enforced.

In New York State, the number of cases of rabies is increasing at an alarming rate, as determined by the examinations made on dogs' heads at the New York State Veterinary College in Ithaca. Whereas a few years ago one suspected case a month was the average number sent in, during this last year, 1909, there have been sent to the laboratory, at times, as many as five or six a day, the number being larger in the warm weather. When the disease appears in the dog, one manifestation of it is that the animal runs over large areas of country, perhaps within a radius of twenty-five or thirty miles, and in this mad race the dog may infect other dogs throughout the entire distance. It is, therefore, of small value to muzzle dogs only in a particular village, since the dogs while muzzled may be bitten by an outsider. There is no reason why the disease could not be stamped out of a state in six months by muzzling all the dogs. But muzzling the dogs in a village here or in a town there is really only temporizing with the trouble.

Hydrophobia in man requires usually from two to six weeks to develop, so that there is a long period in which to utilize preventive measures, and it is on this account that children may be sent, as happens frequently, to New York City or to Paris to be treated by what is known as "Pasteur treatment." This treatment involves the inoculation of the rabies virus which has first been passed through a series of rabbits, in the course of which the virus has become exceedingly strong. The treatment of the [Pg 408] human being consists in successive inoculations with virus of various strengths, beginning with the weakest and ending with the most powerful rabbit virus. After this has been done, the effect of the bite of the mad dog has been neutralized, so that in most cases the disease has been robbed of its power. Of the cases treated at the Pasteur Institute in 1897, numbering 1521, there were six deaths, and these six were among those whose arrival at the Institute was so late that the treatment could not be begun in time.

*Tetanus.*

The fourth disease for which an antidote in the form of antitoxin has been developed is tetanus, commonly known as lockjaw. This is a bacterial disease caused by a specific germ, the peculiarity of which, in its progress, is a long-continued spasm of certain muscles of the body. The germs are commonly found in dirt, garden soil being always full of them, and whenever the skin is broken by any object, such as a rusty nail or a knife not clean, lockjaw may be the result. Rather curiously, it is particularly likely to develop after gunpowder wounds, and the number of cases of tetanus after the Fourth of July is notable. This special prevalence of the disease is so well recognized that health officers usually lay in a large stock of antitoxin about the first of July, awaiting the inevitable demand for it.

The disease is most commonly contracted from wounds which occur in the hands or the feet, although it may be the result of wounds in other parts of the body. Very often the wound may be so insignificant as to escape the attention, as a pin prick, and yet be followed by an attack of tetanus. Formerly, the universal treatment for injuries from which tetanus was feared was to firmly cut out all [Pg 409] portions of the flesh and skin which might have been infected. Sometimes cauterization was employed, as was done also with cases of rabies, and, if it were possible to reach the virus in the wounds before it escaped into the blood, such a method of treatment would be quite reasonable, but it is quite beyond hope to prevent infection in a jagged wound by cutting out adjacent flesh, with no regard to the dissolved poison. The more reasonable treatment is to inject the antitoxin, which neutralizes the poison and prevents, or at least minimizes, the disease.

[Pg 410]

## CHAPTER XXI

## *HYGIENE AND LAW*

One of the fundamental principles of society is that each individual must, in his methods of living, conduct himself with a due regard for the rights, comfort, and health of others in the same society. A single man or a single family living alone on a desert island requires no restrictions of conduct, since there are no fellow-beings on whom his violations of good conduct might react. The inhabitants of small villages with small families on large lots are but little concerned with laws governing social intercourse, since, at best, the amount of that intercourse is inconsiderable. But, as population becomes greater, as congestion increases, and as civilization and its requirements develop, the need for law governing the interrelations of individuals becomes imperative. Such laws deal with the moral life under many phases, and the courts exist for the enforcement of such laws as the people themselves, through their legislatures, demand for their own self-protection.

One of the primitive laws found necessary, even among uncivilized people, is that against theft, and, whether committed in the barbarous tribes of Africa or on the frontier plains of the West, the act is recognized as being contrary to the greatest good of the community, and, if detected, is severely punished. As civilization advances, the code of [Pg 411] laws found necessary becomes more and more complex, and, although use has made obedience to such laws almost second nature, it is hardly possible to-day to escape the immediate restraint of such laws for more than a moment at a time throughout any period of twenty-four hours.

*Principle of laws of hygiene.*

It is particularly the laws which pertain to health and hygiene which we shall consider in this chapter. The principle on which laws relating to hygiene are passed is that while nominally a person is always free to do with his own whatever he may choose, yet as a member of a community he must choose to do only that which shall not injure or affect the health or comfort of his neighbors. This principle was not at first invoked to prevent violations of laws of health, but rather to prevent the inconvenience which might come to a neighbor or to the public at large by some unreasonable though apparently legitimate use of individual property. As an example we may mention the law of New York State requiring each owner of property in the country to cut grass, weeds, and brush along the highway twice each year. Although this interferes with the right of the owner to have the land which belongs to him left as he chooses, it is legal because of the greater convenience and comfort it contributes to the larger number of persons traveling along the highway.

The state does not assume the right to interfere with the acts of individuals so long as such acts affect only their own individual well-being, but when those actions affect others, then the police power of the state may be invoked. It is on this principle that the law prohibits suicide, assuming that no man can live or die without affecting the interests [Pg 412] of other people. This is plainly so in the case of the head of a family or in the case of a man upon whom others are dependent and whose death removes their support and causes those supported to become dependent upon the state or county. This principle has been extended so as to include the cases where a method of living, a lack of care, or even a mere appearance in public may adversely affect the health of others in the same community. If, for example, a member of a family has diphtheria or smallpox, and such a child is isolated so that no danger of the spread of the disease exists, the state would not, in general, insist upon the use of any preventive or curative inoculation; but if a child with incipient diphtheria or whooping cough goes to school where other children may be infected and the disease spread, the state, acting through its Board of Education, would have a perfect right to send the child home and prevent its enjoying school privileges until recovery from the disease.

It is on this principle that the state says that no child in New York State may attend school unless vaccinated, the law reading, "No child, not vaccinated, shall be admitted into any of the public schools of the state, and the trustees of the schools shall cause this provision of law to be enforced." This law has been questioned and brought before the Supreme Court for review, and it was held by the judges that the protection to the community implied is of sufficient importance to justify its enactment.

For like reason, other restrictions governing the control of contagious diseases is a function of the police power of the state in which the rights of the individual must yield to the greater good of the community. The writer remembers [Pg 413] a particularly malignant case of smallpox where the efforts of the local Board of Health had been concentrated on the enforcement of quarantine, and where by the aid of policemen, day and night, it was hoped that the disease was being confined in the one house; yet, after the death of the patient, and when apparently efforts for protection might be relaxed, a wake was held in the house, in the very room of the patient, which might have resulted in the spread of the disease through the entire town. Regulations, therefore, covering the conduct of funerals and of burials should be agreed to, since they are intended to prevent the spread of disease.

*Self-interest the real basis of law.*

Many practices which are required by law in cities where the population is crowded are not required or are not enforced in country districts, since there the failure to carry out protective measures reacts only on those immediately concerned. Disinfection of rooms in which contagious diseases have occurred is one such provision. It rarely happens that a health officer of a country community concerns himself with seeing that a case of scarlet fever, for example, is prevented from spreading by a thorough disinfection of the rooms. That seems to be left to the good sense of the individual. It is hardly conceivable that a mother with three or four children (when one child has been sick with a contagious disease) will neglect ordinary and reasonable precautions to prevent the spread of that disease to the rest of the family.

It is inconceivable, when the small amount of trouble and expense is considered, that the parents of a family, after a case of diphtheria, will neglect to fumigate and disinfect [Pg 414] the clothing and bedding which may be thus infected, particularly if such clothing or bedding is to be used by other members of the family; and yet instances are recorded where a child has died of scarlet fever and a year later another child, perhaps wearing some of the clothes of the previous victim, has been seized with the disease and has followed its brother or sister to the grave. Cases of tuberculosis have been known to follow each other almost year after year, as one member of a family after another occupied a room where the infection persisted, either in the carpet or furniture, which was never properly disinfected. Such cases must be left to the good sense, intelligence, and understanding of the persons concerned. The police power can never in this age take the place of an enlightened sense in the community, nor are laws, as a matter of fact, of any use except as they are sustained and enforced by public sentiment.

QUALITY OF WATER

There is another way in which the police power of the state exercises control over rural communities, and that is in the matter of food which the country generally supplies to the city. Perhaps the pollution of water, which is, after all, one kind of food, is as important as any matter covered by health laws.

In most cities to-day the pollution of streams is prohibited on two grounds, first, that the streams are public property, even though for a part of their course they may be owned individually. The sum of the parts making up the whole stream involves so many individuals as to imply public ownership, and inasmuch as one individual is limited in [Pg 415] his uses of the stream by the principle already referred to, he cannot, even on his own land, do what he pleases with a stream or with its waters. When streams are navigable, according to the law of this country, no private ownership can exist, for the waters are controlled and owned by the federal government. This latter body, in general, does not undertake to control the quality of such waters, but there are many laws covering the quantity of water in such streams, limiting the amounts that can be withdrawn, restricting the filling up or silting of such streams, and qualifying the bridging or damming of such waterways. In small streams, such as are generally found in rural communities, the vital principle of ownership is always limited by the requirement that no owner shall so interfere with the normal quantity or quality of water in the stream as to prevent their full enjoyment by the next man downstream whose rights are equal with his own. This means, in the matter of quantity, that while one individual may water stock in a stream or may pump water from a stream for household use, he may not withdraw from the stream the entire volume to use for irrigation, nor may he, as a riparian owner, sell the water to some city near by which might take out all the water of the stream.

The quality of a stream, likewise, may only to a certain extent be interfered with. If a stream flows through a meadow, cows pastured in the meadow have a natural right to wade in the brook, and if, in so doing, a certain amount of pollution is added to the waters of the brook, no one downstream can justly complain.

If, however, a sewer is carried from barns or houses into a brook which is later used for drinking purposes, the quality [Pg 416] of the water is affected, and such a discharge is so revolting to the senses that complaint to the courts would result in an order to find some other method of disposing of such wastes.

In New York State, the legislature has delegated to the Department of Health certain rights in the matter of the protection from pollution of the waters of the state, particularly when those waters are used for drinking purposes. Upon application from the water company, this department, having carefully inspected the watershed, will prepare a complete and elaborate series of rules, giving in detail just what an individual may or may not do on the watershed, and, when enacted, these rules have all the force of law. They are, however, like all laws, subject to the constitutional limitations, and particularly to the clause of the constitution which provides that "no state shall make or enforce any law which shall deprive any person of property without due process of law." This means that if any law prevents an individual enjoying reasonable use of his own property, or if the deprivation of such use is for the special benefit of some special community or company, then that special body must be prepared to make compensation for that deprivation, although if it were for the general good of the community of which the individual was a member, no compensation might be required.

## REGULATIONS GOVERNING FOODS

Laws covering the sale of adulterated foods are of two kinds, namely, those enacted by the national government at Washington, and those enacted by the local authorities, either state or municipal. The laws enacted by the national government, which are comprehended in the recently [Pg 417] enacted National Pure Food Law, deal particularly with the adulteration and misbranding, not only of foods, but of all sorts of medicines and liquor. Their effect, however, is limited entirely to such articles as make up interstate commerce. If an article is made and sold within the boundaries of any single state, it is not subject to the national law, nor could this national law be applied to the production or sale of any article from a farm unless that article was well enough known to be generally distributed. For example, maple sirup, widely advertised and generally sold, would be subject to the provisions of the national law. Butter and cheese, sold locally, would not be subject to such a law. It is evident, therefore, that this law does not usually apply to farm products, unless, as in the case of some sausages, for example, a widely advertised campaign has been instituted to promote their sale.

There are, however, in the different states, laws which do apply locally and which prohibit adulteration of all sorts. In New York State, for example, the law says that no person shall, within the state, manufacture, produce, compound, brew, distill, have, sell, or offer for sale any adulterated food or product, and the law further specifies that an article shall be deemed to be adulterated: —

"1. If any substance or substances has or have been mixed with it so as to reduce or lower or injuriously affect its quality or strength.

"2. If any inferior or cheaper substance or substances have been substituted wholly or in part for the article.

"3. If any valuable constituent of the article has been wholly or in part abstracted.

"4. If it be an imitation or be sold under the name of another article. [Pg 418]

"5. If it consists wholly or in part of diseased or decomposed or putrid or rotten animal or vegetable substance, whether manufactured or not, or in the case of milk, if it is the produce of a diseased animal.

"6. If it be colored, or coated, or polished, or powdered, whereby damage is concealed, or it is made to appear better than it really is, or of greater value.

"7. If it contain any added poisonous ingredient, or any ingredient which may render such article injurious to the health of the person consuming it. Provided that an article of food which does not contain any ingredient injurious to health shall not be deemed to have been adulterated, in the case of mixtures or compounds which may be now, or from time to time hereafter, known as articles of food under their own distinctive names, or which shall be labeled so as to plainly indicate that they are mixtures, combinations, compounds, or blends, and not included in definition fourth of this section.

"8. If it contains methyl or wood alcohol or any of its forms, or any methylated preparation made from it."

These provisions, just mentioned, are provisions of the New York State Health Law, and violations are in defiance of that law, the penalties for which are specifically stated to be $100 for every such violation.

There is also in New York a police code that prohibits adulteration of food, and in this code the adulteration of maple sirup or fruit juices or spoiled articles of food of all sorts, of milk from which part of the cream has been removed, and the sale of any article which is printed or labeled in such a way as to misrepresent the article, is called a misdemeanor, the penalty for which is left to the discretion of the judge and which would, under ordinary conditions, be a fine of several hundred dollars or imprisonment in a county jail for a term of months, or both. [Pg 419]

*Basis of pure food laws.*

Adulteration of food may be considered from two points of view, the hygienic and the economic, and, while the laws are generally intended to preserve the public from impure food on account of the economic loss involved thereby, the hygienic aspect is really the more important. Adulterations which are plainly injurious to health are very few in number, and it is rather desirable that the economic phase should be the one to command attention of legislators, since, when that objection to adulteration has been so voiced as to result in laws prohibiting adulteration, the health of the public will be promoted by the elimination of objectionable foodstuffs. The long-continued discussion over the use of benzoate of soda in foods is an example of this twofold aspect; some, arguing against its use, protested that when long continued, it had a decidedly injurious effect upon the health of those eating or drinking it; others objected to the chemical, but contended that its use enabled spoiled fruits, like tomatoes, to be substituted for fresh fruits, and the price of the latter obtained where the value of the former only was given. No one seriously thinks that butter with a small amount of butter color added could have any injurious effect upon the human system, yet it is, in the eyes of the law, an adulteration because its appearance indicates a quality of the butter which it does not naturally possess.

## PROTECTION OF MILK

The one article of food produced on the farm about which the greatest amount of agitation has been centered has been the adulteration of milk, as well as the question of the [Pg 420] production of milk under unclean conditions. The responsibility for pure milk rests on the Department of Agriculture of the State, on the Department of Health of the State, on the Department of Health of the city where the milk is sold, and on the Board of Health in the village or town where the milk is produced. In a way, these four departments divide the responsibility for the milk, and, as in all cases of divided responsibility, the very fact of the number subtracts from their efficiency. The local Board of Health of the village or town where milk is produced is not usually interested or concerned particularly in the question of its quality.

If a case of contagious disease in any farmhouse occurs, the local health officer should see that a proper quarantine is established and that the individuals in such a house are instructed in the danger of contamination and in the necessity of avoiding infection in the dairy. It is, however, the Board of Health in the city where the milk is consumed who have a particular responsibility. Such a board has no jurisdiction or authority over matters outside of their city, so that their executive cannot go out into the country, into the district of another health board, and order improvements made in the methods of production. All that a city board can do is to enact and publish restrictions under which milk must be sold in that city.

This is the method pursued in the city of New York, where tons of milk are consumed every day and where manifestly the jurisdiction of the city officials cannot extend over the thousands of farms located in the five states from which the milk supply is drawn. In New York City the local sanitary code provides that no milk shall be [Pg 421] received, held, kept, offered for sale, or delivered in the city of New York without a permit from the Board of Health, and the Board makes this permit depend upon the sanitary conditions existing at the dairy or farm where the milk is produced or handled. In order to find out whether the conditions at the dairies and farms throughout these five states are in a sanitary condition, the city has a force of twenty-five inspectors who are continually engaged in traveling among the farms and in reporting on their condition. If a farm is found where the cows are diseased, or if the buildings in which the cows are stabled or in which the milk is cooled and strained are not clean or are lacking in proper ventilation or otherwise unhygienic, or if the water-supply is bad, the farmer is notified that conditions are such that the city of New York will refuse to receive his milk. He is not forced to clean up, and no orders are given him, but the attitude of the city authorities is made plain, and then it is left to him to decide whether it may not be wise for him to accept the suggestions made by the inspectors. Dr. Darlington, late Health Commissioner of the city of New York, reported in 1907, after two years of inspection, that out of 35,000 dairies inspected, only 47 were shut out on account of unclean conditions, although many more were warned with the result that remedial measures were at once taken. The same sort of procedure may be adopted by any city, and is, in fact, practiced by a number.

Another method of securing a better grade of milk which results in forcing farmers to clean up the barn and barnyard, at the same time allowing the local official to remain within the strict letter of the law, which gives him no direct [Pg 422] authority over conditions on farms outside a city, is to limit the number of bacteria found in samples of milk supplied by the dealer. A common rule is that no milk shall be distributed which contains more than 50,000 bacteria per c.c., and when milk contains a number in excess of this, the milkman is warned, and if, at the next sampling, the number is still higher, the milkman is notified that his milk will no longer be received. Experience has shown that a reasonable regard for cleanliness in the stable and dairy room, with a prompt cooling of the milk, will limit the bacterial growth to this standard, and the requirement, meaning, as it does, only a decent regard for such cleanliness as a self-respecting dairyman would recognize as essential, works no hardship on any one. New York City prints its dairy rules on linen and has them tacked up in every cow barn concerned in the city milk supply, and while they have merely the force of suggestions only, practically they have the force of law in that a disobedience to these rules is likely to involve the refusal of the milk from that particular dairy.

## LAWS GOVERNING QUARANTINE

It is much to be regretted that, in these days of scientific knowledge, when the exact and fundamental causes and processes of diseases are so clearly known to medical men and when laws based on this knowledge have been enacted for the purpose of reducing mortality and preventing the spread of disease, ignorant individuals should allow their prejudices to stand in the way of compliance with the spirit of these laws.

In New York State, Section 24 of the Public Health Law [Pg 423] requires the local Board of Health to isolate all persons and things infected with or exposed to infectious diseases. They are required to prohibit and prevent all intercourse and communication with or use of infected premises, places, and things, and to require and, if necessary, to provide the means for the thorough purification and cleansing of the same before general intercourse with the same or use thereof shall be allowed. The Penal Code of the state further provides that a person who, having been lawfully ordered by a health officer to be detained in quarantine and not having been discharged, willfully violates any quarantine law or regulation is guilty of a misdemeanor, punishable by fine or imprisonment or both. In spite of this prohibition, it is very rare to find that a person in a quarantined house feels any personal obligation. He stays in or out, if obliged to by a policeman, or, if the sentiment among the neighbors is aroused in favor of quarantine, he waits until dark enough to escape observation.

In New York, two years ago, a case of diphtheria broke out in the family of a Christian Scientist. The health officer visited the house, offered to use antitoxin, which was refused, and instructed quarantine. The mother and one daughter died, and the healer was imprisoned for entering the house in defiance of the quarantine law. This case illustrates how the moral obligation may be distinctly repudiated because of religious prejudice. But even religious belief must be subservient to the laws governing the community in which a man chooses to live, and, so long as the residence continues, the laws governing quarantine, as all other laws, must be obeyed. In this case another count against parents may be found. Section 288 of the [Pg 424] Penal Code provides "that a person who willfully omits without lawful excuse to perform a duty by law imposed upon him to furnish food, clothing, shelter, or medical attendance to a minor is guilty of a misdemeanor." It would seem, therefore, that the law is provided by which fanaticism may be overruled in the interests of the health of children, although it must be said that this phase of the law is generally disregarded. Again, in spite of the ample proof to the contrary, there are to be found persons who refuse to be vaccinated even in the midst of a smallpox epidemic. A law in New York State provides that no unvaccinated child shall attend public schools, the law being mandatory upon the school trustees. If this law were faithfully carried out, smallpox would entirely disappear from the state within a few years.

Other instances might be cited to show how the force of the law is invoked to minimize the effects of unhealthy living and to prevent that perfect individual liberty which a few irresponsible persons would assume to themselves. But it will always remain for the good sense of the individuals to direct their actions in such a way as to inflict no evil on the community. Unfortunately, laws are generally the result of some calamity. A law prohibiting child labor is passed only after the evil effects of such labor have been demonstrated by sad experience. Laws forbidding the sale of diseased meat or of spoiled fruit are passed only after repeated cases of illness have demonstrated the need of such laws. Laws involving quarantine are the result of epidemics which have showed plainly, at the cost of valuable lives, perhaps, the need of such quarantine.

It is the aim of hygiene, whether rural or urban, to raise [Pg 425] the standards of living to such a degree that not only will any violation of health laws seem unreasonable and obnoxious, but also every instinct, of the individual will, even without specific laws, direct him so to live that no hygienic offense will be directed towards those with whom he comes in contact. Only in this way will the present violations of the requirements of hygienic living be avoided, and the normal man be enabled to live as he should in absolute harmony with his environment.